Occupational and Environmental Medicine

Occupational and Environmental Medicine

Editor: Charlotte Lance

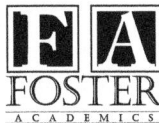

FA
FOSTER
ACADEMICS

www.fosteracademics.com

www.fosteracademics.com

FA FOSTER ACADEMICS

Cataloging-in-Publication Data

Occupational and environmental medicine / edited by Charlotte Lance.
    p. cm.
Includes bibliographical references and index.
ISBN 978-1-63242-791-5
1. Medicine, Industrial. 2. Environmentally induced diseases--Treatment.
3. Occupational diseases. 4. Environmental health. I. Lance, Charlotte.
RC963 .O23 2019
613.62--dc23

Foster Academics,
118-35 Queens Blvd., Suite 400,
Forest Hills, NY 11375, USA

ISBN 978-1-63242-791-5 (Hardback)

Contents

Preface

This book aims to highlight the current researches and provides a platform to further the scope of innovations in this area. This book is a product of the combined efforts of many researchers and scientists, after going through thorough studies and analysis from different parts of the world. The objective of this book is to provide the readers with the latest information of the field.

The field of medicine which deals with the maintenance of health in the workplace is known as occupational medicine. It aims at preventing and treating the injuries and diseases in one's workplace along with the maintenance and increase in the productivity and social adjustment. Some of the common occupational diseases are occupational asthma, contact dermatitis, overuse syndrome, carpal tunnel syndrome, computer vision syndrome, lead poisoning and radiation sickness. Environmental medicine is a sub-field of environmental health. It includes the study of the interactions between the environment and human health. It also studies the role of environment in causing illnesses in humans. This book is compiled in such a manner, that it will provide in-depth knowledge about the theory and practice of occupational and environmental medicine. It is a compilation of chapters that discuss the most vital concepts and emerging trends in the field of occupational and environmental medicine. This book includes contributions of doctors and experts which will provide innovative insights into this field.

I would like to express my sincere thanks to the authors for their dedicated efforts in the completion of this book. I acknowledge the efforts of the publisher for providing constant support. Lastly, I would like to thank my family for their support in all academic endeavors.

Editor

Physicians' working conditions in hospitals from the students' perspective (iCEPT-Study)—results of a web-based survey

Jan Bauer[*] and David A. Groneberg

Abstract

Background: Medical students undergo numerous clinical clerkships. On these occasions they are confronted with current working conditions in hospitals. Because of the many implications of the students' perceptions of these working conditions, it is important to assess those. Hereby the focus was put on the students' perception of their supervising physician.

Methods: This study is a part of a prospective anonymized web-based survey (iCEPT-Study). The study was conducted in Germany among medical students after their clinical rotations. 1587 medical students took part in this study (63,0 % female and 37,0 % male). 11259 were invited to take part (response rate of 14,1 %). In this study a questionnaire was used which was based on the Effort-Reward-Imbalance (ERI) model and the Job-Demand-Control (JDC) model. A mathematical calculated ratio (ER- and JDC-Ratio; combined as 'ER/JDC-Ratio') was used to measure the students' perceptions of working conditions, namely distress (primary outcome). As a secondary outcome perceived job satisfaction was measured.

Results: Distress was perceived by 67.4 % (95 %-CI: 65.1|69.7) of the students. 54.1 % (95 %-CI: 51.7|56.6) of polled students stated that their supervising physician seemed to be very satisfied with his job. Analysis of age distribution revealed that the proportion of students' who perceived their supervising physician as very satisfied with his job dropped from 72.5 % among under 20-year olds to 63.0 % among 20–24-year olds and was at 44.5 % among the over 30-year olds. Looking at the specialty, the specialty of surgery was rated with the highest distress prevalence (ER/JDC-Ratio > 1): 81.3 % of students stated that their supervising surgeon encountered unfavorable working conditions.

Conclusion: Two out of three medical students rated the physicians working conditions as stressful. This implicates that already in this early phase of their career the majority of medical students get to know the hospital as an unfavorable workplace concerning working conditions. To facilitate the transition from medical schools to hospitals working conditions of physicians must be improved.

Keywords: Student, Physician, Hospital, Distress, Satisfaction

Background

There are three important aspects examining physicians' working conditions in the context of medical students: First, the way current working conditions are exemplified to medical students through the physicians. Second, the corresponding students' perception of these working conditions. Third, thereby arising expectations of medical students regarding their future working conditions. The first and latter aspects has already been examined in many studies [1–5]. However research about the second aspect is rare, which is why the study focus has been put on students' perception of physicians' working conditions.

Regarding expectations on working conditions, a survey among German medical students in 2010 [4] showed that the work-life-balance is of outstanding importance: 96 % of respondents stated that combining family and work is important. Furthermore, 60.9 % of respondents would like to work part-time (women: 77.2 %; men: 32.1 %). Regarding

* Correspondence: j.bauer@med.uni-frankfurt.de
Institute of Occupational, Social and Environmental Medicine, Goethe-University Frankfurt, Theodor-Stern-Kai 7, 60329 Frankfurt am Main, Germany

the workplace, 77.7 % of respondents attested the hospital to be an attractive workplace. These trends have been confirmed in several studies [2, 3, 5–7].

In 1996 Bland et al. developed a theoretical model [8] trying to explain the specialty choice of medical students: the so called 'Bland-Meurer model'. Therein the author distinguished two major reasons for a certain specialty choice: On the one hand the 'needs to satisfy' and on the other hand the 'perception of specialty'. Factors playing a role in the perceptions of specialty are workload, patient contact and job satisfaction of the observed physicians.

Taken as a whole, the perception of working conditions (and therefore the specialty choice) is influenced by the direct observation of physicians on the one hand and by information during medical education obtained by fellow students, media or physicians on the other [8–11].

The physicians themselves seemed to show high levels of distress, as shown in several studies [12–14]. However, whether the respective students' perception matches the physicians' self-perception cannot be judged with current literature. Considering the implication the students' perceptions of working conditions have on the specialty choice, a comparative evaluation is of great significance, especially in times of a shortage of qualified physicians. This is the case for example in Germany: The 'deutsche Krankenhausinstitut' [15] predicted further personnel requirements of 37370 physicians until the year 2019. The 'WifOR Institut' in cooporation with PricewaterhouseCoopers [16] forecasted further personnel requirements of 56000 physicians until the year 2020.

Since the polled students of the iCEPT-Study are from Germany some short facts will be presented about German medical students: In Germany there were 82289 medical students in the winter semester of 2011/12 [17]. The number of annual graduates sunk from 11987 to 8659 during the years 1994 to 2006. In the year 2010 there were 9844 graduates [18]. Of the graduates 92 % work as physicians one year after their final exam, according to the 'Medizinerreport 2012' of HIS GmbH [19]. After 10 years only 86 % would work as a physician. Furthermore the official success rate of German medical students from the year 2000 to 2009, meaning the rate of students who graduated successfully, was 95 % [20].

The in the beginning mentioned second aspect, the students' perception of the physicians' working conditions, hasn't been subject of an investigation so far and therefore chosen as study focus.

Methods

This study was part of the iCept-Study (iCept: Neologism of 'i percept'). The respective complete study protocol has already been published [21]. Ethical approval has been obtained.

The iCept-Study used two stress models as the theoretical substructure: The Effort-Reward-Imbalance (ERI) model [22] and the Job-Demand-Control (JDC) model [23, 24]. Both models introduce two parameters, which in case of an imbalance (Ratio > 1) of one parameter ('effort' in the ERI model and 'job-demand' in the JDC model) lead to unfavorable working conditions and therefore distress (defined as negative, chronic stress with negative impact on health) [25]. Therefore distress is present in case of an Effort-Reward (ER)—Ratio > 1 and/or a Job-Demand-Control (JDC)—Ratio > 1. Here both stress models were combined and referred to with the term 'ER/JDC-Ratio' defined by an ER-Ratio > 1 and/or a JDC-Ratio > 1 since thereby a valid decision about the presence of distress can be made.

The iCept-Questionnaire

The iCept-Study has been conceived as an online survey. The items of the iCept-Questionnaire were taken from two established and validated questionnaires: On the one hand the 'Kurz-Fragebogen zur Arbeitsanalyse' (KFZA) of Prümper et al [26] and on the other hand the ERI-Questionnaire of Siegrist et al [27]. Both questionnaires have often been used in hospitals [28–30]. The overall job satisfaction was measured by a single item (JS1) taken from the 'Job Diagnostic Survey' (JDS) of Schmidt et al [31]. A meta-analysis showed that a single-item measure was as reliable and convincing as a scale measure with a correlation of r = 0,67 [32].

Since in this study students were asked to rate the working conditions of physicians, the items had to be adapted to the changed perspective: From first person singular to third person singular. Thus there are only grammatical differences, without changes to content.

Mathematical evaluation

The items of the iCept-Questionnaire were summed up into scales according to the stress models of Siegrist and Karasek. In addition scale values were calculated and thereof a ratio was built. The scale values can vary depending on their respective number of items:

- Scale value 'effort' (x_{eff}): $4 \le x_{eff} \le 16$
- Scale value 'job demand' (x_{job}): $4 \le x_{job} \le 16$
- Scale value 'reward' (x_{rew}): $5 \le x_{rew} \le 20$
- Scale value 'control' (x_{con}): $3 \le x_{con} \le 12$

Because of the varying number of items, corrections factors were introduced: $c_{eri} = 1.25$ (5/4) for the scale 'effort' and $c_{jdc} = 0.75$ (3/4) for the scale 'job-demands'.

$$ER{-}Ratio = \frac{x_{eff}}{x_{rew}} \times c_{eri} \quad JDC{-}Ratio = \frac{x_{job}}{x_{con}} \times c_{jdc}$$

Statistical data analysis

The statistical analysis has been performed using SPSS Version 21. The following tests have been used to test for significant differences: Mann-Whitney-U-Test for two measurement series, Kruskal-Wallis-Test for more than two measurement series and the Chi-Quadrat-Test for categorical criteria. Furthermore the odds ratio respectively the arithmetic average difference has been calculated with the t-test including the 95 %-confidence interval. With these parameters a conclusion could be drawn about strength and direction of differences.

Study participants

For the purposes of the iCept-Study a total number of 11259 medical students in Germany were invited via e-mail to take part in this study. In total 1587 students participated. This corresponds to a response rate of 14.1 % or in relation to all 82289 medical students in Germany (basic sample) to 1.9 %. The Federal Statistical Office of Germany obtains the data used to compare the iCept-sample with the basic sample [17].

In Fig. 1 a comparison of the iCept-sample and the basic sample is given. The average age of the iCept-sample was 25.3 years (SD: 3.6 years), In the basic sample the average age was 25.2 years. Regarding the study phase, 12.1 % of respondents were in their first or second year (1./2. year; i.e. 'preclinical'), 49.7 % of respondents were in the third, fourth or fifth year (3./4./5. year; i.e. 'clinical') and 38.2 % in their final year (6. year; i.e. 'elective year').

Since the students were asked to rate the physicians' working conditions during their internship, the following data analysis do not reflect the students' working conditions but the physicians' working conditions in the perception of medical students.

Results

The analysis of data showed that for 54.1 % (95 %-CI: 51.7|56.6) of polled students their supervising physician seemed to be very satisfied with his job. Unfavorable working conditions in form of an ER/JDC-Ratio > 1 (distress) perceived 67.4 % (95 %-CI: 65.1|69.7) of the students. Furthermore, 41.7 % (95 %-CI: 38.1|44.7) of polled students stated, that their supervising physician seemed to be very satisfied despite distress. In Table 1 an overview of the results is displayed.

The data were analyzed by the following students' characteristics: Gender, age, study phase and specialty.

Gender

There were no significant gender specific differences regarding distress (p = 0,110): 68.8 % of female and 64.9 % of male students rated the physicians working conditions as stressful (ER/JDC-Ratio > 1). Solely the aspect of job satisfaction revealed significant ($p < 0.05$) differences: For 52.0 % of female students and 57.8 % of male students their supervising physician seemed to be very satisfied with his job. This corresponded with an odds ratio of 1.26 (95 %-CI: 1.03|1.55).

Age

Taking the students' age in the focus the data analysis showed a correlation between job satisfaction and the four generated age groups: The proportion of students'

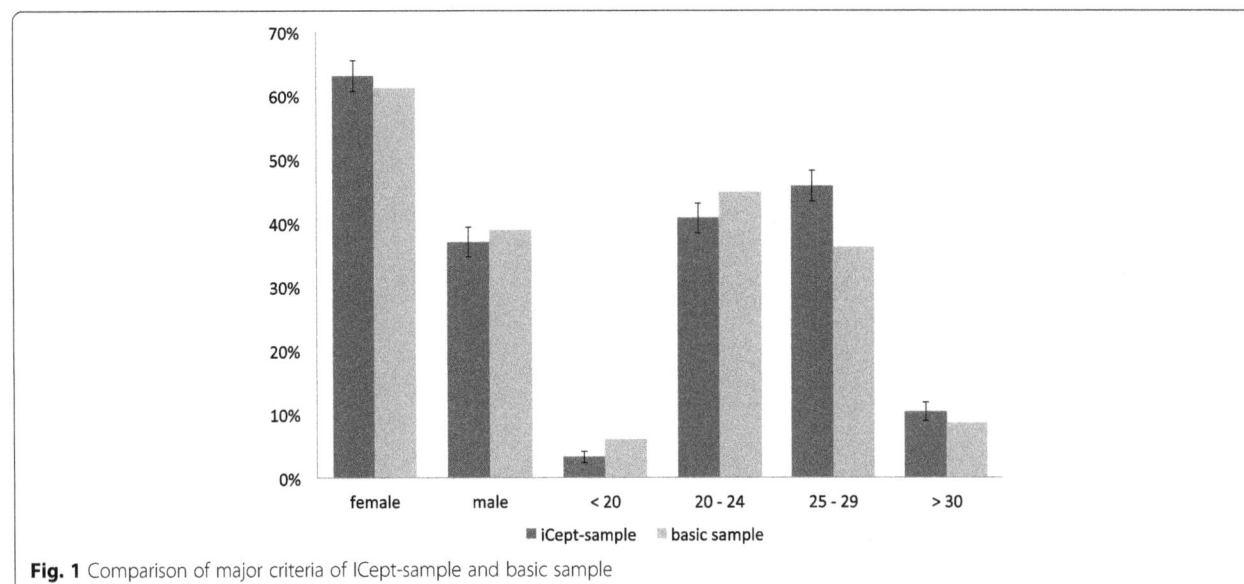

Fig. 1 Comparison of major criteria of ICept-sample and basic sample

Table 1 Overview on results, according to gender, study phase and age; *p < 0.05 **p < 0.01 ***p < 0.001

	Total	Gender – male		Gender – female		Study phase 1/2.		Study phase 3/4./5.		Study phase 6.		Age <20		Age 20 – 24		Age 25 – 30		Age >30	
	n (%)	n (%)	OR (95 %-CI)	n (%)	OR (95 %-CI)	n (%)	OR (95 %-CI)	n (%)	OR (95 %-CI)	n (%)	OR (95 %-CI)	n (%)	OR (95 %-CI)	n (%)	OR (95 %-CI)	n (%)	OR (95 %-CI)	n (%)	OR (95 %-CI)
	n = 1.587	n = 587		n = 1.000		n = 192		n = 788		n = 607		n = 51		n = 646		n = 726		n = 164	
ER- and JDC-Ratio > 1	1.069 (67,4)	381 (64,9)	1	688 (68,8)	1,19 (0,96|1,48)	123 (64,1)	1	517 (65,6)	1,07 (0,77|1,49)	429 (70,7)	1,35 (0,96|1,91)	32 (62,7)	1	420 (65,0)	1,10 (0,60|1,99)	509 (70,1)	1,39 (0,77|2,51)	108 (65,9)	1,15 (0,60|2,20)
			-		-		-		1		1,26 (1,01|1,59)*		-		1		1,26 (1,01|1,58)*		1,04 (0,72|1,49)
			-		-		-		-		-		-		-		1,22 (0,85|1,74)		1
JS1: "very satisfied"	859 (54,1)	339 (57,8)	1,26 (1,03|1,55)*	520 (52,0)	1	129 (67,2)	2,57 (1,83|3,62)***	461 (58,5)	1,77 (1,43|2,19)***	269 (44,3)	1	37 (72,5)	3,30 (1,66|6,55)***	407 (63,0)	2,12 (1,50|3,00)***	342 (47,1)	1,11 (0,79|1,56)	73 (44,5)	1
			-		-		1,45 (1,04|2,03)*		1		-		2,97 (1,58|5,58)***		1,91 (1,54|2,37)***		1		-
			-		-		-		-		-		1,55 (0,82|2,93)		1		-		-

who perceived their supervising physician as very satisfied with his job dropped from 72.5 % among under 20-year olds to 63.0 % among 20–24-year olds, to 47,1 % among 25–30-year olds and was at 44.5 % among the over 30-year olds. Therefore the odds ratio of under 20-year olds to over 30-year olds was 3.30 (95 %-CI: 1.66|6.55). Regarding distress prevalence only the 25–30-year olds had a significant higher distress compared to the 20–24-year olds (65.0 % to 70.1 %). This corresponded with an odds ratio of 1.26 (95 %-CI: 1.01|1.58; $p < 0.05$).

Study phase

The analysis of study phases revealed that for first- and second-year students their supervising physician seemed more often satisfied with his job than for students in higher study phases: This statement applied to 67.2 % of first-and second-year students, 58.5 % of third-, fourth- and fifth-year students and 44.3 % of final-year students. The odds ratio of third-, fourth- and fifth-year students to final-year students was 2.57 (95 %-CI: 1.83|3.62; $p < 0.001$). Concerning distress prevalence, the third-, fourth- and fifth-year

students perceived their supervising physician less often stressed out (ER/JDC-Ratio > 1) with a prevalence of 65.6 % compared to 70,7 % of final-year students who stated this. With an odds ratio of 1.26 (95 %-CI: 1.01|1.59; $p < 0.05$) this finding was significant.

Specialty

This chapter focuses on working conditions in different specialties from the students' perspective. The specialty of surgery was rated with the highest distress prevalence (ER/JDC-Ratio > 1): 81.3 % of students stated that their supervising surgeon encountered unfavorable working conditions. Compared to the average of 64.4 % this corresponded with an odds ratio of 1.99 (95 %-CI: 1.51|2.61; $p < 0.001$). The lowest distress prevalence in the perception of students was present in the specialty of anesthesiology with 34.8 % and a corresponding odds ratio to the average of 0.24 (95 %-CI: 0.17|0.36; $p < 0.001$). Also a significant lower prevalence was present in the specialty of psychiatry (45.2 %) and radiology (48.3 %). More details and specialties are displayed in Fig. 2. As this figure

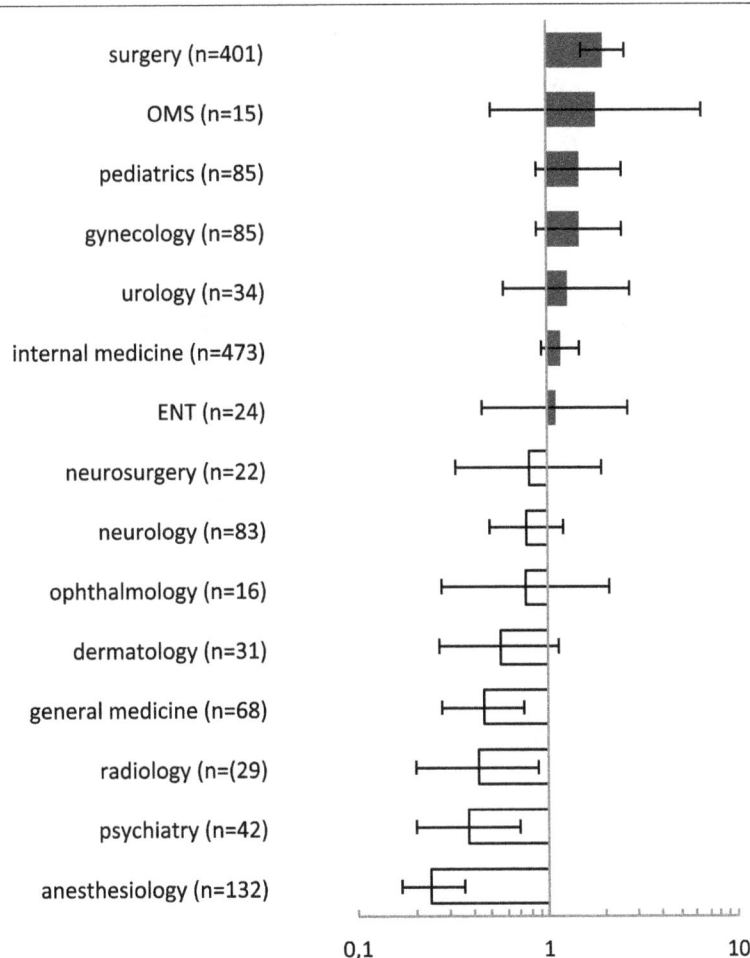

Fig. 2 Odds ratio of distress prevalence compared to the average, according to specialty; ENT (ear-nose-throat), OMS (oral and maxillofacial surgery)

indicates, there were substantial differences between specialties compared to the average and even more if compared directly: The odds ratio of anesthesiology to surgery regarding distress was 0.12 (95 %-CI: 0.08|0.19).

The further analysis of specialties regarding job satisfaction revealed similar differences: From the students' perspective the neurosurgeons seemed to be significantly more often satisfied with their job. 77.3 % of students stated that their supervising neurosurgeon was very satisfied with his job. Compared to the average of 54.1 % this corresponded with an odds ratio of 2.94 (95 %-CI: 1.08|8.01; $p < 0.05$). In the specialty of anesthesiology 72.0 % of students stated this with an odds ratio to the average of 2.22 (95 %-CI: 1.50|3.29; $p < 0.001$). Physicians in the specialty of internal medicine seemed to be less often satisfied: 43.8 % of students stated that their supervising physician was very satisfied with his job. Again compared to the average this corresponded with an odds ratio of 0.67 (95 %-CI: 0.55|0.83; $p < 0.001$). If compared to neurosurgery this corresponded with an odds ratio of 0.23

(95 %-CI: 0.08|0.63; $p < 0,001$). More specialties are displayed and compared to the average in Fig. 3.

Discussion

Whether the iCEPT-data can be seen as representative will be discussed first: Considering the response rate of 14.1 %, a selection-bias due to non-responder is possible. The response rate is relatively low compared to other web-based studies [33], raising the question of reliability. However the absolute number of 1587 participants is relatively high. Although there is a relatively high absolute number of participating students (1587) the representativeness of the data must be considered as critical. However, there are high congruencies of the iCEPT-sample in major characteristics with the basic sample, which could be seen as an indicator of representativeness.

As in the introduction indicated, there is a lack of sufficient international and national data regarding students' perception of working conditions (according to gender, age or study phase) to compare these results with.

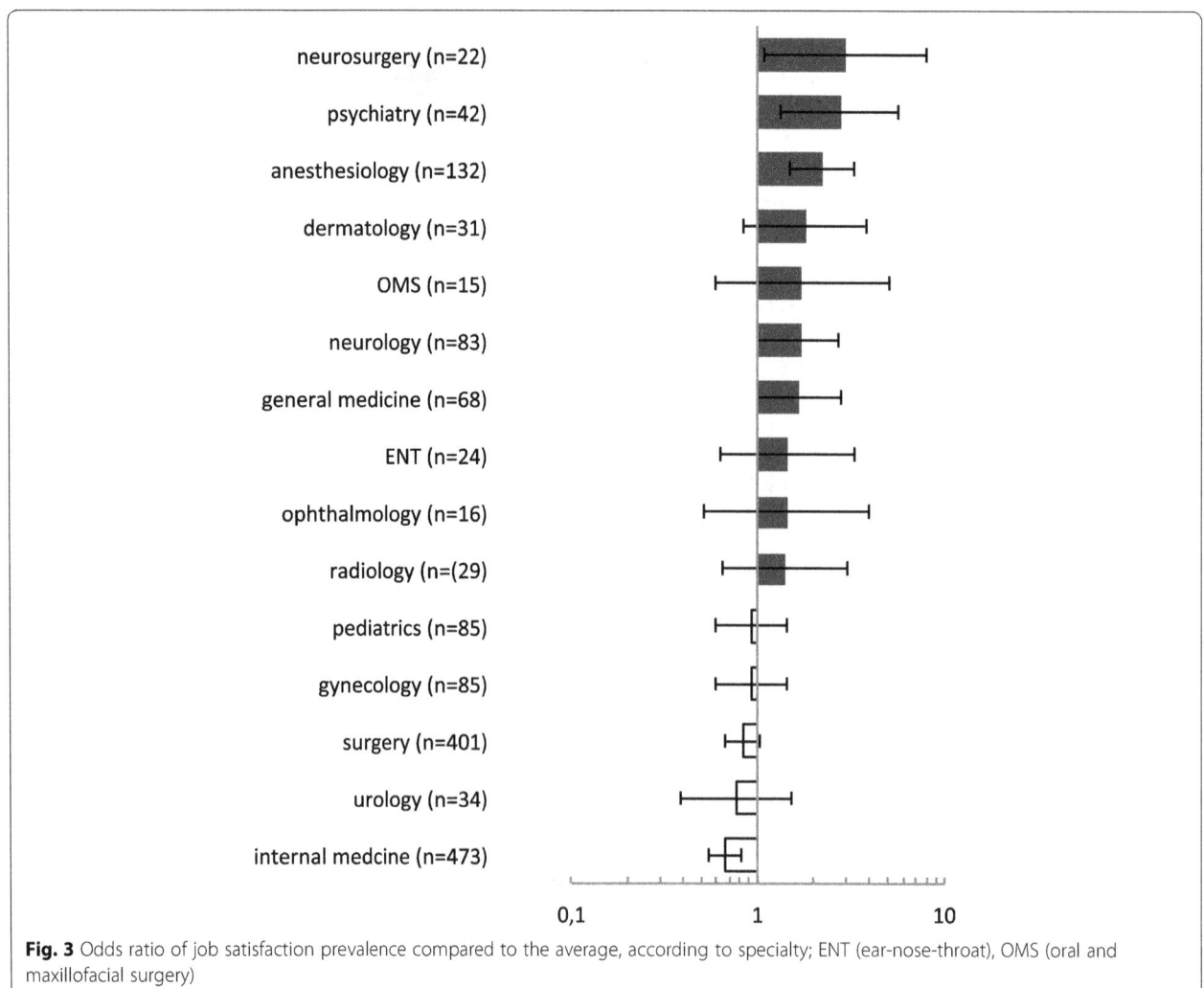

Fig. 3 Odds ratio of job satisfaction prevalence compared to the average, according to specialty; ENT (ear-nose-throat), OMS (oral and maxillofacial surgery)

Discussing the data according to specialty, the data will be compared to the specialty registration of physicians from the year 2013 in Germany [34]. This will be taken as an indirect indicator of students' perception of working conditions. In the iCEPT-Study the specialty of anesthesiology had relatively high job satisfaction prevalence and at the same time relatively low distress prevalence. The proportion of anesthesiology registration compared to all specialty registrations was 8.5 % and therefore anesthesiology came third. This seems to confirm the results of the iCEPT-study. On the other hand, first in specialty registration was internal medicine and second surgery. Both had relatively high distress prevalences and low job satisfaction prevalences in the iCEPT-Study. This seems to call the data into question. But there are multiple factors limiting this comparison: First the time lag of the final study exam to the specialty registration (at least 4–6 years). Second, there are many factors to be considered when making a specialty choice, the students' perception of working conditions only being one of them [8]. Still the perception of working conditions plays an important role: In a study from the year 2011 which focused on specialty choice of medical students, working conditions were the number two reason for students to choose their specialty [35]. However, the focus of our study was the perception of working conditions and not specialty choice, therefore despite similarities, the comparison of both studies has limitations.

The outlined results of students' perspective on physicians' working conditions will now be compared to the physicians' view on their own working conditions. For this purpose data of 7090 physicians from another published part of the iCEPT-study will be taken as the comparative data [14, 36–38]. Therefore the reference value of job satisfaction and distress among physicians is as followed: 53.9 % of polled physicians encountered distress (ER/JDC-Ratio > 1) and 55.8 % were very satisfied with their job. For these data the comparison with the students' data is indicated by the odds ratio: Among students there seem to be higher distress prevalences present than among physicians with an odds ratio of 1.76 (95 %-CI:1.57|1.98; $p < 0,001$). Especially female students seemed to rate the working conditions more often in form of an ER/JDC-Ratio > 1 (OR: 1.88; 95 %-CI:1.64|2.17; $p < 0.001$). Regarding the age, the 25-30-year old students stated a significant higher distress prevalence than physicians themselves (OR: 2.00; 95 %-CI:1.70|2.36; $p < 0.001$). The overall job satisfaction seemed to be perceived similarly among students and physicians, since there was no significant difference. Solely female students in contrast to male students seemed to perceive the physicians less often as satisfied with their job than the physicians themselves. The analysis of students' age regarding perception of job satisfaction revealed that especially for the under 20-year old students

their supervising physician seemed more often satisfied than the physicians stated themselves (OR: 2,09; 95 %-CI: 1,13|3,88; $p < 0.001$). Studies [39] have shown that there is a strong correlation between job stressors such as lack of leader support and low job satisfaction. The gender differences in the perception of working conditions could be explained by differing expectations of working conditions resulting in differing numbers regarding part-time: in 2013 30,4 % of all female physicians in Germany worked part-time, whereas 11,8 % of male physicians worked part-time [40]. Also during medical education gender issues arise which could influence the perception of working conditions [41]. In regard to differences among the age groups, the cumulative time spent in hospitals as well as personal experiences could affect the perception. However in the presented study no causal factors were investigated and therefore no conclusion can be drawn about causal factors.

In an Australian study comparing the perception of students and consultants in the field of emergency medicine there were also significant differences: 22.4 % of students and 50.0 % of consultants ($p < 0.05$) said that the workload would be too high. Furthermore 95.5 % of consultants and 64.9 % of students ($p < 0.001$) said that being an emergency physician would be a rewarding career [42].

Conclusion
The data set provided is valid and objective, giving clear insight on the students' perception of working conditions. So far this is among the first studies focusing explicit on external perception of working conditions. Two out of three medical students rated the physicians working conditions as stressful. This implicates that already in this early phase of their career the majority of medical students get to know the hospital as an unfavorable workplace concerning working conditions. In order to keep medical employees interested in the hospital, this has to be changed. However, the supervising physicians still seemed to be quite often very satisfied with their job. The discrepancy of satisfaction and working conditions illustrate the need for more research on this topic. Focusing on specialties, there are substantial differences regarding distress and job satisfaction. Taking the implications into account which go along with the perception of working conditions for the future career and/or specialty choice of medical students, it is crucial to improve the very same. Hence the displayed data can be used for creating balanced working conditions according to the respective stress models.

Competing interests
The authors declare that they have no competing interests.

Authors' contribution
JB conceived and designed the study and wrote the manuscript. DAG contributed to its final version. All authors read and approved the final manuscript.

Acknowledgements
This study was supported by the "Marburger Bund" and the German Medical Association. We want to thank Prof. Dr. med Ulrich Montgomery for his support.

References

1. Schmidt CE, Möller J, Schmidt K, Gerbershagen MU, Wappler F, Limmroth V, et al. Generation Y : recruitment, retention and development. Anaesthesist. 2011;60:517–24.
2. Gedrose B, Wonneberger C, Jünger J, Robra BP, Schmidt A, Stosch C, et al. Do female medical graduates have different views on professional work and workload compared to their male colleagues? Dtsch Med Wochenschr. 2012;137:1242–7.
3. Götz K, Miksch A, Hermann K, Loh A, Kiolbassa K, Joos S, et al. Aspirations of medical students: "planning for a secure career" - results of an online-survey among students at five medical schools in Germany. Dtsch Med Wochenschr. 2011;136:253–7.
4. Heinz A, Jacob R. Medical students and their career choices. Preferred specialty, where and how to work. Bundesgesundheitsblatt Gesundheitsforschung Gesundheitsschutz. 2012;55:245–53.
5. Buxel H. Motivation, job satisfaction and specialty choice of junior doctors and medical students. Münster: University of Applied Science in Münster; 2009.
6. Hermann K, Buchholz A, Loh A. Entwicklung, faktorenanalytische Überprüfung und psychometrische Evaluierung eines Fragebogens zur Gebietswahl von Medizinstudierenden. Gesundheitswesen. 2012;74:426–34.
7. Kiolbassa K, Miksch A, Hermann K, Loh A, Szecsenyi J, Joos S, et al. Becoming a general practitioner–which factors have most impact on career choice of medical students? BMC Fam Pr. 2011;12:25.
8. Bland CJ, Meurer LN, Maldonado G. Determinants of Primary Care Specialty Choice: A Non-statistical Meta-analysis of the Literature. Acad Med. 1995;70:620–41.
9. Holmes D, Tumiel-Berhalter L, Zayas L, Watkins R. "Bashing" of medical specialties: students' experiences and recommendations. Fam Med. 2008;40:400–6.
10. Jerant A, Srinivasan M, Bertakis KD. Attributes affecting the medical school primary care experience. Acad Med. 2010;85:605–13.
11. Phillips J, Weismantel D, Gold K, Schwenk T. How do medical students view the work life of primary care and specialty physicians? Fam Med. 2012;44:7–13.
12. Gulalp B, Karcioglu O, Sari A, Koseoglu Z. Burnout: need help? J Occup Med Toxicol. 2008;3:32.
13. Kersten M, Kozak A, Wendeler D, Paderow L, Nübling M, Nienhaus A. Psychological stress and strain on employees in dialysis facilities: a cross-sectional study with the Copenhagen Psychosocial Questionnaire. J Occup Med Toxicol. 2014;9:4.
14. Bauer J, Groneberg DA. Stress and job satisfaction in the discipline of inpatient anaesthesiology : Results of a web-based survey. Anaesthesist. 2014;63:32–40.
15. Blum K, Löffert S. Ärztemangel im Krankenhaus - Ausmaß, Ursachen, Gegenmaßnahmen. Deutsches Krankenhausinstitut: Düsseldorf; 2010.
16. WifOR-Institut. Fachkräftemangel: Stationärer und ambulanter Bereich bis zum Jahr 2030. Ostwald DA, Ehrhard T, Bruntsch F, Schmidt H, Friedl C, editors. Frankfurt am Main: PricewaterhouseCoopers AG Wirtschaftsprufungsgesellschaft; 2010.
17. Statistisches Bundesamt. Studierende an Hochschulen - Wintersemester 2011/12. Fachserie 11 R 41. Wiesbaden: German Federal Bureau of Statistics; 2012. 1–459
18. Statistisches Bundesamt. Bildung und Kultur: Prüfungen an Hochschulen. Fachserie 11 R 42. Wiesbaden: German Federal Bureau of Statistics; 2011. 244.
19. Schwarzer A, Fabian G. Medizinerreport 2012 – Berufsstart und Berufsverlauf von Humanmedizinerinnen und Humanmedizinern. Hochschul-Informations-System gmbH. Hannover: Hochschul-Informations-System GmbH (HIS); 2012.
20. Statistisches Bundesamt. Bildung und Kultur: Erfolgsquoten 2010. Wiesbaden: German Federal Bureau of Statistics; 2012.
21. Bauer J, Groneberg DA. Perception of stress-related working conditions in hospitals (iCept-study): a comparison between physicians and medical students. J Occup Med Toxicol. 2013;8:3.
22. Siegrist J. Adverse health effects of high-effort/low-reward conditions. J Occup Health Psychol. 1996;1(1):27–41.
23. Karasek RA. Job demands, job decision latitude and mental strain: Implications for job redesign. Adm Sci Q. 1979;24:285–308.
24. Karasek RA, Theorell T. Healthy work: stress, productivity and the reconstruction of working life. New York: New York Basic Books; 1990.
25. Peter R, Siegrist J, Hallqvist J, Reuterwall C, Theorell T. Psychosocial work environment and myocardial infarction: improving risk estimation by combining two complementary job stress models in the SHEEP Study. J Epidemiol Community Heal. 2002;56:294–300.
26. Prümper J, Hartmannsgruber K, Frese M. KFZA. Kurz-Fragebogen zur Arbeitsanalyse. Zeitschrift fur Arbeits- und Organisationsphsychologie. 1995;39:125–32.
27. Siegrist J, Starke D, Chandola T, Godin I, Marmot M, Niedhammer I, et al. The measurement of effort-reward imbalance at work: European comparisons. Soc Sci Med. 2004;58:1483–99.
28. Voltmer E, Rosta J, Siegrist J, Aasland OG. Job stress and job satisfaction of physicians in private practice: comparison of German and Norwegian physicians. Int Arch Occup Env Heal. 2012;85:819–28.
29. Siegrist J, Shackelton R, Link C, Marceau L, von dem Knesebeck O, McKinlay J. Work stress of primary care physicians in the US, UK and German health care systems. Soc Sci Med. 2010;71:298–304.
30. Lau B. Effort-reward imbalance and overcommitment in employees in a Norwegian municipality: a cross sectional study. J Occup Med Toxicol. 2008;3:9.
31. Schmidt K-H, Kleinbeck U. Job Diagnostic Survey (JDS - deutsche Fassung). In: Ulich E, editor. Dunkel,H Handb Psychol Arbeitsanalyseverfahren Schriftenr Mensch-Technik-Organisation. Band 14. Zürich: vdf Hochschulverlag AG; 1999. p. 205–30.
32. Wanous JP, Reichers AE, Hudy MJ. Overall job satisfaction: how good are single-item measures? J Appl Psychol. 1997;82:247–52.
33. Cummings SM, Savitz LA, Konrad TR. Reported Response Rates to Mailed Physician Questionnaires. Health Serv Res. 2001;35:1347–55.
34. German Medical Association. Ärztestatistik [Internet]. 2015. Available from: http://www.bundesaerztekammer.de/ueber-uns/aerztestatistik/aerztestatistik-2014/.
35. Orbach-Zinger S, Rosenblum R, Svetzky S, Staiman A, Eidelman L. Attitudes to anesthesiology residency among medical students in the American and the Israel programs at Sackler Faculty of Medicine, Tel Aviv University. IMAJ. 2011;13:485–7.
36. Bauer J, Groneberg DA. Distress Among Surgeons - a Study in German Hospitals. Zentralbl Chir. 2014 [Epub ahead of print]; Available from: http://www.ncbi.nlm.nih.gov/pubmed/24399503
37. Bauer J, Groneberg DA. Distress among physicians in hospitals - an investigation in Baden-Württemberg, Germany. Dtsch Med Wochenschr. 2013;138:2401–6.
38. Bauer J, Groneberg DA. Distress and job satisfaction among hospital physicians in internal medicine. Internist (Berl). 2014;55(10):1242–50.
39. Sterud T, Hem E, Lau B, Ekeberg O. A comparison of general and ambulance specific stressors: predictors of job satisfaction and health problems in a nationwide one-year follow-up study of Norwegian ambulance personnel. J Occup Med Toxicol. 2011;6:10.
40. German Federal Bureau of Statistics. Employees in the health care sector [Internet]. 2015 [cited 2015 Dec 29]. Available from: http://www.gbe-bund.de/oowa921-install/servlet/oowa/aw92/dboowasys921.xwdevkit/xwd_init?gbe.isgbetol/xs_start_neu/&p_aid=3&p_aid=26339847&nummer=96&p_sprache=D&p_indsp=-&p_aid=46264559
41. Risberg G, Johansson EE, Westman G, Hamberg K. Attitudes toward and experiences of gender issues among physician teachers: a survey study conducted at a university teaching hospital in Sweden. BMC Med Educ. 2008;8:10.
42. Celenza A, Bharath J, Scop J. Improving the attractiveness of an emergency medicine career to medical students: An exploratory study. Emerg Med Australas. 2012;24:625–33.

2

An evaluation of the protective role of vitamin C in reactive oxygen species-induced hepatotoxicity due to hexavalent chromium in vitro and in vivo

Xiali Zhong[1†], Ming Zeng[1†], Huanfeng Bian[2], Caigao Zhong[1] and Fang Xiao[1*]

Abstract

Backgroud: Drinking water contamination with hexavalent chromium [Cr (VI)] has become one of the most serious public health problems, thus the investigation of Cr (VI)-induced hepatotoxicity has attracted much attention in recent years.

Methods: In the present study, by determining the indices of hepatotoxicity induced by Cr (VI), the source of accumulated reactive oxygen species (ROS), and the protective effect of the antioxidant Vitamin C (Vit C), we explored the mechanisms involved in Cr (VI)-induced hepatotoxicity in vitro and in vivo.

Results: We found Cr (VI) caused hepatotoxicity characterized by the alterations of several enzymatic and cytokine markers including aspartate aminotransferase (AST), alanine aminotransferase (ALT), interleukine-1β (IL-1β), and tumor necrosis factor-α (TNF-α), etc. ROS production after Cr (VI) exposure was origins from the inhibition of electron transfer chain (ETC) and antioxidant system. Vit C inhibited ROS accumulation thus protected against Cr (VI)-induced hepatotoxicity in L-02 hepatocytes and in the rat model.

Conclusions: We concluded that ROS played a role in Cr (VI)-induced hepatotoxicity and Vit C exhibited protective effect. Our current data provides important clues for studying the mechanisms involved in Cr (VI)-induced liver injury, and may be of great help to develop therapeutic strategies for prevention and treatment of liver diseases involving ROS accumulation for occupational exposure population.

Keywords: Hexavalent chromium [Cr (VI)], Reactive oxygen species (ROS), Hepatotoxicity, Vitamin C (Vit C), Mitochondrial respiratory chain complex I (MRCC I)

Background

Chromium (Cr) is commercially used in various industrial processes such as leather tanning, stainless steel welding and chrome plating [1]. The pollution of hexavalent chromium [Cr (VI)] has become one of the most serious public health problems worldwide and the serious pollution incidents have dramatically increased in the last few years. The adverse health effects following occupational or accidental exposures of Cr (VI) and its compounds include a range of slight gastrointestinal reactions such as nausea and vomiting to more serious effects including hepatic damage, primary liver cancers, and even death [2]. Now we have to pay attention that not only the Cr-operating workers, but also the general population may also be at risk because Cr (VI) and the compounds are now widespread in our intimately related environment even in the food [3]. It is known that Cr (VI) enters the target cells and then undergoes metabolic reduction to pentavalent chromium [Cr (V)], tetravalent chromium [Cr (IV)] and trivalent chromium [Cr (III)], causing the accumulation of reactive oxygen species (ROS) [4]. ROS, including hydroxyl radicals (OH·), hydrogen peroxide (H_2O_2), and superoxide anion radical ($O_2^{·-}$), are the molecules that contain an odd number of electrons.

* Correspondence: fangxiao@csu.edu.cn
†Equal contributors
[1]Department of Health Toxicology, Xiangya School of Public Health, Central South University, NO. 238 Shangmayuanling Road, Kaifu District, Changsha 410078, Hunan, People's Republic of China
Full list of author information is available at the end of the article

The main sources of intracellular ROS are enzymatic reactions, nicotinamide adenine dinucleotide phosphate-oxidase (NADPH oxidase), and mitochondrial respiration [5]. Mitochondrial respiratory chain complexes (MRCCs), whose inhibition may cause the escape of electrons from electron transfer chain (ETC), are the most important source of heavy metal-induced ROS accumulation [6]. The major sites of ETC for ROS production remained controversial, and it is reported by others that MRCC III from the ETC is the major site for ROS production [7]. The members of antioxidant system including superoxide dismutase (SOD) and glutathione (GSH) are known as ROS scavenging enzymes whose function are associated with the elimination of excess ROS. ROS play an important role in various cellular signaling processes at low levels while exert a cytotoxic effect by damaging macromolecules such as proteins, lipids and nucleic acids. The reduction of Cr (VI) results in the formation of free radicals which induce a cascade of cellular events including apoptosis, genotoxicity and carcinogenicity, but the related mechanisms of the accumulated free radicals still remain unclear. In the present study we hypothesize that the accumulation of free radicals after Cr (VI) exposure is associated with both the burst generation and the decreased elimination of ROS.

Since there is accumulating evidence indicating a possible causative involvement of ROS in liver injury [8], the anti-oxidative therapy may be of great importance for the established Cr (VI)-associated liver diseases. Vitamin C (Vit C), also known as ascorbic acid, is necessary for the body and widely found in fruits and vegetables. Vit C plays a role as an essential coenzyme in the oxidative stress (OS) pathways, and is an important antioxidant and ROS scavenger. Therefore, Vit C is potentially useful as a therapeutic agent in the treatment of the disorders that associated with free radicals. The liver, an important body organ for its involvement in the biotransformation of various xenobiotics, plays crucial roles in metal homeostasis and detoxification. Although Cr (VI) has been reported to induce hepatotoxicity and natural and synthetic antioxidants have been shown to exert protective effects, the related molecular and cellular mechanisms as well as the potential anti-hepatotoxic protective effect of Vit C on Cr (VI)-induced hepatotoxicity both in vitro and in vivo remain to be fully elucidated. Therefore, we aimed to explore the underlying mechanism of Cr (VI)-induced hepatotoxicity and the possibility that the administration of Vit C would have a beneficial effect on Cr-induced hepatic injuries for the occupation exposure population. The present work was undertaken to study the liver injury by detecting the enzymatic and cytokine markers, to examine the possible sources of the elevated ROS, and to investigate the protective effect of Vit C on Cr (VI)-induced hepatotoxicity both in L-02 hepatocyte and in the rat model.

Materials and methods

Cell line

Human L-02 hepatocyte line was obtained from Type Culture Collection of Chinese Academy of Sciences, Shanghai, China. Cells were cultured as previously described [9].

Animals

The adult Sprague-Dawley (SD) rats aged about 2 months with the average body weight of 180 ± 20 g were purchased from the animal center of Central South University (Changsha, Hunan, China). All rats were housed at the temperature of 22 ± 2 °C and a humidity of 55 ± 5% in a 12h light/dark cycle in standard clear plastic cages with food and water. All animal experiments were performed in accordance with the guidelines of China Council on Animal Care and Use. All animal procedures carried out in this study were reviewed, approved, and supervised by the Animal Care and Use Committee of Central South University.

Animal experiment design

Sixty SD rats were randomly divided into 6 groups, each with 10 animals. Group 1 was the control group, and received normal saline (NS); group 2 was treated with low dose of Cr (VI) (8.84 mg/kg.Bw) (potassium dichromate ($K_2Cr_2O_7$) was dissolved in NS and then was configured to various test doses); group 3 received high dose of Cr (VI) (17.68 mg/kg.Bw); group 4 received Vit C alone (500 mg/kg.Bw); group 5 was treated with the combination of Vit C (500 mg/kg.Bw) plus Cr (VI) (8.84 mg/kg.Bw); group 6 was treated with the combination of Vit C (500 mg/kg.Bw) plus Cr (VI) (17.68 mg/kg.Bw). All rats were given the drugs by gavage at a dose of 0.5 ml/100 g body weight daily for a week (7 consecutive days). Group 1, 2 and 3 were firstly treated with NS by gavage, half an hour later, group 1 received NS and group 2 and 3 received Cr (VI); group 4, 5 and 6 were firstly treated with Vit C by gavage, half an hour later, group 4 received NS and group 5 and 6 received Cr (VI).

Sample collection and preparation

One week later and at the end of the experiment, the urine and stool of the last 24 h treatment of all rats were collected. The urine was precipitated to remove residue, and the stool was dried to constant weight. Blood samples (4 ml of each rat) collected from the femoral artery were allowed to coagulate for 30 min and centrifuged at 2500 rpm for 15 min to separate the serum for biochemical analysis as described below. The rats were sacrificed using ether anesthesia. For each rat, liver specimen (1 g) was collected and then was suspended in ice-cold NS and homogenized in a polytron homogenizer to obtain

10 ml liver tissue suspension. All the samples were stored at −80 °C for further analysis.

Materials

$K_2Cr_2O_7$ and Vit C were purchased from Sigma (St. Louis, MO, USA). RPMI-1640 culture medium, fetal bovine serum (FBS), and trypsin were obtained from Solarbio (Beijing, China). All chemicals and solvents were of analytical grade or the best pharmaceutical grade.

The detection of enzymatic makers of liver injury

The supernatant from treated hepatocytes and serum samples from rats in groups 1 to 6 were analyzed for aspartate aminotransferase (AST) and alanine aminotransferase (ALT) activities spectrophotometrically using the detection kits (Jiancheng Institute of Biological Products, Nanjing, China). The experiments were performed according to the manufacturer's protocols.

The detection of cytokines and LTB4 levels

The levels of leukotriene B4 (LTB4) and the cytokines including interleukine-1β (IL-1β), tumor necrosis factor-α (TNF-α), interferon-γ (IFN-γ), and interleukine-10 (IL-10) were examined using the enzyme linked immunosorbent assay (ELISA) detection kits (Huamei Institute of Biological Products, Wuhan, China). The experiments were performed according to the manufacturer's protocols.

ROS detection

ROS levels were evaluated using fluorescent probe 5-(and 6)-chloromethyl-2′, 7′-dichlorodihydrofluorescein diacetate (CM-H2DCFDA, Molecular Probers, USA). Briefly, after the treatment of various compounds as indicated in the legends to figures, cells of each group were incubated with 10 μM CM-H2DCFDA and analyzed by fluorescence microscope and flow cytometry (Ex 485 nm and Em 535 nm). 2′, 7′-dichlorofluorescein (DCF) is the oxidized product of CM-H2DCFDA. Intracellular ROS level was considered to be directly proportional to the fluorescence intensity of the oxidized product DCF after CM-H2DCFDA treatment. Three independent experiments were performed for each assay condition.

Superoxide anion production detection

Superoxide anion production was assessed by dihydroethidium (DHE) staining. The cells were cultured and treated as above. After rinsed twice with phosphate buffered saline (PBS), the cells were incubated in the dark with 5 μM DHE (Sigma-Aldrich, St Louis, MO) for 30 min. In the presence of superoxide anion, DHE can be oxidized to ethidium bromide (EtBr) (Ex 488 nm and Em 610 nm) which expressing red fluorescence. Thus the amount of EtBr is well correlated to the level of cellular superoxide anion. Superoxide anion in the cells

was analyzed by flow cytometry and presented by the percentage of positively staining cells.

Mitochondria isolation

Mitochondria were isolated as described previously [10]. Cells were washed twice with cold PBS, and resuspended with 5 ml buffer A (250 mM sucrose, 20 mM 4-(2-hydroxyethyl)-1-piperazineethanesulfonic acid (HEPES), 10 mM KCl, 1.5 mM $MgCl_2$, 1 mM ethylene diaminetetra acetic acid (EDTA), 1 mM ethylene glycol-bis (2-aminoethylether)- N, N, N ′, N ′-tetraacetic acid (EGTA), 1 mM dithiothreitol, 0.1 mM phenylmethylsulfonyl fluoride, pH 7.5). Cells were homogenized and centrifuged twice at 750×g for 10 min. Mitochondria pellets were obtained after centrifugation at 10,000×g for 15 min. Isolated mitochondria were used immediately for the measurement of complexes activity. In order to confirm the purity and functionality of the purified mitochondria, transmission electron microscope was used to observe the ultra-structure at magnification of 300,000 times and Clark-type oxygen electrode was used to detect the respiratory function.

Measurement of MRCC activities

The activities of MRCC I-IV were determined using MRCC activity assay kits (Genmed Scientifics, shanghai, China) and were quantified using an UV-9100 spectrophotometer. MRCC I (Nicotinamide adenine dinucleotide (NADH) CoQ oxidoreductase) activity was measured following the oxidation of NADH at 340 nm and expressed as nmol oxidized NADH/min/mg prot; MRCC II (succinate: 2, 6-Dichloroindophenol (DCIP) oxireductase) activity was measured following the reduction of DCIP at 600 nm and expressed as nmol reduced DCIP/min/mg prot; MRCC III (ubiquinol: cytochrome c (Cyt c) reductase) activity was measured following the reduction of Cyt c at 550 nm and expressed as nmol reduced Cyt c /min/mg prot, and MRCC IV (Cyt c oxidase) activity was measured following the oxidation of Cyt c at 550 nm and expressed as nmol oxidized Cyt c/min/mg prot. All measurements were performed at least three times.

Real-time quantitative PCR

Total RNA was extracted from L-02 hepatocytes treated with different concentrations of Cr (VI) using the RNeasy Mini Kit (QIAGEN, Hilden, Germany). Then the total RNA (5 μg) from each treatment group was reverse-transcribed by the PrimeScript RT reagents kit (Takara, Dalian, China) according to the standard protocol. cDNAs were analyzed immediately for Real-time PCR assay using SYBR®Premix Taq™ (Takara, Dalian, China) with Applied Biosystems 7900HT Fast Real-Time PCR System (Applied Biosystems, Inc., Foster City, CA, USA) to observe the mRNA levels of targeted genes. The primer sequence of MRCC I [NADH dehydrogenase [ubiquin-one] iron-sulfur protein 3 (NDUFS3)]: 5'- atgttgcc caaactggtctc –3 (forward primer), 5'- tcactgccttcccagagagt –3' (reverse primer).

Measurement of GSH, SOD, Trx, MDA cellular levels and protein levels

The assessments of the GSH, SOD, and malondialde-hyde (MDA) levels were conducted by using the stand-ard kits (Jiancheng Bioengineering Institute, Nanjing, China). And the examination of thioredoxin (Trx) level was also using the kit (Huamei Bioengineering Institute, Wuhan, China). GSH level was examined by the amount of total non-protein sulfhydryl groups, SOD level was examined based on the inhibitory effect of SOD on nitro blue tetrazolium (NBT), Trx level was examined by a double antibody sandwich ELISA method, and MDA level was examined by thiobarbituric acid reactive sub-stances (TBARS).

Protein levels were determined by Western Blotting. Cell lysate was prepared by lysing the cells and then the protein was electrophoretically transferred onto polyvi-nylidene difluoride (PVDF) membranes and immuno-blotted with the antibodies GSH-1 (H-41) (sc-292,189), SOD-1 Antibody (FL-154) (sc-11,407), and Trx (FL-105) (sc-20,146) (Santa Cruz Biotechnology, USA). After in-cubated with second antibodies, the membranes were developed with the detection system and exposed to films.

Measurement for cell survival rate

Three-(4,5-dimethylthiazol-2yl-)-2,5-diphenyl tetrazolium bromide (MTT) assay was used to evaluate cell survival rate. Briefly, the hepatocytes were seeded at a density of 1×10^4 cells/well in the 96-well plate. Vit C of indicated final concentrations were added to the cultures. Control cells and medium controls without cells received DMSO. The cells were incubated at 37 °C in 5% CO_2 saturated at-mosphere and then were washed twice with PBS. Cells were treated with 5 µl 5 mg/ml MTT solution for additional 4 h at 37 °C, and then were lysed in PBS containing 20% Sodium dodecyl sulfate (SDS) and 50% N, N-dimethylformamide (pH 4.5). MTT conversion was quantified by a multiwell ELISA reader Versamax (Molecular Devices, Sunnyvale, CA, USA) at 570 nm.

Histopathological examination of liver

Liver tissue samples were fixed overnight with 10% neutral buffered formalin and then were rinsed for 2 h using running water. The tissues were dehydrated with different concentrations of ethanol and dimethyl-benzene and then were embedded in paraffin, sec-tioned at a thickness of 4 µm, and stained with

hematoxylin and eosin (H&E). The specimens were then examined under light microscopy.

Measurement of Cr content

The chromium contents of the samples were determined using the flame atomic absorption spectrometry (F-AAS) method as described earlier [11]. Briefly, prepare chro-mium standard solution (10 µg/l) and add with 1% spectra pure HNO_3. Then determine the absorbance of different concentrations of standard chromium solution (0, 0.2, 0.5, 1.0, 2.0, 4.0 µg/l) and draw the standard curve. Cr con-tents of stool, urine, liver and plasma samples were then measured at a wavelength of 357.9 nm.

Measurement of free radical scavenging capacity

The assay was based on benzoic acid hydroxylation method with slight modification. Briefly, in a colorimet-ric tube, 20 µl $FeSO_4$ (20 mM) and 20 µl EDTA (3 mM) were added. Then, 100 µl sample solution and 1840 µl PBS (pH 7.4) and 20 µl benzoic acid (10 g/l) were added to give a total volume of 2 ml. The reaction mixture was incubated in 37 °C water bath for 90 min. Then the fluorescence was measured at excitation/emission wave-lengths of about 305/410 nm. Free radical scavenging capacity % = 100% × [Fs-(Ft-Fc)]/(Fs-Fc). Fs is the fluor-escence intensity of the colorimetric tube without the adding of liver sample solution, Ft is the fluorescence in-tensity of the colorimetric tube with the adding of liver samples from different treatment groups, and Fc is the fluorescence intensity of the colorimetric tube without the adding of $FeSO_4$ or liver sample solution.

Statistical analysis

The results are expressed as mean ± standard deviation (SD). Normal distribution test and Levene's test were performed for Equality of Variances. Significant differ-ences were calculated by one-way analysis of variance (ANOVA) (data fitting normal distribution) or Kruskal-Wallis rank test (data not fitting normal distribution). All statistical analyses were performed using SPSS 19.0. The level of significance was set at $p < 0.05$.

Results

Cr (VI) induced hepatotoxicity in vitro

AST and ALT levels are widely used enzymatic markers of hepatotoxicity. The Cr (VI) treatment groups (8 and 16 µM) showed considerable increase in AST and ALT activities compared with that of the control group (Fig.1a). IL-1β is a potent pro-inflammatory cytokine and IL-10 is an anti-inflammatory cytokine. TNF-α and IFN-γ are also the members of cytokine family that involved in systemic inflammation. IL-10 possesses a hepatic protective effect on proliferation, and it has been shown to inhibit the production of pro-inflammatory

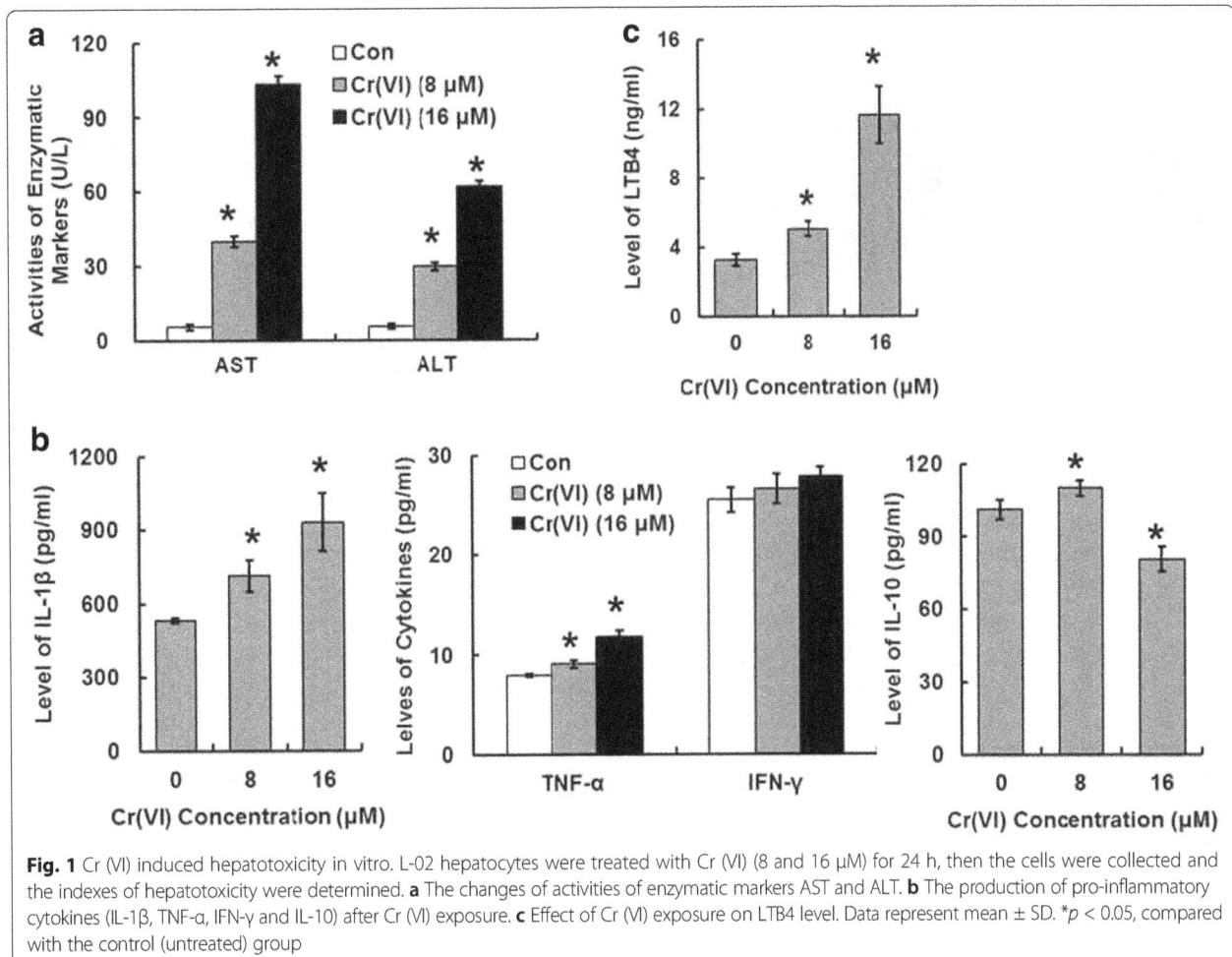

Fig. 1 Cr (VI) induced hepatotoxicity in vitro. L-02 hepatocytes were treated with Cr (VI) (8 and 16 μM) for 24 h, then the cells were collected and the indexes of hepatotoxicity were determined. **a** The changes of activities of enzymatic markers AST and ALT. **b** The production of pro-inflammatory cytokines (IL-1β, TNF-α, IFN-γ and IL-10) after Cr (VI) exposure. **c** Effect of Cr (VI) exposure on LTB4 level. Data represent mean ± SD. *$p < 0.05$, compared with the control (untreated) group

cytokines, such as TNF-α and IL-1β during the acute inflammation. As shown in Fig. 1b, after Cr (VI) exposure, IL-1β and TNF-α production were increased obviously compared with control, while IFN-γ level showed no obvious change. IL-10 level was increased at the Cr (VI) treatment concentration of 8 μM and decreased at 16 μM. Fig. 1c revealed that Cr (VI) induced increased level of LTB4.

Cr (VI) induced ROS accumulation in the hepatocytes

ROS have been implicated in liver injury. To evaluate the effect of Cr (VI) treatment on intracellular ROS level, we performed the assay by utilizing fluorescent probe CM-H2DCFDA in L-02 hepatocytes treated with different concentrations of Cr (VI) (8 and 16 μM). We identified that compared with control group, Cr (VI) treatment induced higher level of fluorescence signals when observed under microscope (Fig. 2a, left panel). The values of the related DCF fluorescence of each group quantitated by flow cytometry were also shown (Fig. 2a, right panel). DCFH can be oxidized directly by Cr intermediates such as Cr (IV) and Cr (V), thus in the

present study we also used DHE which is insensitive to Cr intermediates to monitor superoxide anion production. Superoxide anion is one of a group of molecules referred to as ROS. It has been confirmed that superoxide anion can be produced by both MRCCs and NADPH oxidase in a highly regulated manner and low amounts of superoxide anion plays critical roles in cell proliferation and apoptosis [12]. Superoxide anion production in the hepatocytes was assessed by DHE staining. We found that the percentage of positive staining cells was obviously higher in Cr (VI)-treated groups than that of the control group (Fig. 2b).

The inhibition of MRCC I and antioxidant system were associated with Cr (VI)-induced ROS accumulation

The enzyme complexes of the ETC locate in the mitochondrial inner membrane and play central roles in energy metabolism and other physiological activities. We inferred that the MRCCs in ETC may be responsible for ROS overproduction because the inhibition of MRCCs could induce increased electron leakage from ETC. We examined the alterations of MRCC I-IV activities in

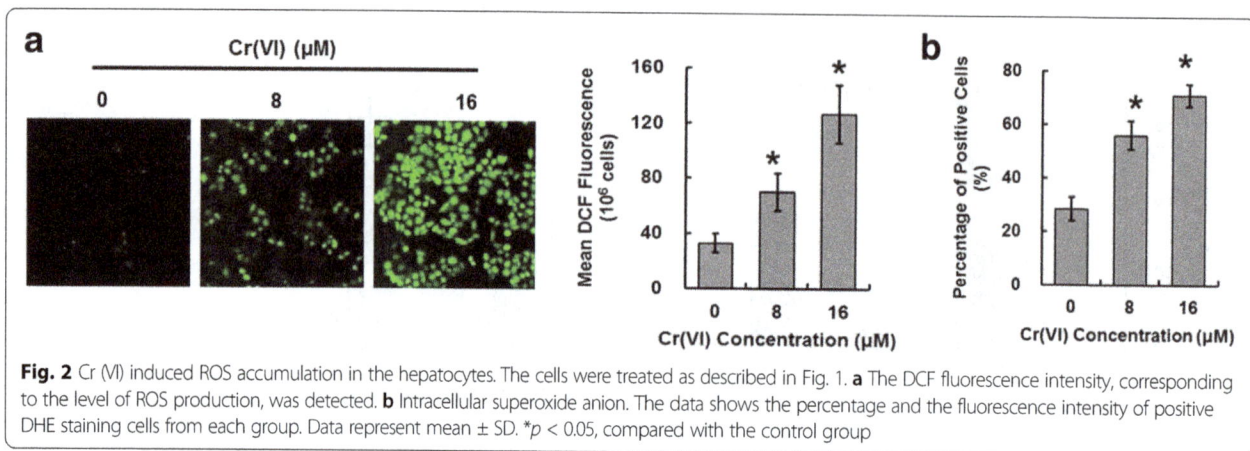

Fig. 2 Cr (VI) induced ROS accumulation in the hepatocytes. The cells were treated as described in Fig. 1. **a** The DCF fluorescence intensity, corresponding to the level of ROS production, was detected. **b** Intracellular superoxide anion. The data shows the percentage and the fluorescence intensity of positive DHE staining cells from each group. Data represent mean ± SD. *$p < 0.05$, compared with the control group

purified mitochondrial fraction. MRCC I appeared to be the most affected one after Cr (VI) exposure. Although complex II was also altered to some extent, the change was not as significant as that of complex I. The activities of MRCC III and IV were not altered compared with control (Fig. 3a). The result suggested that MRCC I and II, especially the former may be the main target of Cr

(VI) to induce mitochondrial ETC dysfunction and ROS accumulation. NDUFS3 encodes one of the iron-sulfur protein components of MRCC I. Mutations or inhibition of this gene are associated with MRCC I deficiency. The results shown in Fig. 3b revealed that Cr (VI) inhibited NDUFS3 at both mRNA and protein levels. GSH, SOD, and Trx are main antioxidative proteins that involved in

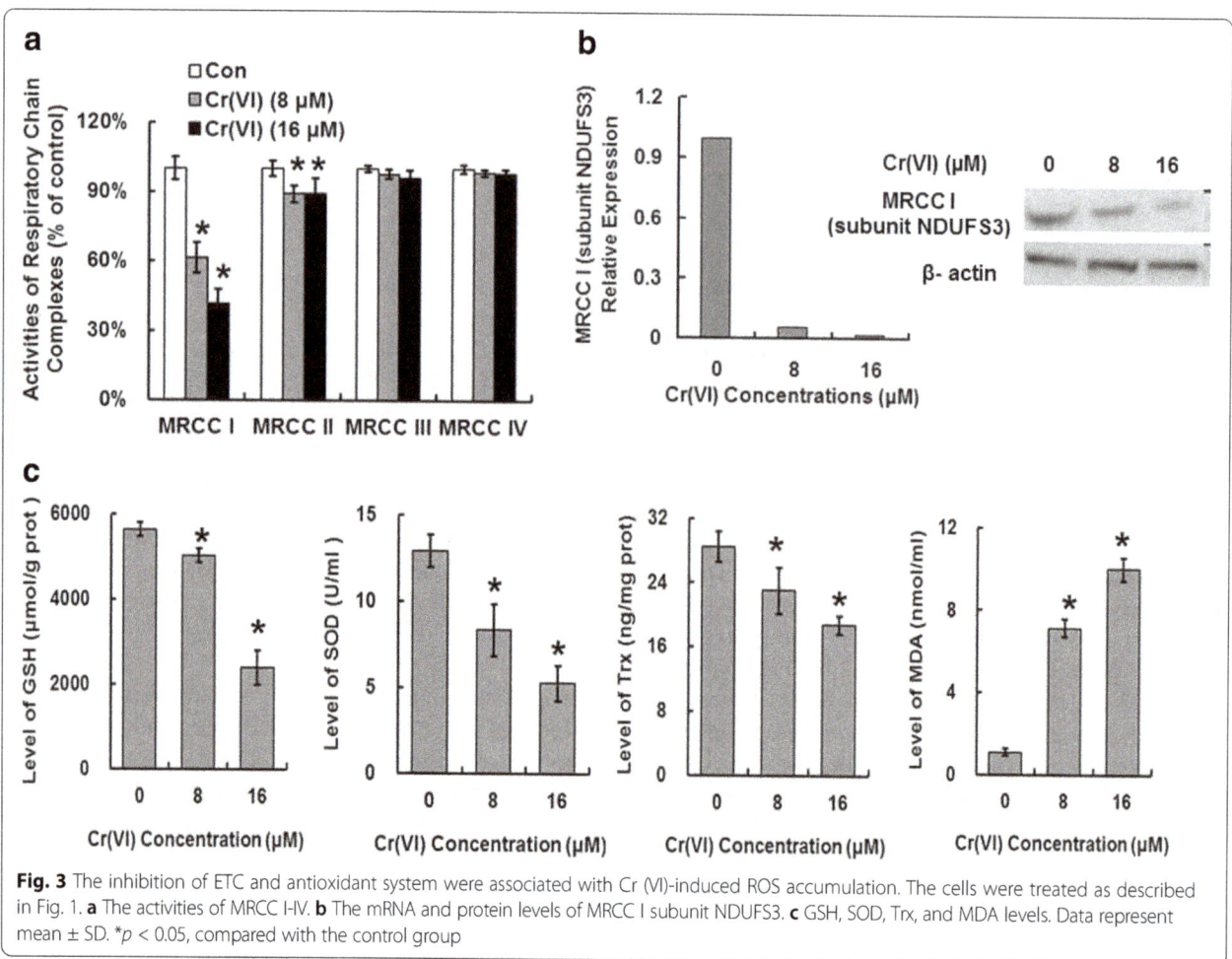

Fig. 3 The inhibition of ETC and antioxidant system were associated with Cr (VI)-induced ROS accumulation. The cells were treated as described in Fig. 1. **a** The activities of MRCC I-IV. **b** The mRNA and protein levels of MRCC I subunit NDUFS3. **c** GSH, SOD, Trx, and MDA levels. Data represent mean ± SD. *$p < 0.05$, compared with the control group

ROS clearance. It is reported that some chemotherapeutic agents cause ROS-dependent cytotoxicity by down-regulating the expression of the antioxidative proteins to facilitate ROS over-production, thus we tested these proteins expressions in Cr (VI)-treated hepatocytes to confirm the resource of ROS. As shown in Fig. 3c, Cr (VI) decreased GSH, SOD and Trx levels in the dose-dependent manner. Cr (VI) also increased MDA level which suggested the occurrence of lipid peroxidation.

Vit C inhibited ROS accumulation

The potential role of free radicals in hepatotoxicity associated with Cr (VI) exposure suggests that antioxidant supplementation may mitigate Cr (VI)-induced toxicity, thus we utilized Vit C in the present study to decrease intracellular ROS level. We analyzed the effect of Vit C (0–2430 μM) on cell survival rate and chose the concentration of 200 μM for the following studies according to the MTT result showed in Fig. 4a. To confirm the antagonistic effect of Vit C on Cr (VI)-induced free radical accumulation, L-02 hepatocytes were pretreated with Vit C (200 μM) for 2 h and then were exposed to Cr (VI) (8 and 16 μM) for 24 h. ROS assay was then performed as described before. As shown in Fig. 4b, Vit C decreased the fluorescence signal levels under microscope and the

DCF fluorescence values by flow cytometry, suggesting the inhibition of Cr (VI)-induced ROS production. The DHE staining also showed that Vit C inhibited superoxide anion production by decreasing the percentage of positive staining cells (Fig. 4c).

Vit C protected against Cr (VI)-induced hepatotoxicity in vitro

The cells were exposed to Cr (VI) (0, 8 and 16 μM) with or without the pretreatment of 200 μM Vit C. Vit C significantly inhibited the increase of Cr (VI)-induced AST/ALT levels (Fig. 5a). We also examined effect of Vit C on other liver injury markers including IL-1β, TNF-α and LTB4 and obtained the similar results (Fig. 5b). Vit C also restrained Cr (VI)-induced antioxidant system dysfunction by inhibiting the decrease of GSH, SOD, and Trx levels (Fig. 5c). Fig. 5d showed the western blotting result. These results confirmed that Vit C exerted protective effect against Cr (VI)-induced hepatotoxicity in the L-02 hepatocytes.

Vit C protected against Cr (VI)-induced hepatotoxicity in vivo

All rats were given the drugs by gavage at a dose of 0.5 ml/100 g body weight daily for a week (seven consecutive

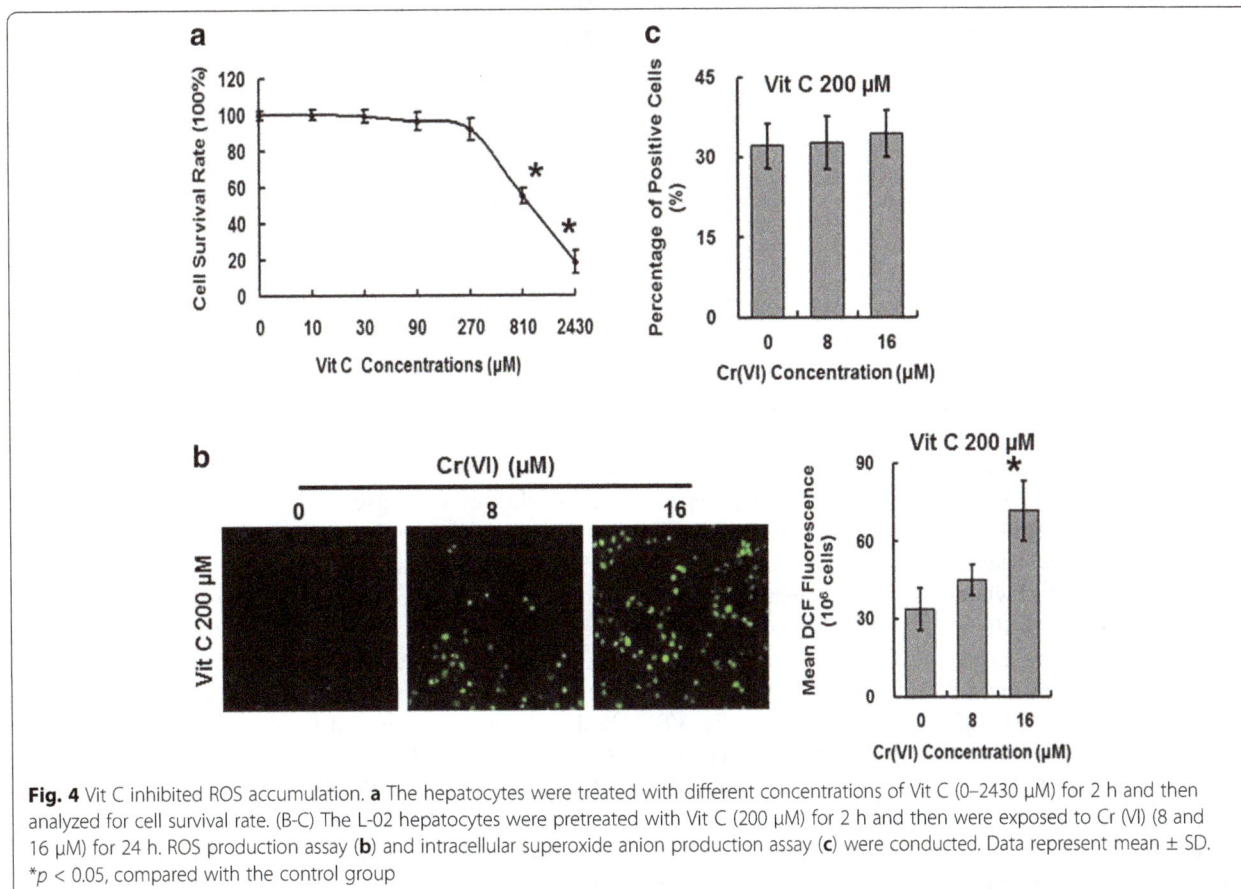

Fig. 4 Vit C inhibited ROS accumulation. **a** The hepatocytes were treated with different concentrations of Vit C (0–2430 μM) for 2 h and then analyzed for cell survival rate. (B-C) The L-02 hepatocytes were pretreated with Vit C (200 μM) for 2 h and then were exposed to Cr (VI) (8 and 16 μM) for 24 h. ROS production assay (**b**) and intracellular superoxide anion production assay (**c**) were conducted. Data represent mean ± SD. *$p < 0.05$, compared with the control group

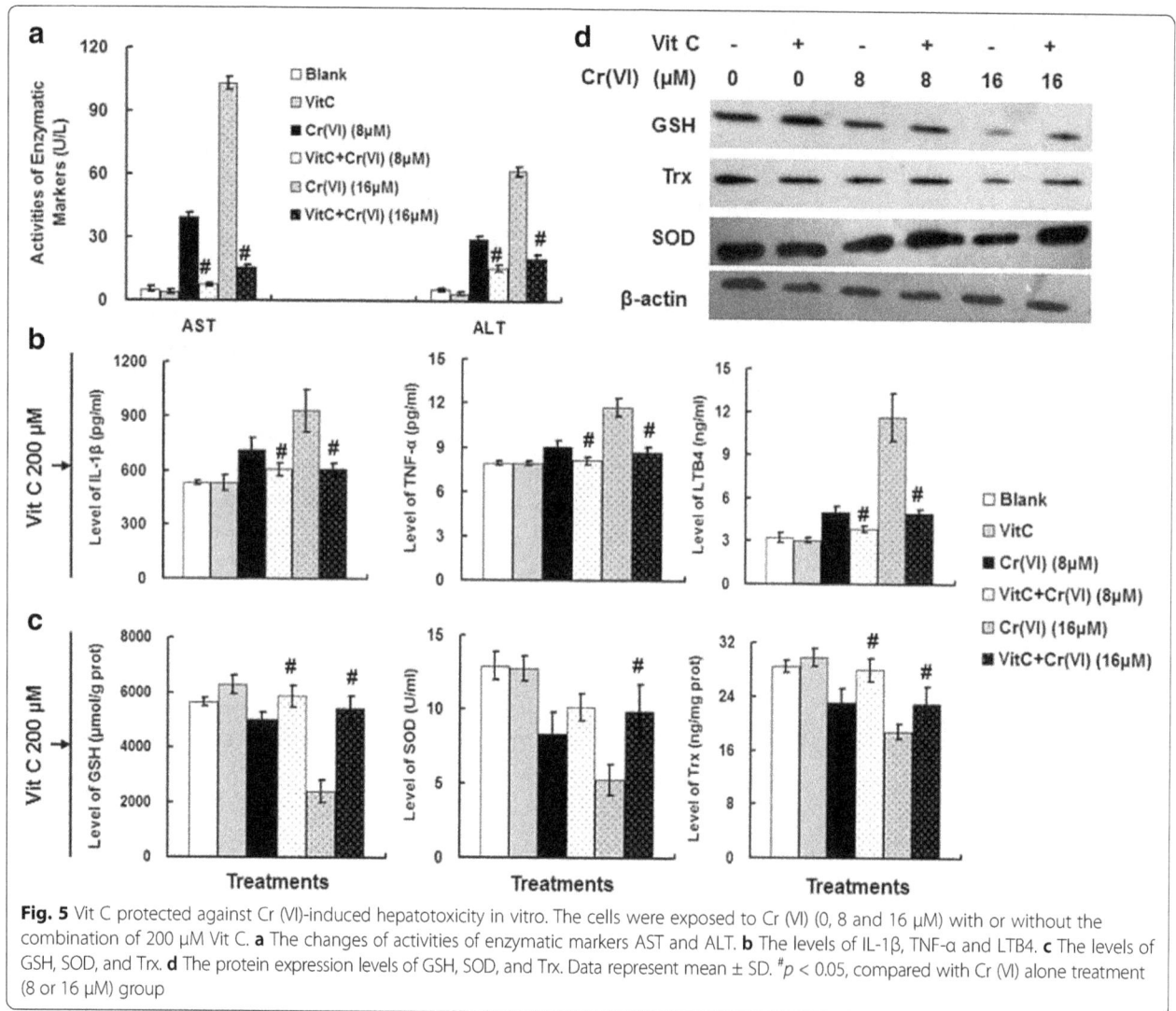

Fig. 5 Vit C protected against Cr (VI)-induced hepatotoxicity in vitro. The cells were exposed to Cr (VI) (0, 8 and 16 μM) with or without the combination of 200 μM Vit C. **a** The changes of activities of enzymatic markers AST and ALT. **b** The levels of IL-1β, TNF-α and LTB4. **c** The levels of GSH, SOD, and Trx. **d** The protein expression levels of GSH, SOD, and Trx. Data represent mean ± SD. #$p < 0.05$, compared with Cr (VI) alone treatment (8 or 16 μM) group

days). Groups are indicated by pretreatment + treatment as follows: Con, Vit C, Cr (VI) (8.84 mg/kg.bw), Vit C+ Cr (VI) (8.84 mg/kg.bw), Cr (VI) (17.68 mg/kg.bw), and Vit C + Cr (VI) (17.68 mg/kg.bw). As shown in Fig. 6a, a microscopic examination of the liver samples from all treatment groups revealed the typical histopathological features. Both the control and the Vit C (500 mg/kg.bw) group represented the normal rat liver showing normal hepatic architecture (H & E, ×200 magnification). The administration of Cr (VI) (8.84 mg/kg.bw) induced focal necrosis in the centrilobular region with infiltration of neutrophils and lymphocytes, while the hepatic lobules were clear and the hepatic cords were arranged in order. The histology of the livers from Vit C (500 mg/kg.bw) pretreatment plus Cr (VI) (8.84 mg/kg.bw) group showed slight inflammatory cell infiltration. And the Cr (VI) (17.68 mg/kg.bw) group revealed moderate to intense cytoplasmic vacuolization, central vein stenosis, and hepatocyte focal necrosis. Vit C (500 mg/kg.bw) pretreatment significantly alleviated Cr

(VI) (17.68 mg/kg.bw)-induced pathological changes. We also examined the effect of Vit C on Cr excretion and Cr content in plasms and liver. Fig. 6b revealed that treatment of Cr (VI) significantly increased Cr content in stool, urine, liver and plasma in a dose-dependent manner. Vit C pretreatment plus Cr (VI) (17.68 mg/kg.bw) group showed higher fecal excretion and lower Cr content in liver and plasma compared with that of the Cr (VI) (17.68 mg/kg.bw) alone treatment group, indicating that Vit C treatment accelerated the fecal excretion of Cr in liver and plasma. High dose of Cr (VI) treatment increased AST activity, and Vit C pretreatment only alleviated high dose of Cr (VI)-induced AST activity elevation. Both low and high dose of Cr (VI) treatments increased ALT activity, and Vit C pretreatment showed obvious inhibitory effect on AST activity elevation (Fig. 6c). The examination of effect of Vit C on Cr (VI)-induced hepatic antioxidant system damage showed that Cr (VI) decreased GSH and SOD levels and increased MDA level, and Vit C

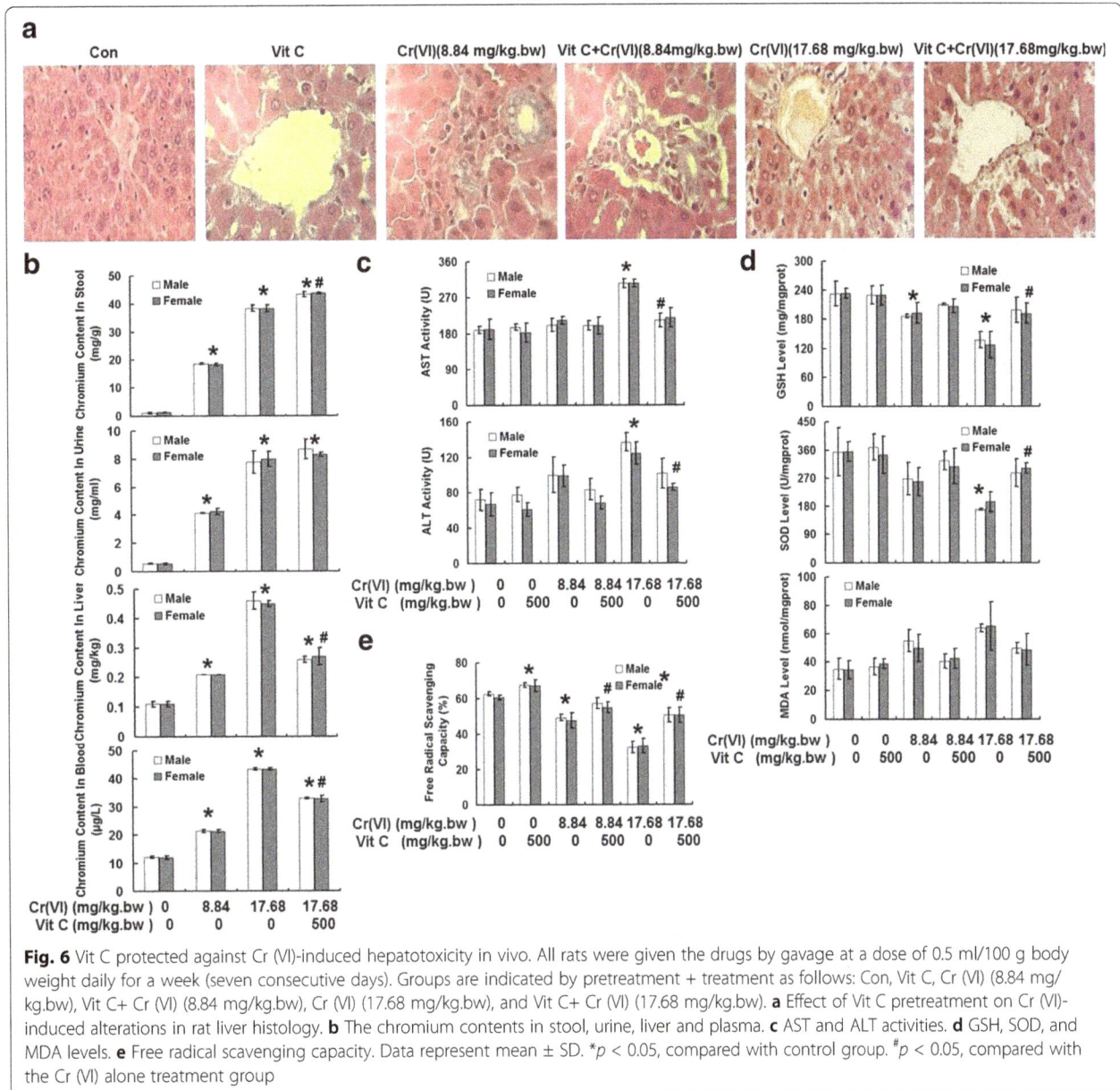

Fig. 6 Vit C protected against Cr (VI)-induced hepatotoxicity in vivo. All rats were given the drugs by gavage at a dose of 0.5 ml/100 g body weight daily for a week (seven consecutive days). Groups are indicated by pretreatment + treatment as follows: Con, Vit C, Cr (VI) (8.84 mg/kg.bw), Vit C+ Cr (VI) (8.84 mg/kg.bw), Cr (VI) (17.68 mg/kg.bw), and Vit C+ Cr (VI) (17.68 mg/kg.bw). **a** Effect of Vit C pretreatment on Cr (VI)-induced alterations in rat liver histology. **b** The chromium contents in stool, urine, liver and plasma. **c** AST and ALT activities. **d** GSH, SOD, and MDA levels. **e** Free radical scavenging capacity. Data represent mean ± SD. *$p < 0.05$, compared with control group. #$p < 0.05$, compared with the Cr (VI) alone treatment group

pretreatment reduced the antioxidant system damage (Fig. 6d). MDA quantification is known as the most widely used method to evaluate lipid peroxidation, the general mechanism accounts for cell injury and other cellular toxic ending. Cr (VI) inhibited free radical scavenging capacity, and Vit C pretreatment also showed the protective effect, suggesting that Vit C rescued the decrease of Cr (VI)-induced free radical scavenging capacity (Fig. 6e). Male and female rats showed similar results. Our present data revealed Vit C pretreatment effectively inhibited Cr (VI)-induced hepatotoxicity in the rat model, and the protective effect of Vit Cwas associated with the inhibition of various enzymatic markers and cytokines as well as the restoration of the antioxidant system function.

Discussion

It is known that heavy exposure to Cr (VI) is closely associated with the increased risk of liver primary cancers [13], thus study on the hepatotoxicity induced by Cr (VI) has become the hot spot in the research field of toxicology. Liver is particularly susceptible to injury for its involvement in xenobiotic metabolism. Under resting conditions the hepatocytes must maintain the critical balance between cellular oxidants and antioxidant defenses. The disruption of this balance may cause the entrance of the cells to an inflammatory state, resulting in the damage of both the cells involved and the surrounding tissues due to the induction of the inflammatory cytokines, the activation of various signaling pathways, and other molecular and cellular modifications. Inflammation is known as the protective mechanism to help the injured or infected organism to initiate cellular repair processes and to restore physiological functions. Liver inflammation has been shown to be associated with elevated production of various cytokines such as IL-1β, TNF-α and IFN-γ, which have been implicated in hepatocarcinogenesis [14, 15]. Although the activities of AST and ALT are the most commonly used and well-known enzymatic markers of liver injury, they only change in late stages and often lack sensitivity in early stages of various liver diseases [16]. IL-1β is known as an initiator cytokine that plays an important role in the regulation of the inflammatory responses [17]. As a major endogenous mediator of hepatotoxicity, TNF-α is a pro-inflammation cytokine that expresses in various liver injuries and plays an important role in tissue damage. Being another pro-inflammatory cytokine, IFN-γ is also a sensitive biomarker as well as a critical mediator of liver damage from several xenobiotic agents [18]. IL-10 is known to have anti-inflammatory effect for its ability to down-regulate the production of pro-inflammation cytokines such as IL-1β and IFN-γ from T cells and exerts its inhibitory effect on several model of liver injury [19]. We found IL-10 level was increased at low dose of Cr (VI) treatment but decreased at high dose of Cr (VI) treatment, indicating that IL-10 played a compensatory role at first, but then showed compensatory failure in severe liver injury. The data indicates that liver damage is likely occurring at the high dose of Cr (VI) treatment because we can speculate that the liver may be able to recover from the injury and regain its normal functions at low dose of Cr (VI) treatment. LTB4, which can be synthesized on activation of 5-lipoxygenase (5-LO), has also been confirmed to participate in different experimental models of liver injury [20].

Cr (VI) could enter the target cells and then undergoes metabolic reduction to Cr (III), causing the accumulation of ROS together with a cascade of various cellular toxic events. MRCC I is a large enzyme complex that embedded in the inner mitochondrial membrane and plays an important role in energy metabolism by proving protonmotive force required for ATP synthesis [21]. While other studies have confirmed that MRCC III is the important source of cellular ROS, in the present study we showed that MRCC I may be the precise site for ROS generation after Cr (VI) exposure. Complex I consists of at least 45 subunits of which 38 subunits are encoded by nuclear genome and 7 are encoded by the mitochondrial genome [22]. In order to investigate how Cr (VI) inhibits MRCC I, we checked the expression levels of all the subunits involved in MRCC I assembly by performing gene chip and RT-PCR. Data revealed that Cr (VI) significantly affected NDUFS3. The mechanisms involved in Cr (VI)-induced

inhibition of MRCC I remain to be fully explored. There is evidence supporting that in hepatocytes, the pro-inflammatory cytokines such as TNF-α and IFN-γ can also induce ROS accumulation [23], but the related mechanism is not clear. ROS exhibit the dual role in biology. When produced by normal cellular metabolism and in limited quantities, ROS exert beneficial effects on mediating signaling pathways and contributing to cellular functions including proliferation and differentiation. However, the over-generation of ROS may act as key players in disease pathogenesis and induce cell and tissue damage by attacking vital cellular components such as DNA, lipids and proteins. OS is the state which can result from the increased formation of ROS and the unbalance between pro-oxidants and antioxidants [24]. Chaverrí et al. has reported that OS is associated with Cr (VI)-induced nephrotoxicity [25]. ROS scavenging enzymes, including SOD and GSH, are the members of antioxidants system whose function is to eliminate excess ROS. SOD is known to facilitate the conversion of superoxide to hydrogen peroxide. And GSH is a tripeptide responsible for protection against free radicals, and the depletion of GSH could decrease cellular antioxidant capacity and induce oxidative stress. It has been reported that infection with hepatitis C is accompanied with the accumulation of ROS and the inhibited antioxidant levels [26], thus we inferred that the decreased levels of antioxidant defenses, which were characterized by the inhibition of GSH, SOD and Trx levels, together with the augmented formation of ROS, appear to play an important part in Cr (VI)-induced liver injury. The role of free radicals in Cr (VI)-induced hepatotoxicity and the capacity of Cr (VI) to promote OS are important areas of research in toxicology, because such information may possess important therapeutic significance to prevent liver injury even cancer progression after Cr (VI) by antioxidants such as Vit C.

Previous reports suggest that Cr (VI) is a hepatotoxin and Cr (VI)-induced hepatotoxicity can be alleviated by several natural and synthetic compounds [27]. We think that free radical accumulation and the occurrence of OS is early event and the main mechanism of Cr (VI)-induced liver damage, thus the administration of antioxidant, especially in the early stage of Cr (VI) exposure, may significantly diminish liver injury and even inhibit hepatocarcinogenesis. The present research we conducted in vivo study. The purpose of utilization of experimental rat model of toxicant-induced hepatotoxicity is to evaluate the biochemical processes involved in various liver diseases and to explore the possible pharmacological effects of the liver protective agents such as Vit C. Based on our results, pretreatment with Vit C inhibited the above-mentioned hepatotoxicity-related alterations both in vitro and in vivo, and accelerated the fecal excretion of chromium in liver and plasma of the rates, indicating the hepatoprotective effect of Vit C against Cr (VI)-induced liver injury. Considering the difference between animals and humans and before we can provide valuable experimental evidence for the anti-oxidative therapy in clinic, we definitely need conduct further study because the effective dose and safe dose, during of treatment, and bio-availability of Vit C require thorough exploration.

The current federal maximum contaminant level for total Cr is 100 μg/l [28]. A 2-year cancer bioassay conducted by the National Toxicology Program (NTP) reported that administration of Cr (VI) in drinking water (in the form of sodium dichromate dihydrate [SDD]) induced tumors in the small intestines of rats at ≥172 mg/l SDD (≥60 mg/l Cr (VI)) [29]. The increasing evidence has suggested that both inflammation and ROS play important role in the induction of the carcinogenic phenotype. It is confirmed that inflammatory cell infiltration during cancer progression is accompanied with the generation of various cytokines, chemokines and growth factors, favoring increased cellular proliferation [30]. ROS generated from ETC and oxidation-reduction system after Cr (VI) exposure could cause oxidative damage to host DNA, resulting in activation of oncogenes and/or inactivation of tumor suppressor genes as well as various epigenetic modifications that favor tumor progression. Although we focused on liver injury and the protective effect of Vit C after Cr (VI) exposure in vitro and in vivo, the present study also provided important experimental evidence for the mechanism and treatment study of Cr (VI)-associated cancers. And in addition to the exploration of Cr (VI)-induced cytotoxicity and carcinogenicity, future attention should also be paid to the development of antioxidant-based strategies for primary prevention of liver injury even primary liver cancers in occupational Cr (VI) exposure individuals.

Conclusions

The present study confirmed that ROS played a role in Cr (VI)-induced hepatotoxicity and Vit C exhibited protective effect. Our current data provides important clues for studying the mechanisms involved in Cr (VI)-induced liver injury, and may be of great help to develop therapeutic strategies for prevention and treatment of liver diseases involving ROS accumulation for occupational exposure population.

Abbreviations

5-LO: 5-lipoxygenase; ALT: alanine aminotransferase; AST: aspartate aminotransferase; Cr (VI): hexavalent chromium; Cyt c: cytochrome c; ETC: electron transfer chain; GSH: glutathione; IFN-γ: interferon-γ; IL-10: interleukine-10; IL-1β: interleukine-1β; LTB4: leukotriene B4; MDA: malondialdehyde; MRCCs: mitochondrial respiratory chain complexes; NADH: Nicotinamide adenine dinucleotide; NADPH oxidase: nicotinamide adenine dinucleotide phosphate-oxidase; ROS: reactive oxygen species; SOD: superoxide dismutase; TNF-α: tumor necrosis factor-α; Trx: thioredoxin; Vit C: Vitamin C

Acknowledgements
Not applicable.

Funding
This research was financially supported by National Natural Science Foundation of China (NO. 81302456) and Natural Science Foundation of Hunan Province, China (NO. 2015JJ3135).

Authors' contributions
FX designed the experiments, supervised the project, and wrote the paper. XLZ, MZ and HFB performed the experiments. CGZ provided advice on technical development. XLZ analyzed the data. All authors read and approved the final manuscript.

Competing interests
The authors have no conflicts of interest to declare in relation to this article.

Author details
[1]Department of Health Toxicology, Xiangya School of Public Health, Central South University, NO. 238 Shangmayuanling Road, Kaifu District, Changsha 410078, Hunan, People's Republic of China. [2]Shajing Institution of Health Supervision of Baoan District, Shenzhen 518104, People's Republic of China.

References
1. Tchounwou PB, Yedjou CG, Patlolla AK, Sutton DJ. Heavy metal toxicity and the environment. EXS. 2012;101:133–64.
2. Sazakli E, Villanueva CM, Kogevinas M, Maltezis K, Mouzaki A, Leotsinidis M. Chromium in drinking water: association with biomarkers of exposure and effect. Int J Environ Res Public Health. 2014;11:10125–45.
3. Zhang X, Zhong T, Liu L, Ouyang X. Impact of soil heavy metal pollution on food safety in China. PLoS One. 2015;10:e0135182.
4. Xiao F, Feng X, Zeng M, Guan L, Hu Q, Zhong C. Hexavalent chromium induces energy metabolism disturbance and p53-dependent cell cycle arrest via reactive oxygen species in L-02 hepatocytes. Mol Cell Biochem. 2012;371:65–76.
5. Xie X, Zhao R, Shen GX. Impact of cyanidin-3-glucoside on glycated LDL-induced NADPH oxidase activation, mitochondrial dysfunction and cell viability in cultured vascular endothelial cells. Int J Mol Sci. 2012;13:15867–80.
6. Belyaeva EA, Sokolova TV, Emelyanova LV, Zakharova IO. Mitochondrial electron transport chain in heavy metal-induced neurotoxicity: effects of cadmium, mercury, and copper. Sci World J. 2012;2012:136063.
7. Chen Q, Vazquez EJ, Moghaddas S, Hoppel CL, Lesnefsky EJ. Production of reactive oxygen species by mitochondria: central role of complex III. J Biol Chem. 2003;278:36027.
8. Kim D, Kim GW, Lee SH, Han GD. Ligularia Fischeri extract attenuates liver damage induced by chronic alcohol intake. Pharm Biol. 2016;54:1–9.
9. Xiao F, Li Y, Luo L, Xie Y, Zeng M, Wang A, et al. Role of mitochondrial electron transport chain dysfunction in Cr (VI)-induced cytotoxicity in L-02 hepatocytes. Cell Physiol Biochem. 2014;33:1013–25.
10. Brustovetsky N, Brustovetsky T, Jemmerson R, Dubinsky JM. Calcium-induced cytochrome c release from CNS mitochondria is associated with the permeability transition and rupture of the outer membrane. J Neurochem. 2002;80:207–18.
11. Suliburska J, Krejpcio Z, Staniek H, Krol E, Bogdanski P, Kupsz J, et al. The effects of antihypertensive drugs on chromium status, glucose metabolism, and antioxidant and inflammatory indices in spontaneously hypertensive rats. Biol Trace Elem Res. 2014;157:60–6.
12. Bedard K, Krause KH. The NOX family of ROS-generating NADPH oxidases: physiology and pathophysiology. Physiol Rev. 2007;87:245–313.
13. Linos A, Petralias A, Christophi CA, Christoforidou E, Kouroutou P, Stoltidis M, et al. Oral ingestion of hexavalent chromium through drinking water and cancer mortality in an industrial area of Greece-an ecological study. Environ Health. 2011;10:50.

14. Sun B, Karin M. Obesity, inflammation, and liver cancer. J Hepatol. 2012;56:704–13.

15. Garcia-Nino WR, Tapia E, Zazueta C, Zatarain-Barron ZL, Hernandez-Pando R, Vega-Garcia CC, et al. Curcumin pretreatment prevents potassium dichromate-induced hepatotoxicity, oxidative stress, decreased respiratory complex I activity, and membrane permeability transition pore opening. Evid Based Complement Alternat Med. 2013;2013:424692.

16. Shih TY, Young TH, Lee HS, Hsieh CB, Hu YP. Protective effects of Kaempferol on Isoniazid- and Rifampicin-induced Hepatotoxicity. AAPS J. 2013;15:753–62.

17. Cover C, Liu J, Farhood A, Malle E, Waalkes MP, Bajt ML, et al. Pathophysiological role of the acute inflammatory response during acetaminophen hepatotoxicity. Toxicol Appl Pharmacol. 2006;216:98–107.

18. Küsters S, Gantner F, Künstle G, Tiegs G. Interferon gamma plays a critical role in T cell-dependent liver injury in mice initiated by concanavalin a. Gastroenterology. 1996;111:462–71.

19. Thompson K, Maltby J, Fallowfield J, Mcaulay M, Millwardsadler H, Sheron N. Interleukin-10 expression and function in experimental murine liver inflammation and fibrosis. Hepatology. 1998;28:1597.

20. Mei Chen BKL, Andrew D, Luster SZ, Murphy RC, Bair AM, Soberman RJ, et al. Joint tissues amplify inflammation and Alter their invasive behavior via Leukotriene B4 in experimental inflammatory arthritis. J Immunol. 2010;185:5503.

21. Efremov RG, Baradaran R, Sazanov LA. The architecture of respiratory complex I. Nature. 2010;465:441–5.

22. Rodenburg RJ. Mitochondrial complex I-linked disease. Biochim Biophys Acta. 1857;2016:938–45.

23. Adamson GM, Billings RE. Tumor necrosis factor induced oxidative stress in isolated mouse hepatocytes. Arch Biochem Biophys. 1992;294:223–9.

24. Halliwell B. Biochemistry of oxidative stress. Biochem Soc Trans. 2007;35:1147–50.

25. Pedraza-Chaverrí J, Barrera D, Medina-Campos ON, Carvajal RC, Hernández-Pando R, Macías-Ruvalcaba NA, et al. Time course study of oxidative and nitrosative stress and antioxidant enzymes in K2Cr2O7-induced nephrotoxicity. BMC Nephrol. 2005;6:4.

26. Lozano-Sepulveda SA, Bryan-Marrugo OL, Cordova-Fletes C, Gutierrez-Ruiz MC, Rivas-Estilla AM. Oxidative stress modulation in hepatitis C virus infected cells. World J Hepatol. 2015;7:2880–9.

27. Boşgelmez İİ, Söylemezoğlu T, Güvendik G. The protective and Antidotal effects of Taurine on Hexavalent chromium-induced oxidative stress in mice liver tissue. Biol Trace Elem Res. 2008;125:46.

28. Thompson CM, Kirman CR, Proctor DM, Haws LC, Suh M, Hays SM, et al. A chronic oral reference dose for hexavalent chromium-induced intestinal cancer. J Appl Toxicol. 2014;34:525–36.

29. Stout MD, Herbert RA, Kissling GE, Collins BJ, Travlos GS, Witt KL, et al. Hexavalent chromium is carcinogenic to F344/N rats and B6C3F1 mice after chronic oral exposure. Environ Health Perspect. 2009;117:716–22.

30. Coussens LM, Werb Z. Inflammation and cancer. Nature. 2002;420:860–7.

3

Acetylsalicylic acid as a potential pediatric health hazard: legislative aspects concerning accidental intoxications in the European Union

Menen E. Mund[1*], Christoph Gyo[1], Dörthe Brüggmann[1,2], David Quarcoo[1] and David A. Groneberg[1]

Abstract

Acetylsalicylic acid is a frequently used medication worldwide. It is not used in pediatrics due its association with Reye syndrome. However, in case of pediatric intoxication, children are more fragile to salicylate poisoning because of their reduced ability of buffer the acid stress. Intoxication leads to a decoupling of oxidative phosphorylation and subsequently to a loss in mitochondrial function. Symptoms of poisoning are diverse; eventually they can lead to the death of the patient. Governmental websites of various EU countries were searched for legal information on acetylsalicylic acid availability in pharmacies and non-pharmacy stores. Various EU countries permit prescription-free sales of acetylsalicylic acid in pharmacies and non-pharmacy stores. In Sweden acetylsalicylic acid 500 mg may be sold in a maximum package size of 20 tablets or effervescent tablets in a non-pharmacy. In the UK a maximum of 16 tablets of acetylsalicylic acid 325 mg is allowed to sell in non-pharmacies. In Ireland acetylsalicylic acid is classified as S2 medication. Subsequently, acetylsalicylic acid is allowed to be sold prescription-free in pharmacies and non-pharmacy stores. In the Netherlands acetylsalicylic acid may only be sold in drug stores or pharmacies. A maximum of 24 tablets of 500 mg is allowed to purchase in a drug store. Several countries in the European Union are permitted to offer acetylsalicylic acid prescription-free in pharmacies and non-pharmacy stores without legal guidance on the storage position within the store. Further research is needed to investigate whether acetylsalicylic acid is located directly accessible to young children within the stores in EU countries which permit prescription-free sales of acetylsalicylic acid.

Keywords: Acetylsalicylic acid, Analgesics, Poisoning, Intoxication, Child, Pediatrics, Legislation, European Union, Non-pharmacy

Background

Recently we published a narrative review about paracetamol as a toxic substance for children [1]. Accordingly, the present review will focus on another important analgesic as a potential pediatric health hazard: acetylsalicylic acid. It is one of the most wildly used analgesic and antiplatelet medication throughout the world. It is commonly known as aspirin, which is the product name introduced by the pharmaceutical company *Bayer AG*. Figure 1 shows the chemical structure of acetylsalicylic acid. In order to avoid Reye syndrome, it is not commonly used in pediatric treatment any more. Nonetheless, acute poisoning in children can occur by accidental ingestion of adult medication [2, 3]. This narrative review summarizes the effects of acetylsalicylic acid intoxication, especially in children. Additionally, it outlines the current legal requirements on acetylsalicylic acid sales in various countries ofthe European Union. The goal was to establish whether the pharmaceutical might be accessible to young children within pharmacies and non-pharmacy stores.

Acetylsalicylic acid toxicity

The acetylsalicylic acid metabolite salicylate affects most organ systems. It decouples oxidative phosphorylations

* Correspondence: menen-mund@t-online.de
[1]Institute of Occupational Medicine, Social Medicine and Environmental Medicine, Departments of Female Health and Preventive Medicine, Goethe University, Frankfurt am Main, Theodor-Stern-Kai 7, Frankfurt 60590, Germany
Full list of author information is available at the end of the article

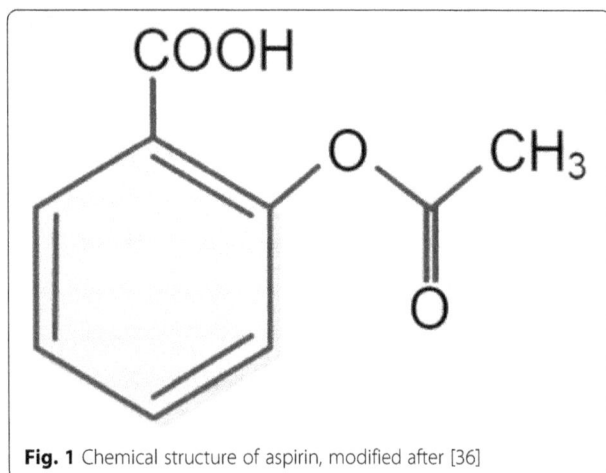

Fig. 1 Chemical structure of aspirin, modified after [36]

like the *Krebs cycle* and amino acid synthesis. On a molecular level it increases oxidative stress and subsequently results in a loss of mitochondrial potential; the consequence is a damaged mitochondrial respiratory function. Initially, acetylsalicylic acid poisoning leads to pure respiratory alkalosis due to activation of the respiratory center in the medulla oblongata. Thereafter, acetylsalicylic acid poisoning causes anaerobic oxidation which results in anion gap metabolic acidosis; the undetected anions include salicylates and lactate [4–6]. The typical triad of acetylsalicylic acid intoxication consists of hyperventilation, tinnitus and gastrointestinal symptoms such as vomiting and nausea. Other early symptoms include hematemesis, deafness, lethargy and confusion. Pulmonary edema, hemorrhages and hyperglycemia have also been observed. Serious poisoning can additionally lead to hepatotoxicity. After severe intoxication, central nervous system (CNS) changes like agitation and confusion might occur with a risk of cerebral edema; these symptoms can lead to coma. Acetylsalicylic acid intoxication can eventually result in the death of the patient [2, 7, 8]. One study reported a case of a child with detected high acetylsalicylic acid blood levels suffering from acute myocarditis. These findings suggest a causal relationship between myocarditis and acetylsalicylic acid overdose [9].

Acetylsalicylic acid intoxication in children
The acetylsalicylic acid metabolite salicylate has been listed amongst the nine pediatric poisons which lead to death in children at low doses [10]. Young children are more fragile to salicylate poisoning because they cannot compensate acid stress as effectively as adults; CNS changes like agitation and restlessness are especially widespread in children [2]. The acute toxic acetylsalicylic acid dosage is considered to be more than 150 mg/kg body weight [8]. Salicylate intoxication is probably under-represented in poison center data because the

symptoms are unspecific and intoxication is often not diagnosed as such [7]. A US study showed that unintentional acetylsalicylic acid poisoning in children was a common problem around 1970. At that time it was the most frequent medicine leading to accidental poisoning in children. Improving child-proof pharmaceutical containers lead to a decrease of acetylsalicylic acid intoxication in children under 5 years [11]. Statistical data on acetylsalicylic acid intoxication in children is unfortunately limited. This particular intoxication is often not registered specifically in central statistical databases. Governmental agencies in various countries published reports on child injury. Data is usually based on hospital statistics and death cause statistics; these statistics inform about diverse child injury mechanisms. Poisoning is generally registered as one of them, but the reports do not provide information about particular drugs. Accordingly, they do not present statistical information about drug poisonings with acetylsalicylic acid in children [12–14]. In all four countries which were included in this study poison control centers are installed; they generally function as advisor for telephone enquiries made by medical professionals or the general public. Poison control centers usually document information about calls, for example the reason for the phone call or whether the patient is a child. However, in these reports poisoning incidences are often registered by substance group, for example analgesics, but do not show data about acetylsalicylic acid specifically [15–18].

Treatment of acute acetylsalicylic acid intoxication
An antidote for acetylsalicylic acid intoxication is not known. Active charcoal should be administered immediately after ingestion to reduce the quantity of absorbed substance. Emesis should not be forced in children suffering from acute acetylsalicylic acid poisoning; whole bowel irrigation or gastric lavage is also not recommended any more [7, 8]. Serum acetylsalicylic acid levels should be identified and blood gas analysis should be performed repeatedly. Severity of intoxication does often not correlate with the absolute serum level; therefore blood analysis should be repeated and used to monitor serum level changes. A nomogram was developed in 1960 by *A.K. Done* to establish a treatment threshold on basis of serum acetylsalicylic acid levels. However, due to serious limitations of the nomogram is not generally used [7]. Further conservative treatments of acetylsalicylic acid poisoning include rehydration and correction of electrolyte aberrations. Urinary alkalinization is important in order to accelerate the ionization of the drug and therefore force renal elimination [19]. Hemodialysis is a treatment which is commonly used in patients after acetylsalicylic acid poisoning, even though no clear regime exists concerning duration and best method. If a

Acetylsalicylic acid as a potential pediatric health hazard: legislative aspects concerning accidental...

23

decision on hemodialysis is made, alkalinization of urine should nevertheless be promptly administered [20, 21]. Mechanical ventilation should not be applied to patients with acetylsalicylic acid intoxication as it results in abolishment of respiratory alkalosis. Mechanical ventilation aggravates the neurological toxic effects because more salicylate can pass to the CNS [22]. It is suggested that balanced glutathione homeostasis in hepatic cells reduces the cytotoxic effects of acetylsalicylic acid [6].

Pharmaceutical legislation in European Union countries
European Union countries receive legislation from two different legislative authorities. On the one hand, national governments enact laws which apply to every distinct country individually. On the other hand, laws in EU countries can be enacted by the EU; the European Commission (EC), the European Parliament (EP) and the European Council form the EU legislative body. The EC proposes legislation which is discussed and eventually enacted by the EP and the European Council. Two different types of legislation are performed by the EU: regulations and directives. An EU regulation is instantly enforced as law in all EU member countries at the same time; it excels national law. EU directives are guidelines with a defined goal and time period in which it has to be incorporated into national law. Legislation processes on EU level are complicated; occasionally it takes a long time until a regulation or directive becomes enforced [23–25]. The EU pharmaceutical law consists of diverse regulations and directives concerning numerous pharmaceutical subjects like pharmacovigilance, falsified medical products, drug marketing or regulatory processes. Accessibility of acetylsalicylic acid however is not regulated by European law but by national law [26]. Information about legal requirements for pharmaceutical sales in EU countries was not found in a systematic search in PubMed database. Therefore, five countries of the EU were pre-selected. They were chosen to investigate a cultural variety within the EU: the UK, Ireland, Sweden, the Netherlands and Spain. Governmental websites were used to gain information. Due to different native languages on governmental websites, no single search term could be used during the search. Spain does only allow pharmacy sales of acetylsalicylic acid and was therefore excluded from the study.

Legislation in Sweden
The *Swedish Medicines Act* enables the *Medical Product Agency* to control and monitor medical items in Sweden. The agency is furthermore entitled to classify drugs into prescription-free and prescription-only medication [27, 28]. The maximum prescription-free package size of acetylsalicylic acid consists of 500 mg per unit with 20 tablets (tab) and 20 effervescent tablets

Table 1 Aspirin availability in Sweden, modified after [29, 37, 38]

Form	Strength	Pack size non-pharmacy	Pack size pharmacy
Tab	250 mg	50 units	50 units
Tab	500 mg	20 units	50 units
TEF	500 mg	20 units	60 units

(TEF) per package and in a non-pharmacy store. In a pharmacy, it is legal to purchase 50 tablets or 60 TEF per package [29] (Table 1).

Legislation in the United Kingdom
The *Medicines and Healthcare Products Regulatory Agency* is an administrative body of the British *Department of Health*; this agency is responsible for admission, monitoring and safety of pharmaceuticals in the United Kingdom. The *Medicines Act* from 1968 constitutes the legislation of pharmaceuticals. Medicines are divided into three different categories [30, 31]:

- Prescription-only medication
- Pharmacy sales medication
- General sales list medication (GSL)

Certain requirements in package size and strength apply for acetylsalicylic acid in order to be listed as GSL (Table 2). A maximum of 16 tablets of acetylsalicylic acid 325 mg may be offered in a non-pharmacy store [31].

Legislation in Ireland
The *Irish Medicines Board* forms the official agency of the *Department of Health and Children*. This agency regulates pharmaceutical matters like drug safety, drug risks and monitoring. The *Medical Product Regulations Law* regulates prescription and supply of pharmaceuticals. Three categories for medication exist in Ireland. Pharmaceuticals are either classified as:

- General sales medication
- Prescription-controlled medication from *schedule 1* (S1)
- Exemption from S1 medication.

These exemptions are either pharmaceuticals listed in *schedule 2* (S2) or S1 pharmaceuticals which are labeled with maximum dose, maximum daily dose or

Table 2 Requirements for aspirin to listed GSL in the UK, modified after [31]

Form	Strength	Pack size
TEF	500 mg	20 units
Powders or granules	650 mg	10 units
Tab or capsules	325 mg	16 units

Table 3 Aspirin availability in the Netherlands, modified after [35]

Form	Strength	Pack size	Status
Tab	500 mg	24 tab	UAD
Tab	500 mg	> 24 tab	UA

maximum treatment period. S2 medication can be offered in non-pharmacies [32]. Acetylsalicylic acid is classified as S2 medication and it is labeled with a maximum daily dose of 4.0 g for patients aged more than 12 years old. Subsequently, acetylsalicylic acid is allowed to be sold prescription-free in pharmacies and non-pharmacy stores [32, 33].

Legislation in the Netherlands
The Dutch medicine law came into effect in 2007 and was enforced by the *Ministry of National Health, Wellbeing and Sports*. This ministry instructs the administrative body *Medicines Evaluation Board* to control pharmaceutical safety and quality. Medications are divided into four different categories in the Netherlands [34]:

- Prescription-only medication (UR)
- Pharmacy-only medication (UA)
- Pharmacy or drug store-only (UAD)
- Open sales medication (AV)

Acetylsalicylic acid does not belong to the AV list; it is not permitted to sell acetylsalicylic acid outside of drug stores or pharmacies. The medication holds UAD status for a maximum pack size of 24 tablets of 500 mg; more than 24 tablets per package may only be sold in pharmacies [35] (Table 3).

Conclusions
Acetylsalicylic acid is a drug which is not commonly used in pediatrics. However, in case of accidental poisoning, it can lead to severe symptoms. Several countries in the European Union are permitted to offer acetylsalicylic acid prescription-free in pharmacies and non-pharmacy stores without legal guidance on the storage position within the store. Further investigation is needed to analyze whether the pharmaceutical is placed in direct accessibility to young children within these stores.

Abbreviations
AV, Open sale medication (*algehele verkoop geneesmiddel*); CNS, Central nervous system; EC, European Commission; EP, European Parliament; GSL, General sales list; S1, Schedule 1; S2, Schedule 2; Tab, tablets; TEF, Effervescent tablets; UA, Pharmacy only medication (*uitsluitend apotheek geneesmiddel*); UAD, Pharmacy or drug store only (*uitsluitend apotheek of drogist geneesmiddel*); UR, Prescription only medication (*uitsluitend recept geneesmiddel*)

Acknowledgements
We thank G. Volante for expert help.

Authors' contributions
MEM, CG, DB, DQ, and DAG have made substantial contributions to the conception and design of the narrative review, acquisition of the review data and have been involved in drafting and revising the manuscript. All authors have read and approved the final manuscript.

Competing interests
The authors declare that they have no competing interests. DAG was member of the Committee for the Assessment of Intoxications of the Federal Institute for Risk Assessment, Federal Republic of Germany.

Author details
¹Institute of Occupational Medicine, Social Medicine and Environmental Medicine, Departments of Female Health and Preventive Medicine, Goethe University, Frankfurt am Main, Theodor-Stern-Kai 7, Frankfurt 60590, Germany. ²Department of Obstetrics and Gynecology, Keck School of Medicine, University of Southern California, Los Angeles, CA, USA.

References
1. Mund ME et al. Paracetamol as a toxic substance for children: aspects of legislation in selected countries. J Occup Med Toxicol. 2015;10:43.
2. Kliegman RM et al. Nelson Textbook of Pediatrics. 18th ed. Philadelphia: Saunders Elsevier; 2007. Chapter 58.
3. Vane JR, Botting RM. The mechanism of action of aspirin. Thromb Res. 2003;110(5-6):255–8.
4. Fertel BS, Nelson LS, Goldfarb DS. The underutilization of hemodialysis in patients with salicylate poisoning. Kidney Int. 2009;75(12):1349–53.
5. Jacob J, Lavonas EJ. Falsely normal anion gap in severe salicylate poisoning caused by laboratory interference. Ann Emerg Med. 2011;58(3):280–1.
6. Raza H, John A. Implications of altered glutathione metabolism in aspirin-induced oxidative stress and mitochondrial dysfunction in HepG2 cells. PLoS One. 2012;7(4):e36325.
7. O'Malley GF. Emergency department management of the salicylate-poisoned patient. Emerg Med Clin North Am. 2007;25(2):333–46. abstract viii.
8. Chyka PA et al. Salicylate poisoning: an evidence-based consensus guideline for out-of-hospital management. Clin Toxicol (Phila). 2007;45(2):95–131.
9. Pena-Alonso YR et al. Aspirin intoxication in a child associated with myocardial necrosis: is this a drug-related lesion? Pediatr Dev Pathol. 2003;6(4):342–7.
10. Michael JB, Sztajnkrycer MD. Deadly pediatric poisons: nine common agents that kill at low doses. Emerg Med Clin North Am. 2004;22(4):1019–50.
11. Scherz RG. Prevention of childhood aspirin poisoning. Clinical trials with three child-resistant containers. N Engl J Med. 1971;285(24):1361–2.
12. Centers for Disease Control and Prevention. Childhood Injury Report. 2008. Accessed on 18.03.2015. Available from: http://www.cdc.gov/safechild/images/CDC-childhoodinjury.pdf.
13. Australian Bureau of Statistics. Children's Injuries. 2015. Accessed on 18.3. 2015. Available from: http://www.abs.gov.au/ausstats/abs@.nsf/Previousproducts/1301.0Feature%20Article152006?opendocument&tabname=Summary&prodno=1301.0&issue=2006&num=&view=#.
14. Statistisches Bundesamt. Unfälle, Gewalt, Selbstverletzung bei Kindern und Jugendlichen. 2011. Accessed on 18.3.2015. Available from: https://www.destatis.de/DE/Publikationen/Thematisch/Gesundheit/Gesundheitszustand/UnfaelleGewaltKinder5230001117004.pdf%3F__blob%3DpublicationFile.
15. Giftnotrufzentrale-Nord. Jahresbericht. 2012. Accessed on 24.02.2015. Available from: http://www.giz-nord.de/cms/images/JaBe/2012/jabe12d.pdf.
16. World Health Organization. World directory of Poison Centers. 2015. Accessed on 24.02.2015. Available from: http://www.who.int/gho/phe/chemical_safety/poisons_centres/en/.
17. Poisons Information Centre of Ireland. Annual Report. 2014. Accessed on 17.03. 2016. Available from: http://www.poisons.ie/docs/Final%20Report%202014.pdf.
18. Swedish Poisons Information Centre. Annual Report. 2014. Accessed on 17. 03.2016. Available from: http://www.giftinformation.se/globalassets/publikationer/arsrapport-2014_engelska.pdf.
19. Basavarajaiah S, Sigston P, Budack K. Severe salicylate poisoning treated conservatively. J R Soc Med. 2004;97(12):587–8.
20. Minns AB, Cantrell FL, Clark RF. Death due to acute salicylate intoxication despite dialysis. J Emerg Med. 2011;40(5):515–7.

Acetylsalicylic acid as a potential pediatric health hazard: legislative aspects concerning accidental...

25

21. Higgins RM, Connolly JO, Hendry BM. Alkalinization and hemodialysis in severe salicylate poisoning: comparison of elimination techniques in the same patient. Clin Nephrol. 1998;50(3):178–83.
22. Stolbach AI, Hoffman RS, Nelson LS. Mechanical ventilation was associated with acidemia in a case series of salicylate-poisoned patients. Acad Emerg Med. 2008;15(9):866–9.
23. Konsolidierte Fassung des Vertrags über die Europäische Union. 2008. Accessed on 16.03.2015. Available from: http://eur-lex.europa.eu/LexUriServ/LexUriServ.do?uri=OJ:C:2008:115:0013:0045:DE:PDF.
24. EU Info Deutschland. Gesetzgebung. Primäres und sekundäres Gemeinschaftsrecht. 2015 [Accessed 18.03.2015]; Available from: http://www.eu-info.de/europa/eu-richtlinien-verordnungen/.
25. Fretten C, Miller V. The European Union: a guide to terminology, procedures and sources. 2005. Accessed on 17.03.2015. Available from: http://www.parliament.uk/business/publications/research/briefing-papers/SN03689/the-european-union-a-guide-to-terminology-procedures-and-sources-house-of-commons-background-paper.
26. The European Commission. DG Health and food safety. News and updates on pharmaceuticals. 2015. Accessed on 18.05.2015. Available from: http://ec.europa.eu/health/documents/eudralex/vol-1/index_en.htm#dir.
27. Medical Products Agency. Legislation within the Swedish Medical Products Agency's area of control. Accessed on 19.11.2014. Available from: http://www.lakemedelsverket.se/english/overview/Legislation/.
28. Swedish Parliament. The Medicines Act. Accessed on 30.11.2014. Available from: https://www.riksdagen.se/sv/Dokument-Lagar/Lagar/Svenskforfattningssamling/Lakemedelslag-1992859_sfs-1992-859/.
29. Medical Products Agency. Detaljinformation Aspirin 500 mg tablett. Accessed on 19.11.2014. Available from: http://www.lakemedelsverket.se/LMF/Lakemedelsinformation/?nplid=19350131000010&type=product.
30. The National Archives. Medicines Act 1968. Accessed on 17.10.2014. Available from: http://www.legislation.gov.uk/ukpga/1968/67/contents.
31. Medicines and Healthcare Products Regulatory Agency. Lists of substances. 2014. Accessed on 17.10.2014. Available from: http://www.mhra.gov.uk/Howweregulate/Medicines/Licensingofmedicines/Legalstatusandreclassification/Listsofsubstances/.
32. Irish Statute Book. S.I. No. 540/2003 - Medicinal Products (Prescription and Control of Supply) Regulations 2003. Accessed on 04.02.2015. Available from: http://www.irishstatutebook.ie/2003/en/si/0540.html.
33. Weedle P, Clarke L. Pharmacy and Medicines Law in Ireland. 1 ed. Pharmaceutical Press; 2011.
34. Inspectie voor de Gesondheidszorg. Ministerie voor Volksgesondheid, Welzijn en Sport. London, UK: Geneesmiddelwet; 2014. Accessed on 18.10.2014. Available from: http://wetten.overheid.nl/BWBR0021505/geldigheidsdatum_18-10-2014#Hoofdstuk5.
35. College ter Beoordeling van Geneesmiddelen. Indelingsoverzicht NSAID. 2009. Accessed on 17.10.2014. Available from: http://www.cbg-meb.nl/NR/rdonlyres/4082C75F-9EF2-4DC8-B513-8FD7DB2DCACA/0/Indelingsoverzicht NSAID.pdf
36. Kleemann A et al. Pharmaceutical substances. 4th ed. Stuttgart: Georg Thieme Verlag; 2001.
37. Medical Products Agency. Receptfria läkemedel tillåtna för försäljning på andra försäljningsställen än apotek. 2014. Accessed on 19.11.14. Available from: http://www.lakemedelsverket.se/upload/apotek-och-handel/OTC%20listor/gk_otc%20detaljhandel%20enl%20lvfs%202009_2014-10-02.pdf.
38. Medical Products Agency. Detaljinformation Albyl minor 250 mg tablet. Accessed on 19.11.2014. Available from: http://www.lakemedelsverket.se/LMF/Lakemedelsinformation/?nplid=19550809000018&type=product.

4

Fungal cell wall agents and bacterial lipopolysaccharide in organic dust as possible risk factors for pulmonary sarcoidosis

Sanja Stopinšek[1], Alojz Ihan[1], Barbara Salobir[2], Marjeta Terčelj[2] and Saša Simčič[1*]

Abstract

Background: Composition of organic dust is very complex, involving particles of microbial, animal and plant origin. Several environmental exposure studies associate microbial cell wall agents in organic dust with various respiratory symptoms and diseases. The aim of the present study was to investigate the in vitro effects of the co-exposure of fungal cell wall agents (FCWAs) and bacterial lipopolysaccharide (LPS) on inflammatory immune responses of peripheral blood mononuclear cells (PBMCs) from patients with pulmonary sarcoidosis.

Methods: PBMCs from 22 patients with pulmonary sarcoidosis and 20 healthy subjects were isolated and stimulated in vitro with FCWAs (soluble and particulate $(1 \rightarrow 3)$-β-D-glucan, zymosan and chitosan) and/or LPS. Subsequently, cytokines were measured by ELISA and the mRNA expression of dectin-1, toll-like receptor 2 (TLR2), TLR4 and mannose receptor (MR) was analysed by real-time RT-PCR.

Results: Patients with sarcoidosis had a significantly higher secretion of inflammatory cytokines tumour necrosis factor-alpha (TNF-α), interleukin-6 (IL-6), IL-10 and IL-12 (1.7-fold, 2.0-fold, 2.2-fold, and 2.8-fold, respectively; all $p < 0.05$) after in vitro co-stimulation of PBMCs with FCWAs and LPS. We showed that PBMCs from patients with sarcoidosis had a higher baseline mRNA expression of dectin-1, TLR2, TLR4 and MR (6-fold, 11-fold, 18-fold, and 4-fold, respectively). Furthermore, we found a reduced expression of dectin-1, TLR2 and TLR4 after stimulation with FCWAs and/or LPS, although the reduction was significantly weaker in patients than in healthy subjects.

Conclusions: In conclusion, co-stimulation with FCWAs and LPS of PBMC from patients with sarcoidosis caused a weaker reduction of dectin-1, TLR2, TLR4 receptors expression, which could increase the sensitivity of PBMCs, leading to excessive inflammatory cytokine responses and result in the development or progression of pulmonary sarcoidosis.

Keywords: Sarcoidosis, Fungi, $(1 \rightarrow 3)$-β-D-glucan, LPS, PBMC, Cytokines, Pattern-recognition receptors

Background

Several environmental exposure studies at workplaces or at homes associate microbial cell wall agents in organic dust with various respiratory symptoms and diseases, although, the immunopathological events involved in these diseases are very complex and not well understood. We hypothesized that exposure to fungal cell wall agents (FCWAs) and bacterial lipopolysaccharide (LPS) in organic dust may represent a risk factor for pulmonary sarcoidosis development or progression.

Sarcoidosis is a chronic granulomatous disease that most commonly affects the mediastinal lymph nodes and lungs [1]. Despite intensive research, the aetiology of sarcoidosis remains unknown. Terčelj et al. proposed a hypothesis that microbial cell wall agents, particularly agents from moulds, even in the absence of clinical infections can cause a late hypersensitivity reaction leading to granulomas [2]. In support of this hypothesis, several epidemiological studies describe the association between sarcoidosis and living in a damp and mouldy

* Correspondence: sasa.simcic@mf.uni-lj.si
[1]Institute of Microbiology and Immunology, Faculty of Medicine, University of Ljubljana, Zaloška 4, SI-1000 Ljubljana, Slovenia
Full list of author information is available at the end of the article

environment [3–8]. Furthermore, in clinical studies in which sarcoidosis was treated with antifungals, greater clinical improvement was reported compared with corticosteroid treatment [9, 10].

Composition of organic dust is very complex, involving particles of microbial, animal and plant origin. In mice models organic dust exposures induced the development of lymphoid aggregates, peribronchiolar or vascular inflammation, comprised of T and B lymphocytes and macrophages with associated neutrophil recruitment [11]. It has been shown that exposure to high levels of fungi and their components present in organic dust represents a risk factor for developing various respiratory symptoms and diseases, such as asthma, hypersensitivity pneumonitis, sick building syndrome and organic dust toxic syndrome [12–14]. Furthermore, bioaerosols with fungi are known to be associated with granulomatous diseases [4, 7, 15].

Bacterial LPS is one of the prime constituent in organic dust. Inhalation studies showed that LPS can cause cough, dyspnoea, nose and throat irritation, mild fever, flu-like symptoms, acute air flow obstruction, airway inflammation or asthma [16]. Furthermore, adverse effects from LPS may also be increased by other dampness-associated agents [17].

In our previous study we focused on the in vitro and in vivo effects of FCWAs in sarcoidosis. The induced in vitro secretion of cytokines from human peripheral blood mononuclear cells (PBMCs) was higher from subjects with sarcoidosis than from controls. A significant relationship was observed between disease severity, measured as chest X-ray scores indicating granuloma infiltration, and the particulate $(1 \rightarrow 3)$-β-D-glucan-induced secretion of cytokines [18–20]. The aim of the present study was to investigate the in vitro effects of the co-exposure of FCWAs and LPS on inflammatory immune responses of PBMCs from patients with sarcoidosis. We evaluated the FCWAs influence on the in vitro cellular cytokine response to an inflammatory challenge with LPS in sarcoidosis and on the mRNA expression of the main pattern-recognition receptors (PRRs) for recognizing FCWAs and LPS, dectin-1, toll-like receptor 2 (TLR2), TLR4 and mannose receptor (MR).

Methods

Subjects

The study group consisted of 22 patients newly diagnosed with pulmonary sarcoidosis stage II and III according to the established criteria by the American Thoracic Society (ATS), European Respiratory Society (ERS) and World Association of Sarcoidosis and Other Granulomatous Disorders (WASOG) [21], recruited at the Department for Respiratory and Allergic Diseases, University Medical Centre Ljubljana, Slovenia in the

period from September 2008 to January 2012. Patient characteristics are shown in Table 1. The exclusion criteria were pulmonary sarcoidosis stage I and IV, CD4/CD8 ratio in the bronchoalveolar lavage (BAL) less than 4, smoking and receiving any immunosuppressive therapy.

The control group consisted of 20 healthy blood-donor volunteers without any respiratory symptoms or diseases, autoimmune diseases or acute infections. The study was approved by the National Medical Ethics Committee of the Republic of Slovenia (number 122/11/08) and written informed consent was obtained from all the participants.

Reagents and preparation of FCWAs and LPS

All reagents were commercially obtained from Sigma-Aldrich Corp. (USA), unless otherwise stated. Reagents and FCWAs were endotoxin-free and were prepared exactly as previously described [18]. Briefly, the soluble and the particulate forms of $(1 \rightarrow 3)$-β-D-glucan (BGS and BGP) consisted of curdlan from *Alcaligenes faecalis* var. *myxogenes* (Wako Pure Chemical Industries, Japan). BGS was prepared from a suspension of curdlan powder in 0.3 M sodium hydroxide (NaOH) heated at 80 °C in a water bath until completely dissolved. The pH of BGS was neutralized with 0.3 M hydrochloric acid before being added to cell cultures. Curdlan resuspended in RPMI-1640 medium supplemented with 25 mM Hepes buffer (RPMI-1640 medium) represented BGP. Zymosan A from *S. cerevisiae* (ZYM) was prepared from a suspension of ZYM powder, boiled in 0.25 M NaOH and resuspended as a 7.5 mg/ml stock solution in RPMI 1640 medium. A low molecular weight (Mw 50–190 kDa) chitosan from crab shells (75–85 % deacetylated chitosan, CHT) was prepared as a 2 mg/ml stock

Table 1 Patient and healthy subject characteristics

Characteristic	Sarcoidosis patients	Healthy subjects
N	22	20
Gender		
female	12	13
male	10	7
Age in years mean (range)	44.7 (28–57)	39.9 (25–52)
Smoking	No	No
CD4/CD8 ratio in BAL mean (SD)	7.5 (3.0)	
Chest X-ray		
Stage I	0	
Stage II	15	
Stage III	7	
Stage IV	0	
Therapy	None	None

solution in 0.2 % acetic acid. The final concentration in the cell cultures of all FCWAs was 200 μg/ml. LPS from *Escherichia coli* (strain 0111:B4) was dissolved as a 1 mg/ml stock solution in water and further diluted in a cell culture medium to the final concentration of 10 ng/ml.

Isolation and stimulation of PBMCs

The model that we previously described was used for in vitro stimulation of PBMCs [18]. Briefly, PBMCs from patients with sarcoidosis and healthy subjects were isolated from freshly drawn venous blood with EDTA by density gradient centrifugation with Ficoll-Paque™ (GE Healthcare, UK). The cells were cultured in RPMI-1640 medium supplemented with 100 U/ml penicillin, 100 μg/ml streptomycin, 2 mM L-glutamine and 10 % heat-inactivated human serum (Sigma-Aldrich Corp., USA). The 1×10^6 cells (final culture volume of 1.5 ml) were seeded in 24-well culture plates (Corning Costar, USA) with medium alone, with LPS (10 ng/ml), with FCWAs, or with LPS and FCWAs at 37 °C in a humidified atmosphere of 5 % CO_2 in air. The cell-free supernatants were collected after 4 and 18 h of incubation and stored at −30 °C before further analysis.

For mRNA expression studies, 1.2×10^5 PBMCs (final culture volume of 180 μl) were plated in 96-well culture plates (Greiner Bio-One GmbH, Germany) in medium alone or with FCWAs (200 μg/ml) in the absence or presence of LPS (10 ng/ml) at 37 °C in a humidified atmosphere of 5 % CO_2 in air for 4 h.

Real-time reverse transcription polymerase chain reaction (RT-PCR)

The mRNA expression studies were performed as previously described [18]. Briefly, the total cellular RNA was extracted on an ABI Prism 6100 Nucleic Acid PrepStation (Applied Biosystems, Foster City, USA) according to the manufacturer's instructions. RNA was eluted in 150 μl of elution solution and stored at −80 °C until required. Ten microliters of total RNA was reverse transcribed in a 27 μl reaction mixture with a High Capacity cDNA Reverse Transcription kit (Applied Biosystems) according to the manufacturer's instructions on an ABI GeneAmp PCR System. Real-time PCR was performed on an ABI StepOnePlus Realtime PCR instrument using a TaqMan® Universal PCR Master Mix with predeveloped TaqMan Gene Expression Assay primers and probes (Dectin-1 Hs00224028_m1, TLR2 Hs00610101_m1, TLR4 Hs01060206_m1 and MR Hs00267207_m1), according to the manufacturer's instructions (Applied Biosystems). The internal endogenous control used was 18S rRNA. Quantification was performed with the comparative $2^{-\Delta\Delta Ct}$ method [22]. The amount of target gene was normalized to the internal control gene (18S rRNA) and the relative expression of target genes in cultured PBMCs was

calculated in relation to the mean values of target gene expression in healthy subjects after 4 h of incubation in medium alone.

Cytokine measurements

Cytokine concentrations in cell culture supernatants were measured by commercially available enzyme-linked immunosorbent assay (ELISA) kits. Tumour necrosis factor-alpha (TNF-α) (Milenia Biotec, Germany) was measured after 4 h of incubation. The concentrations of interleukin-6 (IL-6), IL-10 and IL-12 (Thermo Scientific, USA) were measured after 18 h of incubation.

Statistical analysis

All statistical analyses were performed using PSAW/SPSS for Windows version 18 (SPSS Inc., IBM Company, USA). Results are presented as the mean +/− standard error of the mean (SEM). Statistically significant differences in cytokine concentration or in mRNA gene expression between the two groups of subjects were estimated by the nonparametric Mann-Whitney test. P values less than 0.05 were considered statistically significant.

Results

In vitro inflammatory cytokine response to FCWAs and LPS by PBMCs from patients with sarcoidosis

After co-stimulation of PBMCs with FCWAs and LPS, the production of TNF-α, IL-6, IL-10 and IL-12 was significantly higher in patients with sarcoidosis, compared to healthy subjects (1.7-fold, 2.0-fold, 2.2-fold, and 2.8-fold, respectively; all $p < 0.05$) (Fig. 1). Fold changes are mean values calculated from all four combinations of FCWAs and LPS. Patients with sarcoidosis thus elicited higher levels of in vitro inflammatory cytokine response of PBMCs after co-stimulation with FCWAs and LPS than healthy subjects.

PBMCs mRNA expression of dectin-1, TLR2, TLR4, and MR at baseline and after in vitro stimulation with FCWAs and/or LPS in patients with sarcoidosis

As shown in Fig. 2, baseline dectin-1, TLR2, TLR4 and MR mRNA expression in PBMCs was higher in patients with sarcoidosis than in healthy subjects (6-fold, 11-fold, 18-fold, and 4-fold, respectively).

When PBMCs were stimulated with FCWAs and/or LPS the mRNA expression of dectin-1, TLR2 and TLR4 was lower than at baseline in both groups of subjects. However, the expression was significantly higher in patients compared to healthy, indicating a weaker reduction of PRRs expression upon FCWAs and/or LPS stimulation in patients with sarcoidosis. Similar results were obtained after 4 and 18 h of incubation (data not shown).

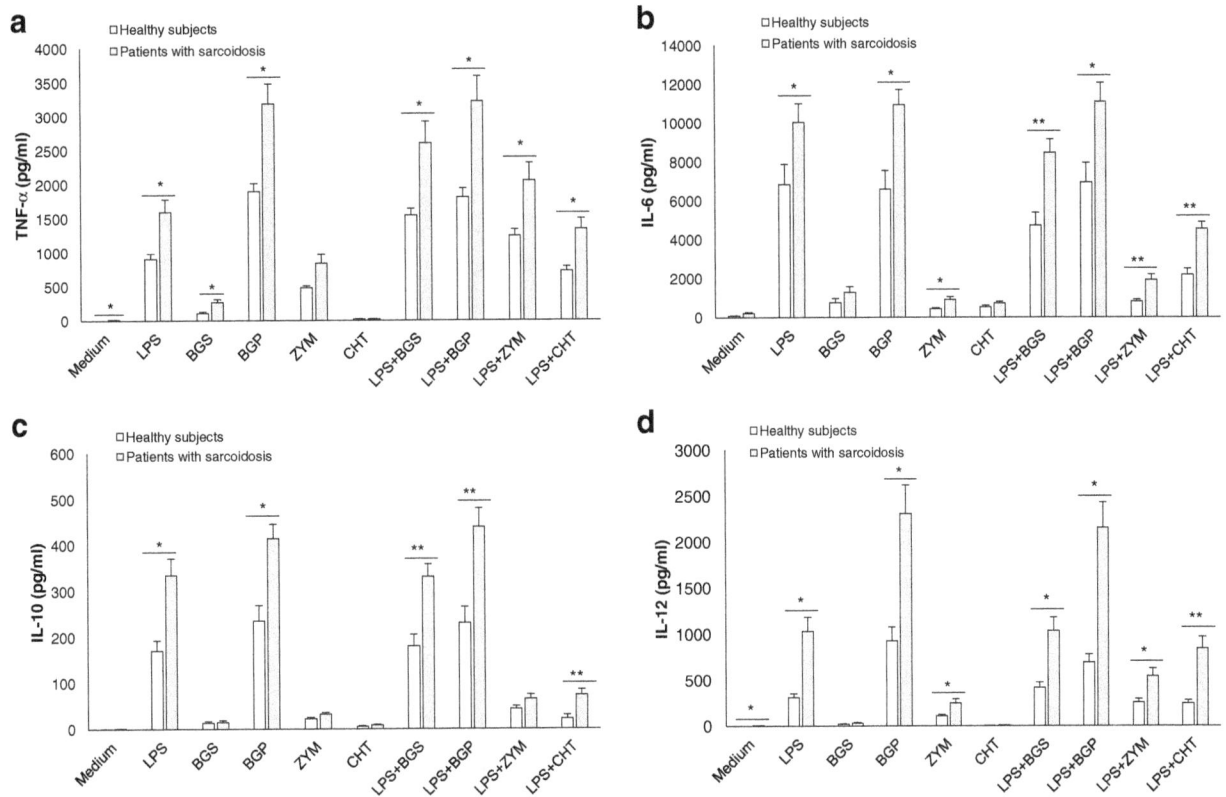

Fig. 1 Cytokine responses of PBMCs after in vitro stimulation with FCWAs and/or LPS. PBMCs (1×10^6 cells/ml) were isolated from venous blood of patients with sarcoidosis ($n = 22$) and healthy subjects ($n = 20$) and incubated with medium alone or stimulated with FCWAs (200 µg/ml) and/or LPS (10 ng/ml). Supernatant TNF-α (pg/ml) (**a**) after 4 h of incubation, IL-6 (pg/ml) (**b**), IL-10 (pg/ml) (**c**) and IL-12 (pg/ml) (**d**) after 18 h of incubation were measured by ELISA. The results are presented as the mean cytokine concentration in culture supernatants with SEM. *$p < 0.05$, **$p < 0.001$: significantly different cytokine production between patients with sarcoidosis and healthy subjects. LPS: lipopolysaccharide, BGS: soluble $(1 \rightarrow 3)$-β D-glucan, BGP: particulate $(1 \rightarrow 3)$-β-D-glucan, ZYM: zymosan, and CHT: chitosan

Discussion

This study was designed to investigate the in vitro effects of the co-exposure of FCWAs and LPS on inflammatory immune responses of PBMCs from patients with sarcoidosis. The main results obtained from this study show that patients with sarcoidosis had a significantly higher secretion of inflammatory cytokines TNF-α, IL-6, IL-10 and IL-12 after in vitro co-stimulation of PBMCs with FCWAs and LPS. We showed that PBMCs from patients with sarcoidosis had a higher mRNA expression of dectin-1, TLR2, TLR4 and MR at baseline. Furthermore, we found a reduced expression of dectin-1, TLR2 and TLR4 after stimulation with FCWAs and/or LPS, although the reduction was significantly weaker in patients than in healthy subjects.

The organic dust we breathe contains particles of animal, plant and microbial origin, of which the most important in relation to respiratory diseases are fungal $(1 \rightarrow 3)$-β-D-glucan and bacterial LPS [14]. We demonstrated previously that after in vitro stimulation of PBMCs with FCWAs alone, the secretion of TNF-α, IL-6, IL-10 and IL-12 was higher in patients with

sarcoidosis compared to healthy subjects [20]. These cytokines have all been implicated in the immunopathogenesis of sarcoidosis [1, 23–25]. Since FCWAs and LPS might have a synergistic effect on the immune responses of patients with sarcoidosis, we investigated in the present study the in vitro synthesis of inflammatory cytokines in PBMCs after co-stimulation with FCWAs and LPS. Our results showed that patients with sarcoidosis, compared to healthy subjects, had a significantly higher secretion of inflammatory cytokines TNF-α, IL-6, IL-10 and IL-12, after co-stimulation of PBMCs with FCWAs and LPS. However, it should be noted that patients with sarcoidosis included in this study had an ongoing inflammatory disease, which may have influenced the immune responses in our in vitro experiments.

In addition to having a strong impact on in vitro human PBMCs inflammatory cytokine responses, FCWAs have been shown to have various biological and immunopharmacological properties (reviewed in [26, 27]). A causal role in the development of respiratory symptoms and diseases associated with fungal exposure has been attributed to β-glucan [12, 28, 29]. β-glucan has also

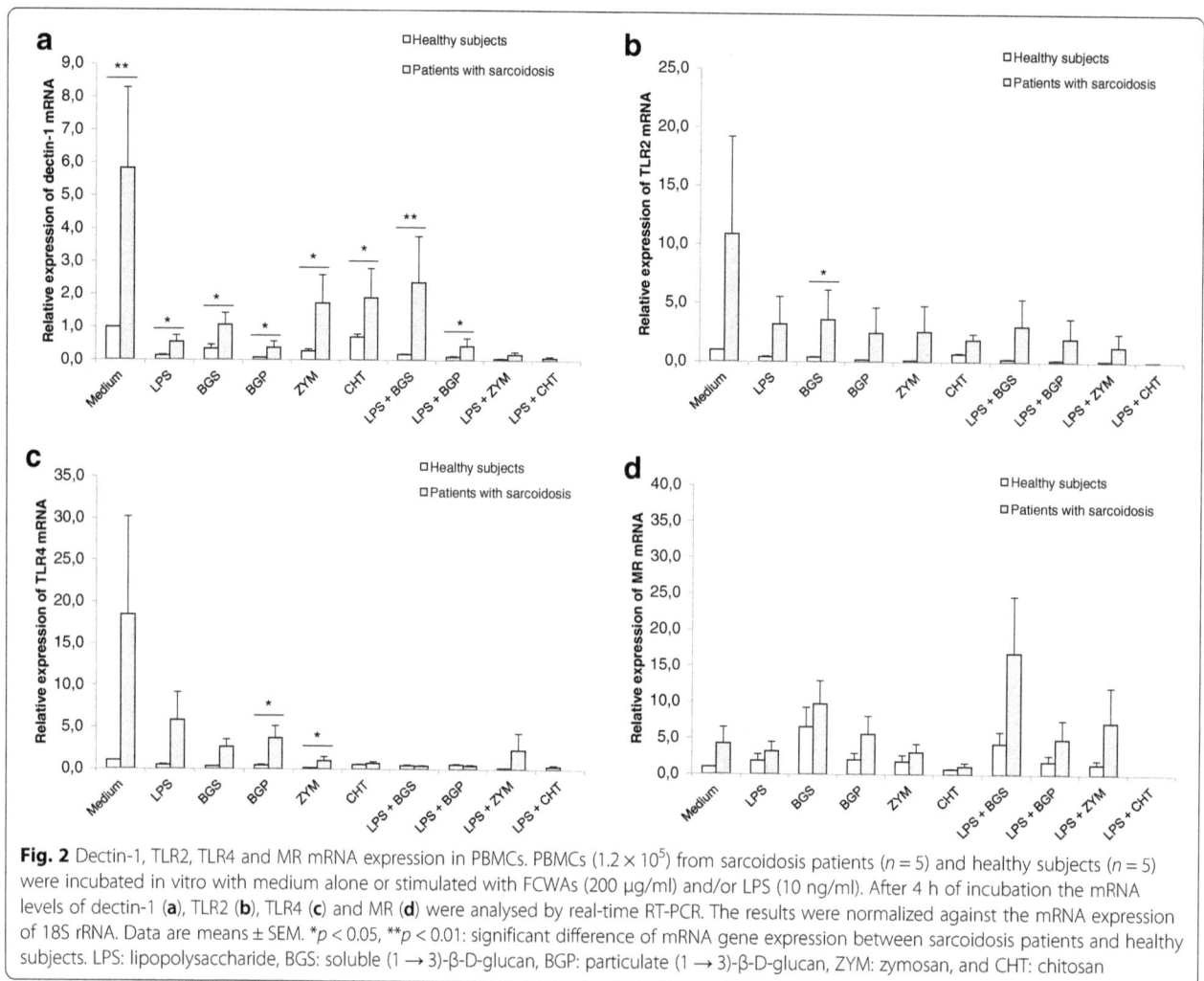

Fig. 2 Dectin-1, TLR2, TLR4 and MR mRNA expression in PBMCs. PBMCs (1.2×10^5) from sarcoidosis patients ($n = 5$) and healthy subjects ($n = 5$) were incubated in vitro with medium alone or stimulated with FCWAs (200 μg/ml) and/or LPS (10 ng/ml). After 4 h of incubation the mRNA levels of dectin-1 (**a**), TLR2 (**b**), TLR4 (**c**) and MR (**d**) were analysed by real-time RT-PCR. The results were normalized against the mRNA expression of 18S rRNA. Data are means ± SEM. *$p < 0.05$, **$p < 0.01$: significant difference of mRNA gene expression between sarcoidosis patients and healthy subjects. LPS: lipopolysaccharide, BGS: soluble $(1 \rightarrow 3)$-β-D-glucan, BGP: particulate $(1 \rightarrow 3)$-β-D-glucan, ZYM: zymosan, and CHT: chitosan

been shown to trigger rheumatoid arthritis in genetically susceptible mice, suggesting that fungal infection may evoke autoimmune conditions in genetically susceptible individuals [30]. Chitin has also been implicated in asthma and allergy [31]. Furthermore, it has been demonstrated that fungi [4, 32, 33] or $(1 \rightarrow 3)$-β-D-glucan itself [34, 35] can trigger granuloma formation. In view of all this, we speculated that FCWAs in combination with LPS may evoke an exaggerated inflammatory reaction in genetically susceptible individuals and lead to sarcoid granuloma formation or progression of the disease.

Recent genetic studies suggest that PRRs might be involved in the pathogenesis of sarcoidosis [36–43]. The central PRRs involved in the recognition of fungi are C-type lectin receptors, such as dectin-1 and MR; TLRs, such as TLR-2, –4 and –9; and the galectin family proteins [44]. The key receptor involved in bacterial LPS recognition is TLR4 [45]. All biological activities of $(1 \rightarrow 3)$-β-D-glucan are mediated by dectin-1, which also collaborates with TLR2 and TLR4. On the other hand, the immunomodulating effects of chitin and its derivatives are

mediated by pathways that involve TLR2, dectin-1 and MR [46]. In our previous study, we examined the in vitro effects of FCWAs alone or in combination with LPS on PRRs mRNA expression in healthy subjects [18]. Since these receptors are suspected of being involved in the pathogenesis of sarcoidosis, we examined the effects of FCWAs and/or LPS on the mRNA expression of these receptors in PBMCs from patients with sarcoidosis.

Our results demonstrated that PBMCs from patients with sarcoidosis had a higher in vitro baseline mRNA expression of dectin-1, TLR2, TLR4 and MR than healthy subjects. The results are in accordance with Wiken et al. [37], who found that TLR2 and TLR4 expression on peripheral blood monocytes at baseline was significantly higher in patients with sarcoidosis than in healthy subjects, as measured by flow cytometry. We found a reduced expression of dectin-1, TLR2 and TLR4 after stimulation with FCWAs and/or LPS, although the reduction was significantly weaker in patients than in healthy subjects. That may indicate a defect in down-regulation of PRRs in sarcoidosis patients when exposed to FCWAs and/or LPS.

Conclusions

In conclusion, microbial cell wall agents are airborne and poorly degradable antigens to which we are constantly exposed. Our study demonstrated that co-stimulation with FCWAs and LPS of PBMC from patients with sarcoidosis caused a weaker reduction of dectin-1, TLR2, TLR4 receptors expression, which could increase the sensitivity of PBMCs, leading to excessive inflammatory cytokine responses and result in the development or progression of pulmonary sarcoidosis.

Acknowledgements
The authors thank Professor Ragnar Rylander and Senior Research Fellow Branka Wraber for their invaluable constructive cooperation in the study.

Funding
This study was supported by a grant from the Slovenian Research Agency, Program Number P3-0083-0381, and by a grant from the Ministry of Higher Education, Science and Technology of the Republic of Slovenia (doctoral fellowship).

Authors' contributions
SS substantially contributed to the concept and design of the study, experimental work (PBMCs cultures, cytokine measurements, gene expression assays), analysis of the results and writing of the manuscript. AI substantially contributed to the concept and design of the study, analysis of the results and writing of the manuscript. BS substantially contributed to the concept and design of the study, experimental work (selection of patients), analysis of the results and writing of the manuscript. MT substantially contributed to the concept and design of the study, experimental work (selection of patients), analysis of the results and writing of the manuscript. SS substantially contributed to the concept and design of the study, experimental work (PBMCs cultures, cytokine measurements, gene expression assays), analysis of the results and writing of the manuscript. All authors read and approved the final manuscript.

Competing interests
The authors declare they have no competing interest.

Author details
[1]Institute of Microbiology and Immunology, Faculty of Medicine, University of Ljubljana, Zaloška 4, SI-1000 Ljubljana, Slovenia. [2]Department for Respiratory and Allergic Diseases, University Medical Centre, Zaloška 2, SI-1000 Ljubljana, Slovenia.

References
1. Baughman RP, Culver DA, Judson MA. A concise review of pulmonary sarcoidosis. Am J Respir Crit Care Med. 2011;183:573–81.
2. Tercelj M, Salobir B, Rylander R. Microbial antigen treatment in sarcoidosis–a new paradigm? Med Hypotheses. 2008;70:831–4.
3. Kucera GP, Rybicki BA, Kirkey KL, Coon SW, Major ML, Maliarik MJ, et al. Occupational risk factors for sarcoidosis in African-American siblings. Chest. 2003;123:1527–35.
4. Newman LS, Rose CS, Bresnitz EA, Rossman MD, Barnard J, Frederick M, et al. A case control etiologic study of sarcoidosis: environmental and occupational risk factors. Am J Respir Crit Care Med. 2004;170:1324–30.
5. Cox-Ganser JM, White SK, Jones R, Hilsbos K, Storey E, Enright PL, et al. Respiratory morbidity in office workers in a water-damaged building. Environ Health Perspect. 2005;113:485–90.
6. Dangman KH, Bracker AL, Storey E. Work-related asthma in teachers in Connecticut: association with chronic water damage and fungal growth in schools. Conn Med. 2005;69:9–17.
7. Laney AS, Cragin LA, Blevins LZ, Sumner AD, Cox-Ganser JM, Kreiss K, et al. Sarcoidosis, asthma, and asthma-like symptoms among occupants of a historically water-damaged office building. Indoor Air. 2009;19:83–90.
8. Tercelj M, Salobir B, Harlander M, Rylander R. Fungal exposure in homes of patients with sarcoidosis - an environmental exposure study. Environ Health. 2011;10:8.
9. Tercelj M, Rott T, Rylander R. Antifungal treatment in sarcoidosis–a pilot intervention trial. Respir Med. 2007;101:774–8.
10. Tercelj M, Salobir B, Zupancic M, Rylander R. Antifungal medication is efficient in the treatment of sarcoidosis. Ther Adv Respir Dis. 2011;5:157–62.
11. Dusad A, Thiele GM, Klassen LW, Gleason AM, Bauer C, Mikuls TR, et al. Organic dust, lipopolysaccharide, and peptidoglycan inhalant exposures result in bone loss/disease. Am J Respir Cell Mol Biol. 2013;49:829–36.
12. Douwes J. (1-> 3)-Beta-D-glucans and respiratory health: a review of the scientific evidence. Indoor Air. 2005;15:160–9.
13. Norback D. An update on sick building syndrome. Curr Opin Allergy Clin Immunol. 2009;9:55–9.
14. Rylander R. Organic dust induced pulmonary disease - the role of mould derived beta-glucan. Ann Agric Environ Med. 2010;17:9–13.
15. Rose CS, Martyny JW, Newman LS, Milton DK, King Jr TE, Beebe JL, et al. "Lifeguard lung": endemic granulomatous pneumonitis in an indoor swimming pool. Am J Public Health. 1998;88:1795–800.
16. Vetvicka V, Novak M. Biology and Chemistry of Beta Glucan: Beta Glucans – Mechanisms of Action. Vol 1. Bussum: Bentham Science Publishers; 2011.
17. Kanchongkittiphon W, Mendell MJ, Gaffin JM, Wang G, Phipatanakul W. Indoor environmental exposures and exacerbation of asthma: an update to the 2000 review by the Institute of Medicine. Environ Health Perspect. 2015;123:6–20.
18. Stopinsek S, Ihan A, Wraber B, Tercelj M, Salobir B, Rylander R, et al. Fungal cell wall agents suppress the innate inflammatory cytokine responses of human peripheral blood mononuclear cells challenged with lipopolysaccharide in vitro. Int Immunopharmacol. 2011;11:939–47.
19. Stopinsek S, Tercelj M, Salobir B, Wraber B, Ihan A, Rylander R, et al. Effects of fungal cell wall polysaccharides and lipopolysaccharide on in vitro tumor necrosis factor alpha production by peripheral blood mononuclear cells of sarcoidosis patients. Zdrav Vestn. 2010;79:684–9.
20. Tercelj M, Stopinsek S, Ihan A, Salobir B, Simcic S, Wraber B, et al. In vitro and in vivo reactivity to fungal cell wall agents in sarcoidosis. Clin Exp Immunol. 2011;166:87–93.
21. Statement on sarcoidosis. Joint Statement of the American Thoracic Society (ATS), the European Respiratory Society (ERS) and the World Association of Sarcoidosis and Other Granulomatous Disorders (WASOG) adopted by the ATS Board of Directors and by the ERS Executive Committee, February 1999. Am J Respir Crit Care Med. 1999;160:736–55.
22. Livak KJ, Schmittgen TD. Analysis of relative gene expression data using real-time quantitative PCR and the 2(−Delta Delta C(T)) Method. Methods. 2001;25:402–8.
23. Gerke AK, Hunninghake G. The immunology of sarcoidosis. Clin Chest Med. 2008;29:379–90. vii.
24. Clementine RR, Lyman J, Zakem J, Mallepalli J, Lindsey S, Quinet R. Tumor necrosis factor-alpha antagonist-induced sarcoidosis. J Clin Rheumatol. 2010;16:274–9.
25. Zissel G. Cellular activation in the immune response of sarcoidosis. Semin Respir Crit Care Med. 2014;35:307–15.

26. Brown GD, Herre J, Williams DL, Willment JA, Marshall AS, Gordon S. Dectin-1 mediates the biological effects of beta-glucans. J Exp Med. 2003;197:1119–24.

27. Muzzarelli RA. Chitins and chitosans as immunoadjuvants and non-allergenic drug carriers. Mar Drugs. 2010;8:292–312.

28. Fogelmark B, Sjostrand M, Rylander R. Pulmonary inflammation induced by repeated inhalations of beta(1,3)-D-glucan and endotoxin. Int J Exp Pathol. 1994;75:85–90.

29. Rylander R, Lin RH. (1– > 3)-beta-D-glucan - relationship to indoor air-related symptoms, allergy and asthma. Toxicology. 2000;152:47–52.

30. Yoshitomi H, Sakaguchi N, Kobayashi K, Brown GD, Tagami T, Sakihama T, et al. A role for fungal {beta}-glucans and their receptor Dectin-1 in the induction of autoimmune arthritis in genetically susceptible mice. J Exp Med. 2005;201:949–60.

31. Brinchmann BC, Bayat M, Brogger T, Muttuvelu DV, Tjonneland A, Sigsgaard T. A possible role of chitin in the pathogenesis of asthma and allergy. Ann Agric Environ Med. 2011;18:7–12.

32. Martin 2nd WJ, Iannuzzi MC, Gail DB, Peavy HH. Future directions in sarcoidosis research: summary of an NHLBI working group. Am J Respir Crit Care Med. 2004;170:567–71.

33. Ezzie ME, Crouser ED. Considering an infectious etiology of sarcoidosis. Clin Dermatol. 2007;25:259–66.

34. Gallin EK, Green SW, Patchen ML. Comparative effects of particulate and soluble glucan on macrophages of C3H/HeN and C3H/HeJ mice. Int J Immunopharmacol. 1992;14:173–83.

35. Tanaka K, Morimoto J, Kon S, Kimura C, Inobe M, Diao H, et al. Effect of osteopontin alleles on beta-glucan-induced granuloma formation in the mouse liver. Am J Pathol. 2004;164:567–75.

36. Schurmann M, Kwiatkowski R, Albrecht M, Fischer A, Hampe J, Muller-Quernheim J, et al. Study of Toll-like receptor gene loci in sarcoidosis. Clin Exp Immunol. 2008;152:423–31.

37. Wiken M, Grunewald J, Eklund A, Wahlstrom J. Higher monocyte expression of TLR2 and TLR4, and enhanced pro-inflammatory synergy of TLR2 with NOD2 stimulation in sarcoidosis. J Clin Immunol. 2009;29:78–89.

38. Hattori T, Konno S, Takahashi A, Isada A, Shimizu K, Shimizu K, et al. Genetic variants in mannose receptor gene (MRC1) confer susceptibility to increased risk of sarcoidosis. BMC Med Genet. 2010;11:151.

39. Margaritopoulos GA, Antoniou KM, Karagiannis K, Samara KD, Lasithiotaki I, Vassalou E, et al. Investigation of Toll-like receptors in the pathogenesis of fibrotic and granulomatous disorders: a bronchoalveolar lavage study. Fibrogenesis Tissue Repair. 2010;3:20.

40. Veltkamp M, Van Moorsel CH, Rijkers GT, Ruven HJ, Van Den Bosch JM, Grutters JC. Toll-like receptor (TLR)-9 genetics and function in sarcoidosis. Clin Exp Immunol. 2010;162:68–74.

41. Wiken M, Idali F, Al Hayja MA, Grunewald J, Eklund A, Wahlstrom J. No evidence of altered alveolar macrophage polarization, but reduced expression of TLR2, in bronchoalveolar lavage cells in sarcoidosis. Respir Res. 2010;11:121.

42. Gabrilovich MI, Walrath J, van Lunteren J, Nethery D, Seifu M, Kern JA, et al. Disordered Toll-like receptor 2 responses in the pathogenesis of pulmonary sarcoidosis. Clin Exp Immunol. 2013;173:512–22.

43. Pabst S, Bradler O, Gillissen A, Nickenig G, Skowasch D, Grohe C. Toll-like receptor-9 polymorphisms in sarcoidosis and chronic obstructive pulmonary disease. Adv Exp Med Biol. 2013;756:239–45.

44. Romani L. Immunity to fungal infections. Nat Rev Immunol. 2011;11:275–88.

45. Park BS, Lee JO. Recognition of lipopolysaccharide pattern by TLR4 complexes. Exp Mol Med. 2013;45, e66.

46. Da Silva CA, Hartl D, Liu W, Lee CG, Elias JA. TLR-2 and IL-17A in chitin-induced macrophage activation and acute inflammation. J Immunol. 2008;181:4279–86.

5

Differential activation of RAW 264.7 macrophages by size-segregated crystalline silica

Steven E. Mischler[1]*, Emanuele G. Cauda[1], Michelangelo Di Giuseppe[2], Linda J. McWilliams[1], Claudette St. Croix[3], Ming Sun[4], Jonathan Franks[4] and Luis A. Ortiz[2]

Abstract

Background: Occupational exposure to crystalline silica is a well-established occupational hazard. Once in the lung, crystalline silica particles can result in the activation of alveolar macrophages (AM), potentially leading to silicosis, a fibrotic lung disease. Because the activation of alveolar macrophages is the beginning step in a complicated inflammatory cascade, it is necessary to define the particle characteristics resulting in this activation. The aim of this research was to determine the effect of the size of crystalline silica particles on the activation of macrophages.

Methods: RAW 264.7 macrophages were exposed to four different sizes of crystalline silica and their activation was measured using electron microscopy, reactive oxygen species (ROS) generation by mitochondria, and cytokine expression.

Results: These data identified differences in particle uptake and formation of subcellular organelles based on particle size. In addition, these data show that the smallest particles, with a geometric mean of 0.3 μm, significantly increase the generation of mitochondrial ROS and the expression of cytokines when compared to larger crystalline silica particles, with a geometric mean of 4.1 μm.

Conclusion: In summary, this study presents novel data showing that crystalline silica particles with a geometric mean of 0.3 μm enhance the activation of AM when compared to larger silica particles usually represented in in vitro and in vivo research.

Keywords: Ultrafine crystalline silica, Alveolar macrophage activation, Size segregation, Occupational aerosols

Background

Occupational exposure to crystalline silica (CS) affects at least 1.7 million US workers [1] and is associated with the development of silicosis, a fibrotic lung disease which is one of the most important occupational diseases worldwide [2–4]. The National Institute for Occupational Safety and Health (NIOSH) reported that 300 silicosis-related deaths occurred each year in the United States between 1991 and 1995 [5]. During those same years China recorded 24,000 silicosis-related deaths per year [6]. These numbers indicate that silicosis remains a fundamental occupational exposure problem in both the developing and developed countries [7].

Exposure to CS occurs in many occupations and industries. The United States Occupational Safety and Health Administration (OSHA) measured detectable levels of respirable CS in samples collected in 255 different industries [1]. In general, silica exposure will occur in any occupation that includes grinding or mechanically breaking material containing silica (mining, construction) or handling fine particles containing silica, such as silica sand (fracking) [4, 8–12].

Although occupational exposure to CS and the related health effects have been well documented in the scientific literature, many uncertainties still exist including the effect of the crystals' surface characteristics, including particle size, on the development of disease [8, 13–

* Correspondence: smischler@cdc.gov
[1]National Institute for Occupational Safety and Health, Office of Mine Safety and Health Research, 626 Cochrans Mill Road, Pittsburgh, PA 15236, USA
Full list of author information is available at the end of the article

18]. Most atmospheric studies suggest that the concentration of smaller particles correlates better with adverse health effects than the concentration of larger particles [16, 19–22]; however, there is little size-dependent toxicity data concerning CS. One difficulty in completing size-dependent toxicity studies with CS is the difficulty in separating the occupational aerosol into distinct size ranges and in necessary quantities for toxicological studies. Recently our group published research on a novel multi-cyclone sampling array which enables the separation of occupational aerosols into distinct size ranges and in quantities needed for toxicological research [23].

Because smaller particles have a higher surface area per unit mass when compared to larger particles, smaller particles may more readily initiate potential negative biological reactions, such as inflammation [24]. Chronic inflammation has been implicated in the pathogenesis of silicosis. In this scenario, the immune cells (alveolar macrophages, epithelial cells, and fibroblasts) are activated and release a host of inflammatory cytokines and generate reactive oxygen species (ROS), resulting in the recruitment of additional inflammatory cells, predominantly alveolar macrophages. The influx of additional inflammatory cells and release of ROS damages pulmonary architecture, causing accumulation of connective tissue products [7, 14, 25–27]. Knowledge of the degree to which particle size affects the activation of macrophages and the resulting ROS generation and inflammatory response is necessary for fully elucidating the mechanisms leading to silicosis from occupational exposure to crystalline silica.

In the present in vitro study, the macrophage response to different-sized crystalline silica particles was evaluated in a well-established murine model [28, 29] using the mouse monocyte-macrophage RAW 264.7 cell line. Airborne CS particles were separated into four distinct size ranges using the multi-cyclone sampling array. The RAW 264.7 macrophages (AM) were exposed to four different sizes of CS and their activation was measured using electron microscopy, mitochondrial ROS (mROS) generation, and cytokine expression.

Methods
Particles used for method evaluation
The crystalline silica (SiO_2 quartz, 99.9%, 1 μm, Stock #: 4807YL) used in this study was purchased from Nanostructured & Amorphous Materials, Inc. (Houston, TX). Before particles were used in the experiment they were baked at 220 °C for 24 h to destroy potential contaminating endotoxins.

Particle separation
The CS particles used in this study were separated into four distinct size ranges as presented in Table 1–

Table 1 Mean particle diameter for each size range using DLS/LLS data

Particle name	Mean (μm)	Standard deviation
Coarse (C)	4.092	2.386
Respirable (R)	2.123	1.146
Submicron (S)	0.716	0.152
Ultrafine (UF)	0.294	0.098

ultrafine (UF), submicron (S), respirable (R), and coarse (C)–using a multi-cyclone sampling array (MCSA).

The MCSA was described in detail previously [23] and particle size ranges are named for consistency with that publication and do not match other established naming conventions found in the literature. Briefly, the MCSA incorporates cyclones in a series of three successive stages. Each cyclone stage is used to capture a specific size range of particles, in decreasing sizes with each stage in the series. The innovative idea in this design is to use the particles collected in the cone and grit pot of each cyclone for characterization and analysis. In this method, three cyclone stages and one filter stage (after the final cyclone) were used to collect size-segregated CS particles. The exhaust from one cyclone was connected to the inlet of the next cyclone in the series using conductive tubing. The mean particle diameter and standard deviation for each size range, measured using light scattering techniques (DLS/LLS), is presented in Table 1 and scanning electron microscope (SEM) photographs at 5,000x magnification of each size range are presented in Fig. 1.

Particle extraction from MCSA
The size-segregated particles were collected from the grit pot of each cyclone using the procedure described in detail in Mischler et al. [23]. Briefly, the grit pot was first inverted and tapped on the outside, allowing the particles to fall out of the grit pot and be collected onto an aluminum collection disk. Any particles which did not fall from the grit pot or particles which remained in the cone were scraped from these surfaces using a plastic or wooden scraping tool. Once the particles were recovered from each cyclone stage, they were stored for later characterization and testing.

The pre-weighed filter, containing the smallest size range of particles, was post-weighed to determine the mass of particles collected on the filter. The particles collected on the filter were then removed using the following procedure: 1) The filter containing the particles was placed in a 15-ml centrifugal test tube, submerged in 5 ml of ultrapure deionized water, and sonicated for five minutes; 2) after sonication, the filter was removed from the first tube and placed in a second tube. Five ml of ultrapure deionized water was added to the second tube, and the

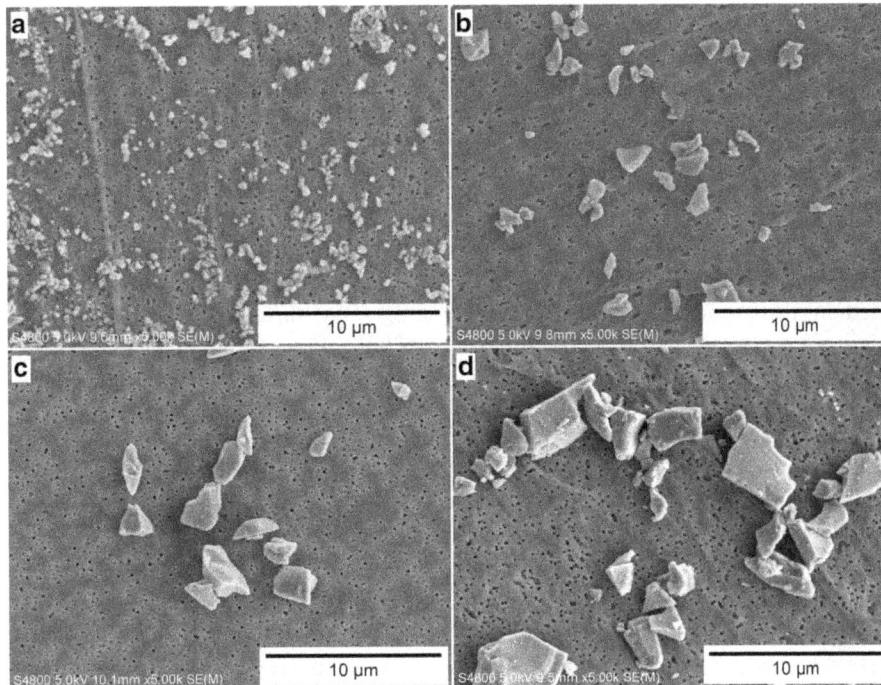

Fig. 1 Comparison of SEM images of the four sizes of crystalline silica particles used for this study, (**a**) Ultrafine (UF), (**b**) Submicron (S), (**c**) Respirable (R), and (**d**) Coarse (C). Images are all at the same magnification (5,000x)

filter was submerged in the water and sonicated for five minutes; 3) after sonication, the water was poured into the first tube, which now contained 10 ml of particle-laden water; 4) another 5 ml of ultrapure deionized water was then added to the tube containing the filter, and the filter was submerged into the water and sonicated for five minutes; 5) after sonication, the 5 ml of water was poured into the first tube, which now contained 15 ml of particle-laden water; 6) the tube containing the 15 ml of particle-laden water was then centrifuged for seven minutes at 3901 relative centrifugal force (RCF); 7) after centrifugation, the supernatant was removed leaving the particles at the bottom of the tube; 8) serum-free Dulbecco's Modified Eagle's Medium (DMEM) was then added to the tube containing the particles to achieve the desired exposure concentration, with the necessary volume for the addition of DMEM calculated based on the post-weight of the filter; 9) once the particles were removed from the filter, the filter was dried and reweighed to verify the mass of particles removed. During this study, the average removal efficiency of the ultrafine CS particles from the filter was 90% as reported previously [23].

Silica particle suspension and characterization

Stock silica suspensions were prepared by adding serum-free DMEM into a measured mass of crystalline silica particles to achieve the desired particle concentrations. For cytokine analysis an exposure concentration of 50 μg/cm^2 was used for all particle sizes, for live-cell experiments and transmission electron microscopy (TEM) analysis an exposure concentration of 16.6 μg/cm^2 was used for all particle sizes. The difference in silica concentrations between these two analyses was necessary because the 50 μg/cm^2 CS concentration completely covered the cells, preventing collection of TEM and live-cell data. 16.6 μg/cm^2 was the highest concentration of UF CS which did not prevent TEM and live-cell data collection. The silica suspensions were used within two hours of mixing with serum-free DMEM. Before each exposure the stock solutions were sonicated for 15 min to ensure adequate distribution of the particles and reduce any agglomeration. After exposure the stock solutions were analyzed with dynamic light scattering, a broadly used and widely accepted method for measuring particle size in solution, to verify particle size distribution, as described previously [23].

Cell cultures

Cells from the mouse monocyte-macrophage RAW 264.7 cell line were purchased from American Type Tissue Culture Collection (ATCC, Rockville, MD) and maintained according to ATCC protocols at 37 °C in a 5% CO$_2$/95% air humidified incubator. Cells were cultured in DMEM with 10% fetal bovine serum (FBS) and penicillin-streptomycin, on 75-cm^2 plates. Approximately 24 h prior to exposure the cells were plated into

6- or 12-well plates. Cells were seeded at a concentration of 1.05×10^5 cells/cm^2 in the indicated culture dishes and the exposure experiments were completed when the cells were at 80% confluency. The use of RAW 264.7 cells is an established murine model in the literature for crystalline silica experiments [28, 29].

TEM analysis

At one, two, and four hours after exposure, cells were fixed in 2.5% glutaraldehyde in phosphate-buffered saline (PBS) and post-fixed in 1% osmium tetroxide in PBS, dehydrated through a graded series of alcohols and embedded in Epon (Energy Beam Sciences, Agawam, MA). Thin (70-nm) sections were cut using a Reichert Ultracut S (Leica, Deerborn, MI), mounted on 200-mesh copper grids and counter-stained with 2% aqueous uranyl acetate for seven minutes and 1% aqueous lead citrate for two minutes. Observation was with a JEOL 1011 transmission electron microscope (Peabody, MA). After TEM images were collected, they were formatted using Adobe Photoshop for brightness and contrast. In addition, during slide preparation, a CS particle could create stretching in the epon resin during the slicing sequence, and when stretching was severe the CS particle could fall out of the resin. During TEM imaging, any areas where the CS particles fell out will show as bright white, causing difficulty in image focusing. These images were corrected by recoloring the white areas back to the color of the silica particles. Importantly, this may result in a slight increase in the CS particle size for the areas that were recolored. In the images at higher magnification, these areas are labelled.

Live-cell analysis

Cells were seeded on 35-mm glass bottom dishes (MatTek Corporation, Ashland, MA) and incubated with the superoxide indicator MitoSOX™ Red (5 μM, Invitrogen, Eugene, OR) for 15 min at 37 °C. Cells were washed with PBS, the media was replaced with exposure media, and the dish was inserted into a closed, thermo-controlled (37 °C) stage top incubator (Tokai Hit Co., Shizuoka-ken, Japan) atop the motorized stage of an inverted Nikon TiE fluorescent microscope (Nikon Inc., Melville, NY) equipped with a 60X oil immersion optic (Nikon, CFI PlanFluor, NA 1.43) and NIS Elements Software. MitoSOX™ Red was excited using a Lumencor diode-pumped light engine (SpectraX, Lumencor Inc., Beaverton OR) and detected using a DsRed longpass filter set (Chroma Technology Corp) and ORCA-Flash4.0 sCMOS camera (HAMAMATSU Corporation, Bridgewater, NJ). Data was collected on approximately 80 to 100 cells per stage position, with eight to ten stage positions in each of the separate experiments for 180 min. Data were analyzed using NIS Elements (Nikon Inc., Melville, NY). Data from three independent analyses

for each particle size were used in the statistical calculations. Stage positions in which the particles did not result in alveolar macrophage (AM) generation of ROS were not used in the statistical analysis.

Cytokine analysis

The effect of particle size on expression of inflammatory cytokines was evaluated using the Bio-Plex multiplex magnetic bead technology (LMC0001, Mouse Cytokine 20-Plex, Invitrogen/Life Technologies, Carlsbad, CA). This assay simultaneously measured the concentration of 20 cytokines in the cellular supernatant. At least three independent experiments were conducted for cytokine expression. Each experiment was conducted using a nested triplicate model where each exposure was run in triplicate and each sample was analyzed in triplicate. For every experiment both a positive and negative control were used. For the negative controls the cells were treated only with serum-free DMEM medium. For the positive control, the cells were treated with serum-free DMEM containing 200 ng/ml of LPS. The effect of CS particles on murine macrophages using control particles such as titanium dioxide or carbon black, is well described in the literature and thus was not repeated in these experiments [30]. In each experiment, cells were exposed to one of four different CS particle stock solutions, described above, for two, four, or eight hours prior to collection of the supernatant. After collection, the supernatant was stored at −80 °C until analysis.

Statistical analysis of ROS measurements

To help understand how CS particle size affects the production of reactive oxygen species in the mitochondria (mROS) in AM, AM were exposed to both UF and C particles over a 3-h exposure period and mROS production was measured using the superoxide indicator Mito-SOX™ Red.

In this study, fluorescence was measured at approximately three-min intervals over a period of 181 min in samples exposed to UF and C particles. Measurements were taken on three samples exposed to each of the two particle sizes at each of the 61 time points. For the purpose of data analysis, the 61 time points were grouped into 30-min periods as shown in Table 2, resulting in a larger sample size for each statistical test, and therefore greater statistical power. Data were analyzed by six independent-samples t-tests comparing mean fluorescence values across the two conditions for each time period. A p-value less than 0.05 was considered to be statistically significant.

Because examination of distributions of fluorescence, using the Shapiro-Wilk test, showed that the values did not follow a normal distribution, data were also analyzed using the Wilcoxin test, which is the non-parametric

Table 2 Grouping of time points for ROS analysis

Time Period	Time points (minutes)	Number of Time Points	Number of Data Points per Condition
1	1, 4, 7, 10, 13, 16, 19, 22, 25, 28, 31	11	33
2	34, 37, 40, 43, 46, 49, 52, 55, 58, 61	10	30
3	64, 67, 70, 73, 76, 79, 82, 85, 88, 91	10	30
4	94, 97, 100, 103, 106, 109, 112, 115, 118, 121	10	30
5	124, 127, 130, 133, 136, 139, 142, 145, 148, 151	10	30
6	154, 157, 160, 163, 166, 169, 172, 175, 178, 181	10	30

counterpart of the t-test. However, since results of the Wilcoxin test agreed with the results of the t-test in every case, only results of the t-tests are reported.

Statistical analysis for cytokine expression

Nonparametric statistical tests, which make no assumption about the distribution of the data, were used to investigate differences of cytokine expression from exposure to the different particle sizes. A p-value less than or equal to 0.10 was considered to be statistically significant to ensure all potentially significant differences were identified. P-values of greater significance are noted in the figures and tables. The Kruskal-Wallis test is the nonparametric alternative to the one-way analysis of variance (ANOVA). This test was used to compare mean ranks among all the samples. When the results of this test were statistically significant the null hypothesis of no difference was rejected and post-hoc tests were run to search for pair-wise differences. For the latter analysis, the Wilcoxon rank sum test, the nonparametric analogue to the t-test for independent samples was used. For both the Kruskal-Wallis and Wilcoxon tests, exact probabilities were calculated [31].

Results

TEM Images of RAW cells after exposure with two sizes of crystalline silica

In order to visualize the difference in the handling of UF particles and C particles by AM, RAW 264.7 AM were exposed to UF and C particles for one, two, and four hours. At the appointed time the cells were fixed and stored until image collection, as discussed in the Methods section.

Figure 2a and b present images (6,000x magnification) of the AM cells after exposure for one hour to C and UF particles, respectively. At this time point, the images show that the UF particles are internalized more quickly and in larger numbers than the coarse particles. This result is consistent with the literature showing faster

uptake of UF particles by AM. In addition, Figure 2b shows phagolysosome (PL) swelling is starting to occur in response to the UF particles. Figure 2c is a higher magnification (20,000x) image of an AM exposed to UF particles for one hour. In this micrograph, the silica particles are marked S, the mitochondria are marked M, and W denotes a white area resulting from particles falling out of the resin, as discussed in the Methods section. In Fig. 2c there is no evidence of UF particles in the cytoplasm or mitochondria.

Figure 3a and b present images (6,000x magnification) of the AM cells after exposure for two hours to C and UF particles, respectively. These micrographs also show that a larger number of UF particles have been internalized by this time point than the C particles, once again consistent with the literature. Figure 3a shows that by the two-hour time period the C particles have been phagocytized by the AM and PL swelling is apparent. Figure 3b shows a cell with up to ten large PLs each containing numerous UF particles. In this figure the PLs are clearly swollen, indicating acidification and enzyme and protease production and delivery. For the C particles, each AM is seen to have phagocytized between one and three particles, whereas as many as 100 UF particles have been phagocytized by this time point. Figure 3c is a higher magnification image of an AM exposed to UF particles for two hours and shows that each PL contains numerous particles. In Fig. 3c there is no evidence of UF particles in the cytoplasm or mitochondria.

Figure 4a and b present images (6,000x magnification) of the AM cells after exposure for four hours to C and UF particles, respectively. These images are similar to two-hour images, where the UF particles have been phagocytized in greater number, resulting in creation of a higher number of PLs. The PLs are swollen but the membrane appears to still be intact. This can be seen more clearly in Fig. 4c, a higher magnification image of an AM exposed to UF particles for four hours. In Fig. 4c there is no evidence of UF particles in the cytoplasm or mitochondria.

Generation of mitochondrial ROS

To help understand how CS particle size affects AM activation, the production of mROS in AM in response to exposure to C and UF particles was measured over a three-hour period. Means and standard deviations of MitoSOX™ Red fluorescence measurements, t-values, and p-values are shown in Table 3. The assumption of equality of variances was not met for several of the tests, and in those cases p-values associated with the Satterthwaite approximation of degrees of freedom are reported. Figure 5 is a representative image from the live-cell experiments taken at 0, 1, 2, and 3 h, for both UF (5A) and C (5B) particles. Increase in mROS can be seen as an increase in

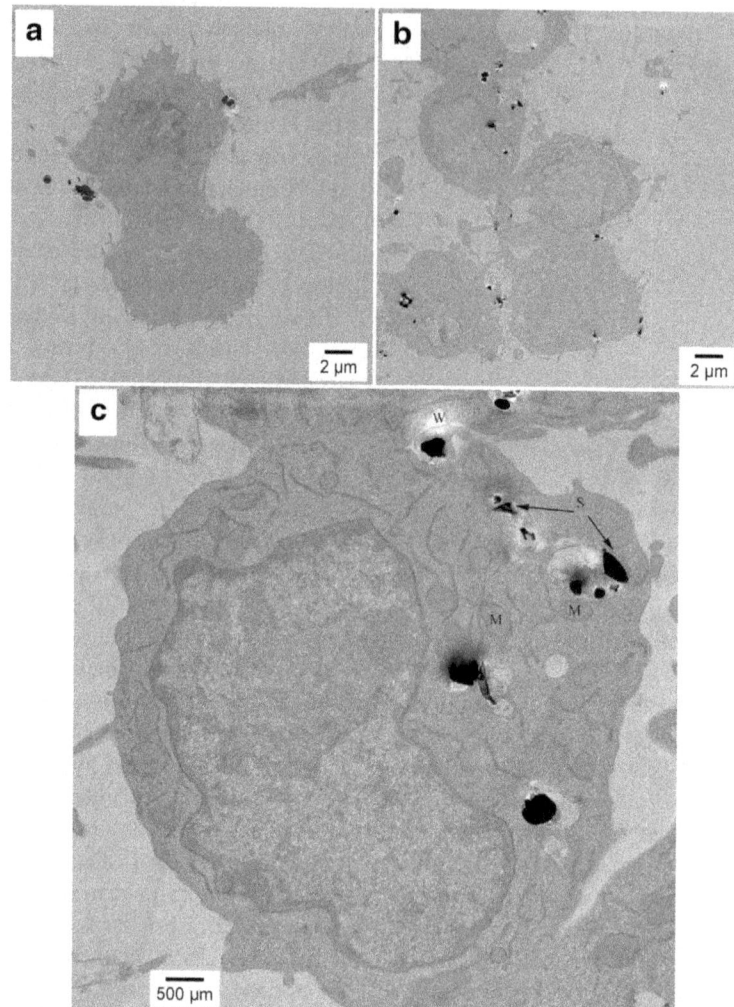

Fig. 2 TEM images of AM after 1-h exposure of AM to (**a**) Coarse particles at 6,000x magnification, (**b**) UF particles at 6,000x magnification, and (**c**) UF particles at 20,000x magnification. In the higher magnification micrograph, the silica particles are marked S, the mitochondria are marked M, and W denotes a white area resulting from particles falling out of the resin. Figures present a representative image of the differences in AM uptake and handling of different sized crystalline silica particles

fluorescence. Figure 6 is a graph of the means reported in Table 3, and shows the increase in AM mROS production resulting from exposure to UF particles, when compared to coarse particles.

As can be seen in Table 3, differences between the UF and C particle size conditions were significant at the 0.01 level for Time Period 1 and significant at the 0.001 level for all other time periods. Mean fluorescence levels were consistently higher for samples exposed to UF particles.

It can be seen in Fig. 6 that fluorescence values increase over time in both conditions. However, the increase appears to be both more gradual and more linear in samples exposed to C particles than in samples exposed to UF particles. This data corroborates what was seen in the TEM images since the PL formation should correspond to the mROS generation.

Expression of inflammatory cytokines

As a way of elucidating the differences in expression of inflammatory cytokines based on exposure to different sized CS particles, we exposed AM to UF, S, R, and C particles for two-, four- and eight-hour exposure periods. A Luminex 200 (Bio-Plex200, Bio-Rad) was used to measure the following cytokines in cell culture supernatant: FGF-basic (fibroblast growth factor 2); GM-CSF (granulocyte-macrophage colony-stimulating factor or colony stimulating factor 2); IFN-γ (interferon-gamma); IL-1α, IL-1β, KC (melanoma growth stimulating activity, alpha); IL2, IL4, IL5, IL6, IL10, IL12B, IL13, IL17A, IP-10 (CXCL10); MCP-1 (monocyte chemoattractant protein 1); MIP-1 alpha (macrophage inflammatory protein 1-alpha); MIG (CXCL9); TNF-α (tumor necrosis factor alpha); and VEGFA (vascular endothelial growth factor A). The data show that for each exposure period the

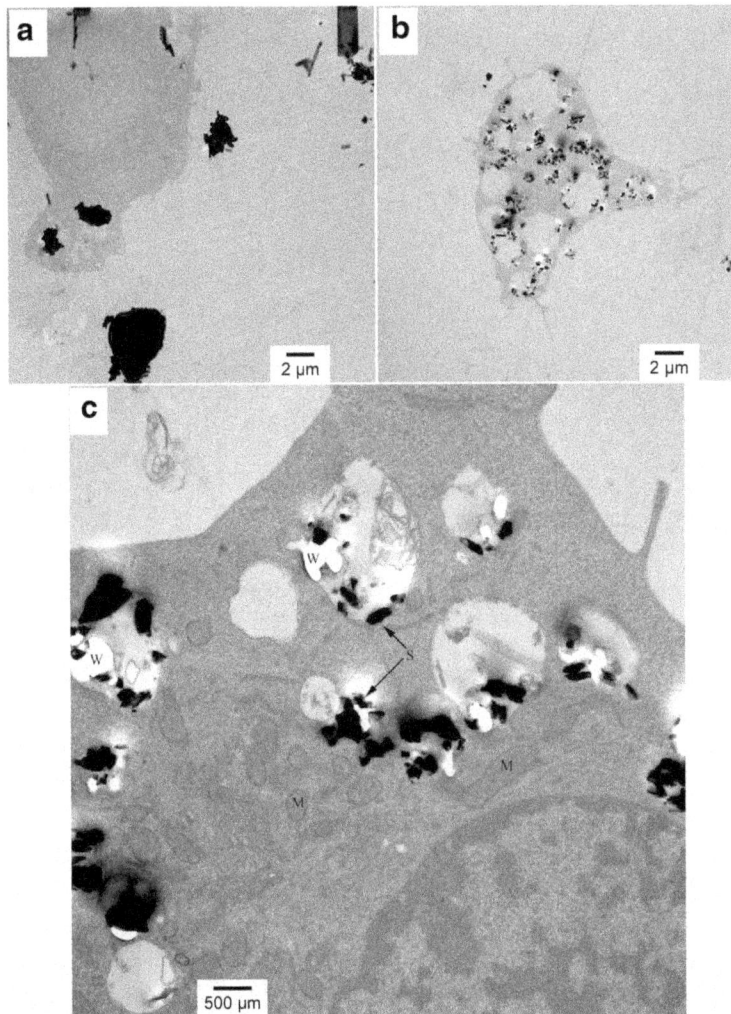

Fig. 3 TEM images of AM after 2-h exposure of AM to (**a**) Coarse particles at 6,000x magnification, (**b**) UF particles at 6,000x magnification, and (**c**) UF particles at 20,000x magnification. In the higher magnification micrograph, the silica particles are marked S, the mitochondria are marked M, and W denotes a white area resulting from particles falling out of the resin. Figures present a representative image of the differences in AM uptake and handling of different sized crystalline silica particles

positive control resulted in significantly elevated expression of the measured cytokines when compared to the CS particle exposures and the negative controls.

The results from the Bio-Plex analysis for the two-hour exposure period are shown for TNF-α in Fig. 7. For this exposure period each CS particle size showed a significant increase in expression of TNF-α when compared to the negative control; however, there was no significant difference on the expression of TNF-α based on CS particle size. Other cytokines measured in the media from the CS particle exposures included IL-5, IL-10, IP-10, MCP-1, and MIP-1A, but no statistical difference based on CS particle size was found for any of these inflammatory cytokines (Data not shown).

The results from the Bio-Plex analysis for the four-hour exposure period are presented for TNF-α in Fig. 8.

At this exposure period each CS particle size showed a significant increase (p-value $<= 0.005$) on expression of TNF-α when compared to the negative control samples. In addition, both the UF and the S particles showed a statistically significant increase in expression of TNF-α when compared to both the C and R particles. Other cytokines measured during this analysis showing a significant difference of expression from exposure to UF versus C particles are as follows: MCP-1 (p-value $= 0.07$); IL-12 (p-value $= 0.003$); IL-5 (p-value $= 0.002$; and IL-6 (p-value $= 0.013$). These data also corroborate those seen in Figs. 2 through 4, since the cytokine production would be expected to be delayed when compared to both PL formation and mROS generation.

The results from the Bio-Plex analysis for the eight-hour exposure period are presented for TNF-α in Fig. 9.

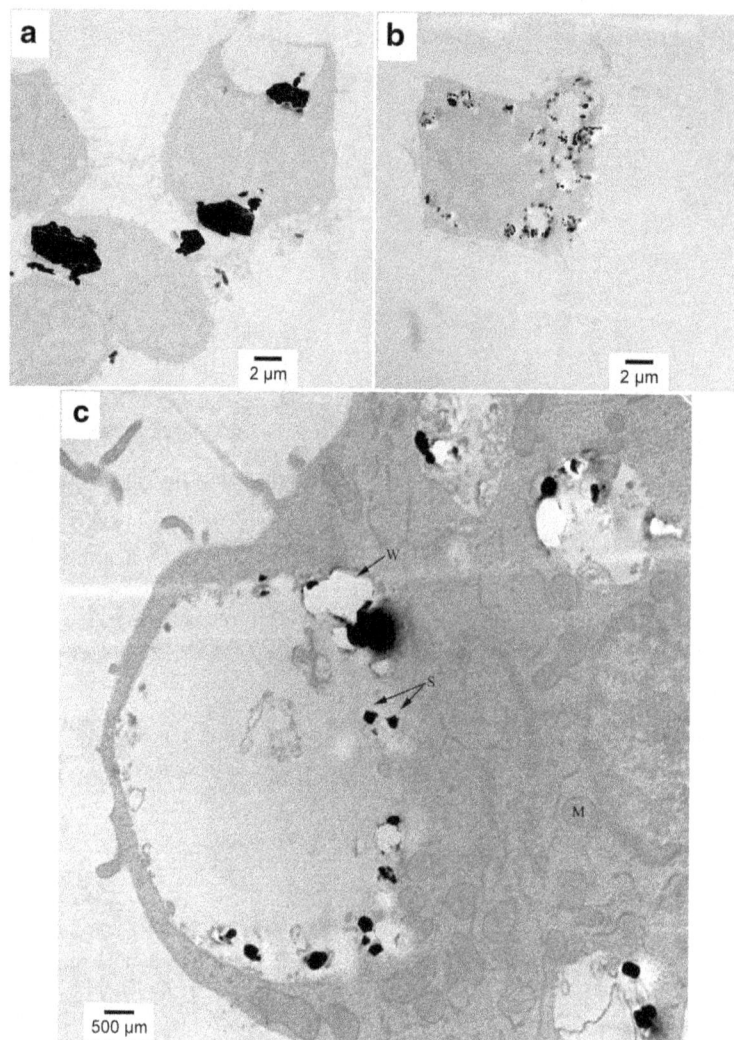

Fig. 4 TEM images of AM after 4-h exposure of AM to (**a**) Coarse particles at 6,000x magnification, (**b**) UF particles at 6,000x magnification, and (**c**) UF particles at 20,000x magnification. In the higher magnification micrograph, the silica particles are marked S, the mitochondria are marked M, and W denotes a white area resulting from particles falling out of the resin. Figures present a representative image of the differences in AM uptake and handling of different sized crystalline silica particles

At this exposure period, each CS particle size showed a significant increase (p-value < = 0.005) on the expression of TNF-α when compared to the negative control samples. Also, the UF particles were found to significantly enhance the expression of TNF-α when compared to the other three particle sizes.

Discussion

This study aimed to understand the effect of different sized crystalline silica particles on the activation and response of murine alveolar macrophages. For this study, the CS was divided into four distinct size ranges-C (4 μm), R (2 μm), S (0.7 μm), and UF (0.3 μm)-using a multi-cyclone sampling array. This method is capable of separating airborne occupational aerosols into distinct size ranges as described in the Methods section. The CS particles at each size range were well defined both in the air and in the culture media.

The results of this study show a consistent relationship between CS particle sizes and AM activation, as measured by TEM imaging, mROS generation, and inflammatory cytokine expression. The TEM data show that a greater number of UF particles are phagocytized in a shorter time period than C particles. In addition, the number of PLs resulting from the UF exposure, the size of the PLs, and the number of particles in each of the PLs is increased for the UF particles when compared to the C particles. The mROS data show both a faster and more intense response from exposure to UF particles versus C particles. Finally, the cytokine measurements

Table 3 Results of independent samples t-tests for mROS production using MitoSOX™ Red fluorescence measurements

Time Period	Particle Size	Mean	SD	t	p
1	Ultrafine	42.55	60.84	3.12	.004[*]
	Coarse	8.98	11.35		
2	Ultrafine	203.81	87.86	8.76	<.0005[*]
	Coarse	51.02	32.47		
3	Ultrafine	297.86	67.92	11.54	<.0005
	Coarse	96.64	67.19		
4	Ultrafine	391.79	49.32	13.43	<.0005[*]
	Coarse	145.69	87.42		
5	Ultrafine	450.25	108.07	9.15	<.0005
	Coarse	196.02	107.24		
6	Ultrafine	477.14	151.41	6.41	<.0005
	Coarse	236.56	139.18		

[*] Based on Satterthwaite approximation

showed that UF particles resulted in a significant increase in TNF-α expression from the AM at four- and eight-hour exposures when compared to C exposure. TNF-α expression is a primary indicator of AM activation [7, 32]. Other cytokines measured during this analysis also show a significant difference in expression between UF exposure versus C exposure at four hours, including MCP-1, IL-12, IL-5, and IL-6. These results agree with previous work discussing cytokine release and AM activation due to silica exposure [28, 33, 34].

Much work, both in vivo and in vitro, is evident in the literature comparing the effect of particle size on biological outcomes. This previous work usually agrees with our data that smaller particles create an enhanced biological response. Typically, this previous work used engineered particles produced in laboratories at specific sizes, such as amorphous silica, titanium dioxide (TiO$_2$), or gold [18, 29, 35, 36]. Oberdorster et al. observed significantly greater pulmonary inflammatory response to ultrafine (20-nm) TiO$_2$ in rats and mice when compared to larger particles (250-nm) [37]. Sager et al. found that ultrafine (21-nm) TiO$_2$ particles caused significantly greater inflammation and were more cytotoxic than fine (1-μm) TiO$_2$ particles when instilled into rats [38]. Also, Leclerc et al. investigated in vitro the rate of macrophage uptake and toxicity of fluorescent silica particles ranging from 850 to 150 nm and found that the smallest particles were internalized in greater quantities [18].

Despite the above work, there are relatively few studies comparing biological effects from different sizes of crystalline silica. Wiessner et al. showed that a 1-μm fraction was more lytic to red blood cell membranes than larger fractions; however, the larger size fractions resulted in a greater in vivo inflammatory response [13]. In this study, the 1-μm fraction was the smallest used. Kajiwara et al.

demonstrated that a 1.8-μm size fraction more intensely affected the lungs of mice than a 0.7-μm size fraction [16]. The major differences between our current study and these previous studies are the size ranges of the particles used for exposure and the procedure for separating the particles into these distinct size ranges. The particles sizes used in these previous studies ranged from 1.8 to 0.7 μm whereas the range for our study was 4 μm to 0.3 μm. Wang et al. showed that silica particles in the size fraction <200 nm were both cytotoxic and genotoxic to human cells [17]. However, this study did not compare the effects of particle size and did not use AM, so no activation criteria were reported.

Each of these previous studies used separation technologies that allowed particle crossover between size ranges such that smaller particles are present in larger particle ranges and vice versa. The biological effects measured in these experiments may have been influenced by the presence of these crossover particles. In the present study, the MCSA was used to separate the crystalline silica particles into distinct size ranges with little crossover between ranges. In addition, the MCSA method allows for the particle separation to occur from the air in concentrations found in occupational environments. Because the particles are separated from the air, they are unaffected by the handling steps necessary for other separation techniques [23].

In addition to showing the significance of particle size on the activation of AMs, our study also sheds some light on the molecular mechanisms behind this activation. The inflammatory effect was shown to be mediated from the recruitment of the NALP3 inflammosome [30, 39, 40]; however, the mechanism of this recruitment and silica-induced toxicity is still in question [27, 35]. In this study we provide data to indicate that mROS production occurs very early in the AM reaction to silica and coincides with the PL formation and swelling in the AM. In addition, the cytokine expression is delayed when compared to the mROS production. In our data, we see a significant difference in mROS generation based on exposure to UF particles versus C particles, with the greatest difference between 2 and 2.5 h. However, at the two-hour time point we see no difference in cytokine expression between these particle sizes. By four hours, a significant difference in cytokine expression between the UF and C particle exposures appears. The TEM images show an increased number of UF particles being phagocytized at two hours and some swelling of the PLs is occurring. By the four-hour time period, there are noticeably more PLs and they are noticeably swelling, when compared to the same time after C particle exposure and as the number of PLs increases the generation of mROS increases. Cassel et al. showed that cellular ROS signaling is occurring upstream of the NALP3 inflammasome activation. Dostert et al.

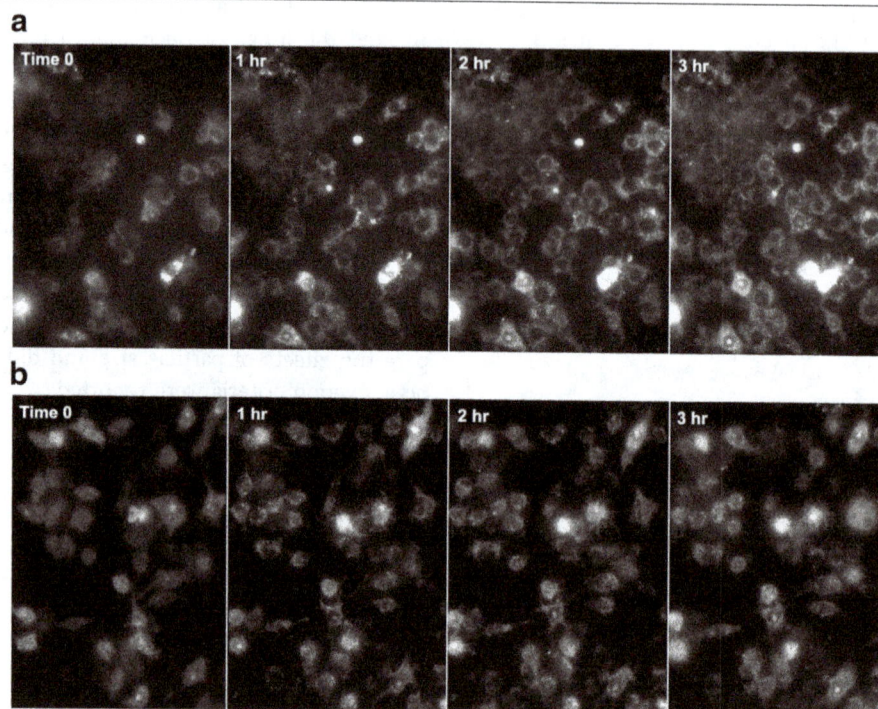

Fig. 5 To help understand how particle size affects the production of reactive oxygen species in the mitochondria (mROS) in AM we exposed AM to both UF (**a**) and C (**b**) particles over a 3-h exposure period and measured mROS production using the superoxide indicator MitoSOX™ Red. mROS production is demonstrated over three hours in these representative images using original magnification x10, of the live cell experiment collected at 0, 1, 2 and 3 h, by increase in fluorescence

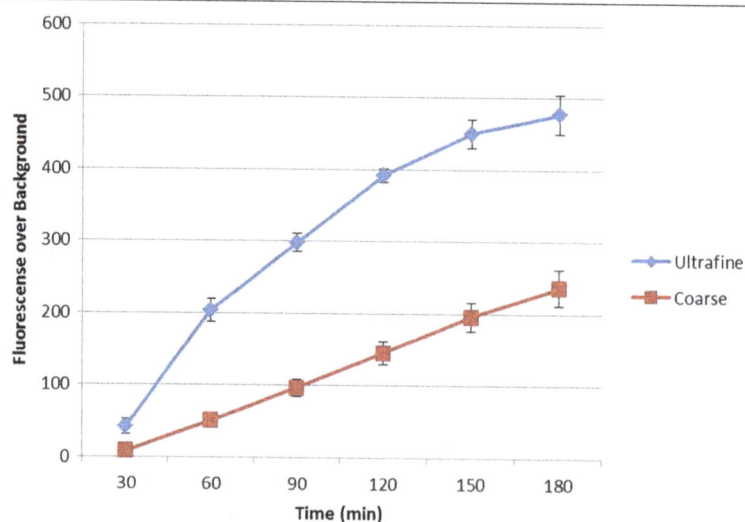

Fig. 6 Increase in AM mROS production resulting from exposure to UF particles, when compared to coarse particles, was confirmed using MitoSOX™ Red fluorescence. Data was collected on approximately 80 to 100 cells per stage position, with eight to ten stage positions in each of the separate experiments for 180 min. Data were analyzed using NIS Elements (Nikon Inc., Melville, NY). Data from three independent analyses for each particle size were used in the statistical calculations. Stage positions in which the particles did not result in AM generation of ROS were not used in the statistical analysis

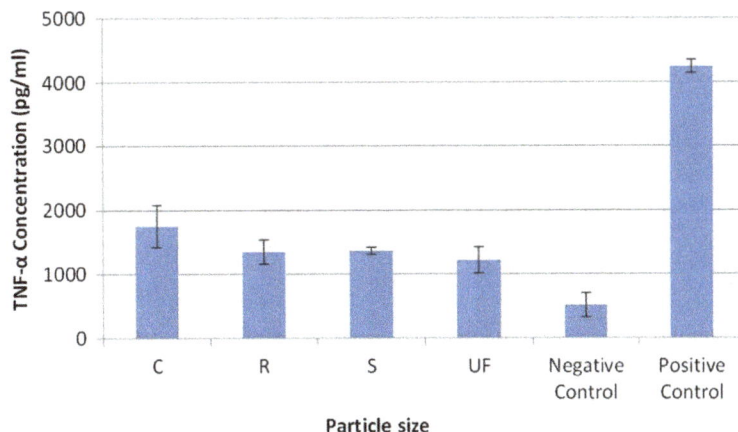

Fig. 7 TNF-α expression after 2-h exposure to four sizes of Crystalline Silica, showing that for a 2-h exposure period each particle size creates a significant increase in expression of TNF-α when compared to the negative control; however, there was no significant difference on the expression of TNF-α based on particle size

suggested that these inflammasome activating cellular ROS are generated by NADPH oxidase complexes on the phagolysosome membrane [40].

The above information, along with the data presented in this study, lends further definition to the pathway recently outlined by Lueng [4]. In this process, cellular ROS is generated by both the mitochondria and the NAPDH oxidase after phagocytosis and this process happens quickly after exposure. The cellular ROS then activates the NALP3 inflammasome, leading to expression of inflammatory cytokines. Our data supports this mechanism since the UF particles are more quickly incorporated into PLs and there are a greater number of PLs formed, corresponding to an increase in mROS generation and ultimately to

elevated expression of inflammatory cytokines. Since only mROS was measured in this study, our data suggest that the increase in cellular ROS, as described earlier, is at least partly caused by generation of ROS in the mitochondria.

A second possibility resulting in inflammation is the activation of the NFκB pathway by cellular ROS. This pathway has been shown to be activated by CS [14, 41], resulting in the expression of TNF-α. Our data also supports this pathway, since TNF-α production continues to increase as the number of PLs and mROS generation increase in the AM. Scarfi et al. add a slightly different perspective on this mechanism [32] by showing that cellular ROS generation and TNF-α expression occur in the absence of phagocytosis. In this case the plasma

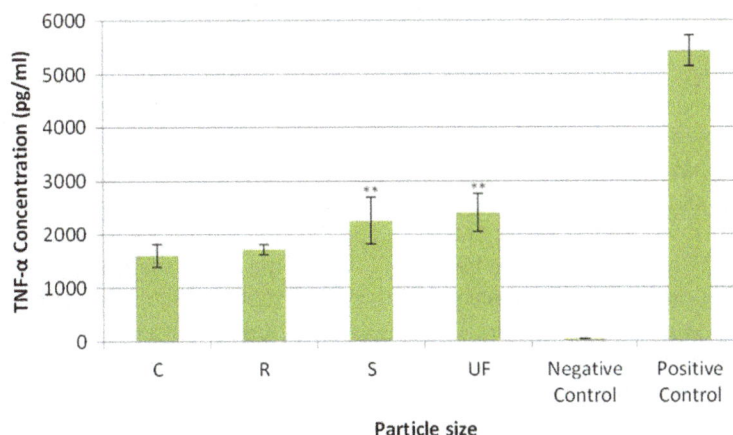

Fig. 8 TNF-α expression after 4-h exposure to four sizes of Crystalline Silica, showing that for a 4-h exposure period each particle size created a significant increase (p-value $<= 0.005$) in expression of TNF-α when compared to the negative control samples. In addition, both the UF and the S particles showed a statistically significant increase in expression of TNF-α when compared to both the C and R particles (p-value $= 0.005$). ** Significant difference from C exposure at p-value $= 0.005$

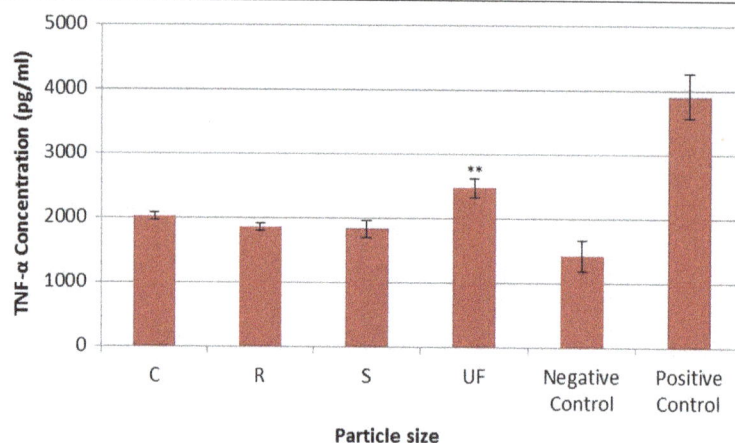

Fig. 9 TNF-α expression after 8-h exposure to four sizes of Crystalline Silica, showing that for an 8-h exposure period, each particle size created a significant increase (p-value $< = 0.005$) in the expression of TNF-α when compared to the negative control samples. In addition, the UF particles were found to significantly enhance the expression of TNF-α when compared to the other three particle sizes (p-value $= 0.0001$). ** Significant difference from C exposure at p-value $= 0.0001$

membrane appears to play a key role in the cellular ROS generation.

Taken together, these data suggest that two potential pathways, independent of each other, lead to the inflammatory response in AM. The first pathway was suggested by Scarfi et al. where the cellular ROS generation results from the CS interaction with the plasma membrane prior to phagocytosis, as a result of lipid peroxidation. Our data show mROS generation occurring with the introduction of the CS particles and TNF-α expression measured at two hours after exposure. In addition, our data show that the mROS production and TNF-α expression increase more quickly corresponding to an increase in the number of PLs formed. In this case, the mROS generation would result from the PL membrane disruption caused by CS and add to the cellular ROS generated from the plasma membrane. Since there are a greater number of PLs created in response to the UF particle exposure, the difference in mROS generation between the two exposure scenarios, as well as the resulting TNF-α expression, should increase as the PLs are formed. This is exactly what our data show. In this slightly delayed scenario the inflammatory response would result from PL generated mROS either through the activation of the NALP3 inflammasome or through the initiation of the NFκB cascade. In both scenarios, the UF particles should cause an enhanced response due first from plasma membrane interaction with a larger number of CS particles and then from the formation of a greater number of PLs after phagocytosis.

Conclusions

The aim of this research was to determine the effect of the size of crystalline silica particles on the activation of macrophages. This study provided novel data showing that UF silica particles enhance the activation of AM when compared to larger silica particles usually represented in in vitro and in vivo research. These data identified differences in particle uptake and formation of subcellular organelles based on particle size. In addition, these data show that the smallest particles, with a geometric mean of 0.3 μm, significantly increase the generation of mitochondrial ROS and the expression of cytokines when compared to larger crystalline silica particles, with a geometric mean of 4.1 μm. However, these data are only meaningful if it can be shown that UF silica particles are a relevant occupational exposure. Recently it was shown that nanoparticles, ranging from 850 to 100 nm inhaled by rats were found in the alveolar macrophages of these animals [42] providing evidence that particles as small as 100 nm can be incorporated into AMs. Furthermore, it has been shown that in occupational environments there is significant variation in particle size and size-related silica content [8], and that as the average particle size of the sample decreases, the percent silica of the sample may increase [43]. Because such substantial differences in particle size and CS content of occupational aerosols have been shown to occur and because we have shown in this study that UF CS particles enhance the activation of AM compared to larger CS particles, more research is needed to more fully define this exposure and potential adverse biological outcomes of UF silica particles. In addition, the results of this study lend support to the growing chorus of researchers calling for regulations based on metrics capable of measuring UF and nanoparticles, to help better protect workers from this exposure.

Abbreviations
AM: Alveolar macrophage; ATCC: American type tissue culture collection; C: Coarse; CS: Crystalline silica; DMEM: Dulbecco's modified eagle's medium;

FBS: Fetal bovine serum; MCSA: Multi-cyclone sampling array; mROS: Mitochondrial reactive oxygen species; OSHA: United states occupational safety and health administration; PBS: Phosphate buffered saline; PL: Phagolysosome; R: Respirable; RCF: Relative centrifugal force; ROS: Reactive oxygen species; S: Submicron; SEM: Scanning electron microscope; TEM: Transmission electron microscopy; UF: Ultrafine particles

Acknowledgements
We thank Joe Archer for his expertise in using the Marple chamber and his aid in collecting samples. We also thank Dr. Keflai Bein for his guidance and advice and Shannon Mischler for her extensive language skills. This work was funded by the National Institute for Occupational Safety and Health, Office of Mine Safety and Health Research, and by NIEHS grant R01ES010859 to LAO.

Funding
National Institute for Occupational Safety and Health - General Project Funds. National Institute of Environmental Health Sciences - R01ES010859 to LAO.

Authors' contributions
SEM, EC, MDG, performed experimental work; MG, JS, CSC performed microscopy work; SEM, LOA, MDG, CSC evaluated data; SEM, EC provided size-segregated particles; LM provided statistical analysis; SEM, LOA, MDG conceived the study; SEM, LOA, JS, CSC wrote and edited the manuscript. All authors read and approved the final manuscript.

Competing interests
The authors declare that they have no competing interests.

Disclaimer
The findings and conclusions in this report are those of the author (s) and do not necessarily represent the views of the National Institute for Occupational Safety and Health (NIOSH). In addition, mention of any company or product does not constitute endorsement by NIOSH.

Author details
[1]National Institute for Occupational Safety and Health, Office of Mine Safety and Health Research, 626 Cochrans Mill Road, Pittsburgh, PA 15236, USA. [2]Department of Environmental and Occupational Health, University of Pittsburgh, Pittsburgh, PA, USA. [3]Center for Biological Imaging, Environmental and Occupational Health, University of Pittsburgh, Pittsburgh, PA, USA. [4]Center for Biological Imaging, University of Pittsburgh, Pittsburgh, PA, USA.

References
1. NIOSH. NIOSH Hazard Review; Health Effects of Occupational Exposure to Respirable Crystalline Silica, DHHS (NIOSH) Publication NO.2002-129. Department of Health and Human Services,CDC,NIOSH, Publication NO.2002-129. 2002.
2. Greenberg MI, Waksman J, Curtis J. Silicosis: a review. Dis Mon. 2007;53:394–416.
3. The Global Occupational Health Network Newsletter: elimination of silicosis [http://www.who.int/occupational_health/publications/newsletter/gohnet12e.pdf]. Accessed 9 Dec 2016.
4. Leung CC, Yu IT, Chen W. Silicosis. Lancet. 2012;379:2008–18.
5. Work-Related Lung Disease Surveillance System (eWoRLD); Silicosis Mortality [http://www2a.cdc.gov/drds/worldreportdata/SubsectionDetails.asp?ArchiveID=1&SubsectionTitleID=8]. Accessed 9 Dec 2016.
6. Silicosis Fact Sheet N° 238 [http://www.nzdl.org/gsdlmod?e=d-00000-00—off-0cdl-00-0——0-10-0—0—0direct-10—4————0-1l-11-en-50—20-about—00-0-1-00-0-4——0-0-11-10-0utfZz-8-00&cl=CL1.242&d=HASHf58c7c472d6ca58330314f.2&x=1]
7. Huaux F. New developments in the understanding of immunology in silicosis. Curr Opin Allergy Clin Immunol. 2007;7:168–73.
8. Sirianni G, Hosgood 3rd HD, Slade MD, Borak J. Particle size distribution and particle size-related crystalline silica content in granite quarry dust. J Occup Environ Hyg. 2008;5:279–85.
9. Beaudry C, Lavoue J, Sauve JF, Begin D, Senhaji Rhazi M, Perrault G, Dion C, Gerin M. Occupational exposure to silica in construction workers: a literature-based exposure database. J Occup Environ Hyg. 2013;10:71–7.
10. Hall RM, Achutan C, Sollberger R, McCleery RE, Rodriguez M. Exposure assessment for roofers exposed to silica during installation of roof tiles. J Occup Environ Hyg. 2013;10:D6–10.
11. McKinney W, Chen B, Schwegler-Berry D, Frazer DG. Computer-automated silica aerosol generator and animal inhalation exposure system. Inhal Toxicol. 2013;25:363–72.
12. Sauve JF, Beaudry C, Begin D, Dion C, Gerin M, Lavoue J. Silica exposure during construction activities: statistical modeling of task-based measurements from the literature. Ann Occup Hyg. 2013;57:432–43.
13. Wiessner JH, Mandel NS, Sohnle PG, Mandel GS. Effect of particle size on quartz-induced hemolysis and on lung inflammation and fibrosis. Exp Lung Res. 1989;15:801–12.
14. Fubini B, Hubbard A. Reactive oxygen species (ROS) and reactive nitrogen species (RNS) generation by silica in inflammation and fibrosis. Free Radic Biol Med. 2003;34:1507–16.
15. Bodo M, Muzi G, Bellucci C, Lilli C, Calvitti M, Lumare A, Dell'Omo M, Gambelunghe A, Baroni T, Murgia N. Comparative in vitro studies on the fibrogenic effects of two samples of silica on epithelial bronchial cells. J Biol Regul Homeost Agents. 2007;21:97–104.
16. Kajiwara T, Ogami A, Yamato H, Oyabu T, Morimoto Y, Tanaka I. Effect of particle size of intratracheally instilled crystalline silica on pulmonary inflammation. J Occup Health. 2007;49:88–94.
17. Wang JJ, Sanderson BJ, Wang H. Cytotoxicity and genotoxicity of ultrafine crystalline SiO2 particulate in cultured human lymphoblastoid cells. Environ Mol Mutagen. 2007;48:151–7.
18. Leclerc L, Rima W, Boudard D, Pourchez J, Forest V, Bin V, Mowat P, Perriat P, Tillement O, Grosseau P, et al. Size of submicrometric and nanometric particles affect cellular uptake and biological activity of macrophages in vitro. Inhal Toxicol. 2012;24:580–8.
19. Churg A, Brauer M. Ambient atmospheric particles in the airways of human lungs. Ultrastruct Pathol. 2000;24:353–61.
20. Donaldson K, MacNee W. Potential mechanisms of adverse pulmonary and cardiovascular effects of particulate air pollution (PM10). Int J Hyg Environ Health. 2001;203:411–5.
21. Knol AB, de Hartog JJ, Boogaard H, Slottje P, van der Sluijs JP, Lebret E, Cassee FR, Wardekker JA, Ayres JG, Borm PJ, et al. Expert elicitation on ultrafine particles: likelihood of health effects and causal pathways. Part Fibre Toxicol. 2009;6:19.
22. Pope 3rd CA, Burnett RT, Krewski D, Jerrett M, Shi Y, Calle EE, Thun MJ. Cardiovascular mortality and exposure to airborne fine particulate matter and cigarette smoke: shape of the exposure-response relationship. Circulation. 2009;120:941–8.
23. Mischler SE, Cauda EG, Di Giuseppe M, Ortiz LA. A multi-cyclone sampling array for the collection of size-segregated occupational aerosols. J Occup Ind Hyg. 2013;10(12):685–93.
24. Monteiller C, Tran L, MacNee W, Faux S, Jones A, Miller B, Donaldson K. The pro-inflammatory effects of low-toxicity low-solubility particles, nanoparticles and fine particles, on epithelial cells in vitro: the role of surface area. Occup Environ Med. 2007;64:609–15.
25. Mossman BT, Churg A. Mechanisms in the pathogenesis of asbestosis and silicosis. Am J Respir Crit Care Med. 1998;157:1666–80.
26. Rimal B, Greenberg AK, Rom WN. Basic pathogenetic mechanisms in silicosis: current understanding. Curr Opin Pulm Med. 2005;11:169–73.
27. Hamilton Jr RF, Thakur SA, Holian A. Silica binding and toxicity in alveolar macrophages. Free Radic Biol Med. 2008;44:1246–58.
28. Gozal E, Ortiz LA, Zou X, Burow ME, Lasky JA, Friedman M. Silica-induced apoptosis in murine macrophage: involvement of tumor necrosis factor-alpha and nuclear factor-kappaB activation. Am J Respir Cell Mol Biol. 2002;27:91–8.
29. Sandberg WJ, Lag M, Holme JA, Friede B, Gualtieri M, Kruszewski M, Schwarze PE, Skuland T, Refsnes M. Comparison of non-crystalline silica nanoparticles in IL-1beta release from macrophages. Part Fibre Toxicol. 2012;9:32.

30. Cassel SL, Eisenbarth SC, Iyer SS, Sadler JJ, Colegio OR, Tephly LA, Carter AB, Rothman PB, Flavell RA, Sutterwala FS. The Nalp3 inflammasome is essential for the development of silicosis. Proc Natl Acad Sci U S A. 2008;105:9035–40.

31. Rosner B. Fundamentals of Biostatistics. 3rd ed. Boston: PWS-Kent Publishing Company; 1990.

32. Scarfì S, Magnone M, Ferraris C, Pozzolini M, Benvenuto F, Benatti U, Giovine M. Ascorbic acid pre-treated quartz stimulates TNF-alpha release in RAW 264.7 murine macrophages through ROS production and membrane lipid peroxidation. Respir Res. 2009;10:25.

33. Driscoll KE, Hassenbein DG, Carter JM, Kunkel SL, Quinlan TR, Mossman BT. TNF alpha and increased chemokine expression in rat lung after particle exposure. Toxicol Lett. 1995;82–83:483–9.

34. Balduzzi M, Diociaiuti M, De Berardis B, Paradisi S, Paoletti L. In vitro effects on macrophages induced by noncytotoxic doses of silica particles possibly relevant to ambient exposure. Environ Res. 2004;96:62–71.

35. Winter M, Beer HD, Hornung V, Kramer U, Schins RP, Forster I. Activation of the inflammasome by amorphous silica and TiO2 nanoparticles in murine dendritic cells. Nanotoxicology. 2011;5:326–40.

36. Downs TR, Crosby ME, Hu T, Kumar S, Sullivan A, Sarlo K, Reeder B, Lynch M, Wagner M, Mills T, Pfuhler S. Silica nanoparticles administered at the maximum tolerated dose induce genotoxic effects through an inflammatory reaction while gold nanoparticles do not. Mutat Res. 2012;745:38–50.

37. Oberdorster G, Finkelstein JN, Johnston C, Gelein R, Cox C, Baggs R, Elder AC. Acute pulmonary effects of ultrafine particles in rats and mice. Res Rep Health Eff Inst. 2000;13(7):823–39.

38. Sager TM, Kommineni C, Castranova V. Pulmonary response to intratracheal instillation of ultrafine versus fine titanium dioxide: role of particle surface area. Part Fibre Toxicol. 2008;5:17.

39. Hornung V, Bauernfeind F, Halle A, Samstad EO, Kono H, Rock KL, Fitzgerald KA, Latz E. Silica crystals and aluminum salts activate the NALP3 inflammasome through phagosomal destabilization. Nat Immunol. 2008;9:847–56.

40. Dostert C, Petrilli V, Van Bruggen R, Steele C, Mossman BT, Tschopp J. Innate immune activation through Nalp3 inflammasome sensing of asbestos and silica. Science. 2008;320:674–7.

41. Cox Jr LA. An exposure-response threshold for lung diseases and lung cancer caused by crystalline silica. Risk Anal. 2011;31:1543–60.

42. Morfeld P, Treumann S, Ma-Hock L, Bruch J, Landsiedel R. Deposition behavior of inhaled nanostructured TiO2 in rats: fractions of particle diameter below 100 nm (nanoscale) and the slicing bias of transmission electron microscopy. Inhal Toxicol. 2012;24:939–51.

43. Page SJ. Comparison of coal mine dust size distributions and calibration standards for crystalline silica analysis. AIHA J (Fairfax, Va). 2003;64:30–9.

6

Awareness of occupational hazards and associated factors among welders in Lideta Sub-City, Addis Ababa

Sebsibe Tadesse[1]*, Kassahun Bezabih[2], Bikes Destaw[1] and Yalemzewod Assefa[1]

Abstract

Background: Welding is a manufacturing industry where workers could be exposed to several hazards. However, there is a dearth of studies clarifying the situation in Ethiopia. The present study determined the level of awareness of occupational hazards and associated factors among welding employees at Lideta Sub-City, Addis Ababa, Ethiopia.

Methods: A work site-based cross-sectional study was conducted among welding employees Lideta Sub-City, Addis Ababa, Ethiopia from April to May 2015. Stratified sampling followed by simple random sampling techniques was used to select the study participants. A pilot tested and structured questionnaire was used to collect data. Multivariable analyses were employed to see the effect of explanatory variables on workers' awareness of occupational hazards.

Results: According to our criteria of awareness 86.5 % of surveyed workers were aware of occupational hazards. A higher work experience, presence of work regulation, job satisfaction, being married, being single, and a higher educational status were factors significantly associated with workers' awareness of occupational hazards.

Conclusion: This study revealed that the level of awareness of occupational hazards among welders was high. However, this does not mean that there will be no need for further strengthening of the safety measures as significant proportions of the workers still had low awareness. Interventions to boost workers awareness of occupational hazards should focus on areas, such as provision of safety trainings, promotion of safety advocacy, and enforcement of appropriate workplace safety regulation.

Keywords: Hazard awareness, Welding, Workplace factors, Workplace safety

Background

The number of occupational accidents and diseases are increasing in developing countries. It has been estimated that over 120 million occupational accidents with over 200,000 fatalities occur each year in these countries [1]. Subsaharan Africa appears to have the greatest rate followed by Asia [2]. There were an estimated 42 million occupational accidents with over 54,000 fatalities annually [3]. In Ethiopia there were an estimated 4.3 million occupational accidents with over 5596 fatalities annually. This gave accident and fatality rate of 16,426 and 21.5 per 100,000 workers, respectively [3].

Welding is one of the occupations that contribute to work-related accidents and diseases in the context to developing countries [4]. The process remains the most common method of joining metals today and is a part of the art of metal fabrication that involves the building of metal structures by cutting, bending and joining. Polishing, painting or coating of the metal pieces also goes along with the other processes [3, 4]. Welding hazards such as the bright and blinding light of the welding arc, the hazardous composition of the welding fumes, the sharp metal edges as well as the hot and flying molten metal particles, fast moving machinery, noise, and vibration may lead to acute and chronic health effects [5, 6]. The acute symptoms may consist of metal fume fever (flu-like symptoms with alternating chills and high fever that last for a few days), irritation of the eyes, nose, chest and respiratory tract causing cough, wheezing, breathlessness, bronchitis, pulmonary edema, pneumonitis and gastrointestinal effects, such as nausea, loss of appetite,

* Correspondence: sbsbtadesse90@gmail.com
[1]Institute of Public Health, the University of Gondar, Gondar, Ethiopia
Full list of author information is available at the end of the article

vomiting, cramps and slow digestion [7, 8]. Chronic health effects include increased risk of lung cancer, cancer of the larynx and urinary tract, hypertension, varieties of respiratory problems, such as bronchitis, asthma, pneumonia, emphysema, pneumoconiosis, decreased lung capacity, silicosis and siderosis. Other chronic effects include heart and skin diseases, hearing loss, chronic gastritis, gastroduodenitis, ulcer of the stomach and small-intestine, kidney damage, and damage to the reproductive system leading to reduction in sperm count and fecundity. Musculoskeletal problems, such as back injuries, shoulder pain, tendonitis, reduced muscle strength, carpal tunnel syndrome, white finger, and knee joint diseases are the other health problems [9–12]. Physical and accidental risks, like burns, cuts, lacerations, and fall injuries are also common [4, 13].

Industrial safety and health problems are becoming major challenges in Ethiopia because of low occupational hazards awareness, lack of workplace safety and health policy, and inefficient safety management system. Due to these employers, workers and the government are losing measurable costs. There is an information gap on occupational hazards in welding industries in the country. Therefore, the aim of this research is to assess the level of awareness of occupational hazards and associated factors among welders at Lideta Sub-City, Addis Ababa, Ethiopia. Such information is vital in understanding the extent of the problem and may be useful when designing intervention strategies targeted at promoting and upholding good health and safety standards in this important working group.

Methods
Study design, area and period
A work site-based cross-sectional study was conducted to assess level of awareness and factors associated with occupational hazards among welders at Lideta Sub-City, Addis Abba, the capital city of Ethiopia, from April to May 2015.

Participants and data collection
All employees who directly involved in the process of welding were included in the study until the required sample size was obtained. Workers who were absent from work due to different reasons during the time of data collection were excluded from the study. A pilot tested and structured interview questionnaire was used to collect the data. Six trained people with first degree in public health administered the questionnaire. The questionnaire contained detailed information on socio-demographic, behavioral and workplace factors that could have association with hazard awareness.

Sample size calculation
A single population proportion to size formula was used to determine the sample size of the study. The total sample size was determined to be 567 by taking 95 % confidence interval, 34.2 % expected proportion (P) [14], 4 % margin of error (W), 5 % non-response rate. That is, Sample size $= \frac{\left(\frac{\alpha}{2}\right)^2 * P(1-P)}{W^2} = \frac{3.842*0.225}{0.0016} \approx 540$. Adding 5 % non-response rate gives 567.

Sampling procedure
Stratified sampling followed by simple random sampling techniques was used to select the study participants. That is, the industries were stratified into three scales, namely large (employed ≥50 workers), medium (employed 10–49 workers) and small (<10 workers) [15]. Then, the total of 567 samples was proportionally allocated to each industry. That is, 99 to large scale (N1 = 184), 195 to medium scale (N2 = 363), and 273 to small scale (N3 = 507). The participants were drawn from the industries' list of workers using simple random sampling.

Data quality control
The training of data collectors and supervisors emphasized issues such as data collection instrument, field methods, inclusion–exclusion criteria, and record keeping. The investigators and supervisors coordinated the interview process, spot-checked and reviewed the completed questionnaire on a daily basis to ensure the completeness and consistency of the data collected. The interview questionnaire was pilot tested on 29 respondents in order to identify potential problem areas, unanticipated interpretations, and cultural objections to any of the questions.

Data management and statistical analyses
Data entered and cleaned using Epi info version 3.5.1 statistical software were analyzed on SPSS version 20. Frequency distribution, mean, standard deviation, and percentage, were employed for most variables. All independent variables were fitted separately into bivariate logistic model to evaluate the degree of association with hazard awareness. Then, variables with a p-value < 0.20 were exported to multivariable logistic regression model to control confounders. The odds ratio (OR) with a 95 % confidence interval (CI) was used to test the statistical significance of variables.

Operational definitions
Awareness of occupational hazards
Summary score was calculated for the participants' awareness of hazards that were potentially related to their work based on ten questions. These were: can weld cause 1) arc eye injury; 2) foreign body enter into eye; 3) breathlessness 4) chronic cough; 5) metallic fume fever;

6) injuries to the body; 7) burns to the body; 8) explosion; 9) back pain; 10) hearing impairment. The mean score for awareness of hazards was taken as a cut-off point and those who scored above the mean were considered as having awareness.

Job satisfaction
Was a self-reported felling of participants about their job as it was pleasurable for them.

Personal protective equipment (PPE)
Workers were observed for their utilization of specialized clothing or equipment for protection against health and safety hazards at the time of interview. The observation was made for about 5 min just before starting administration of the questionnaire.

Permanent employee
Any contract of employment between employee and employer concluded for an indefinite period [16].

Temporary employee
Any employment contract between employee and employer made for definite period [16].

Ethical considerations
The study protocol was reviewed and approved by the Institutional Review Board of the University of Gondar via the Institute of Public Health. Permission was obtained from Lideta Sub-City's large, medium and small scale industry offices prior to data collection. Study participants were interviewed after informed written consent was obtained. They were also informed that their participation was voluntary and that they could withdraw from the interview at any time without consequences. The participants were assured that their responses would be treated confidentially through the use of strict coding measures.

Results
Socio-demographic characteristics
A total of 555 employees completed the questionnaire making response rate 97.9 %. Of whom 98.2 % were males. The majority, 85.9 %, of the employees belonged to the age group of 30–53 years. Half, 48.8 %, of them were married. Regarding educational status 44.0 % attended secondary education (Table 1).

Workplace and behavioral characteristics
Three-fourths, 75.1 %, of the participants were permanent employees. About thirty eight percent served for less than 5 to 9 years. Regarding hours spent on work 95.9 % of the employees had worked for more than 40 h per week. Nearly three-fourths, 72.1 %, were satisfied with

Table 1 Socio-demographic characteristics of welders at Lideta Sub-City, Addis Ababa, Ethiopia, 2015

Variables	Number	Percent
Sex		
Male	545	98.2
Female	10	1.8
Age (in years)		
18–29	53	9.5
30–41	332	59.8
42–53	145	26.1
≥54	25	4.5
Marital Status		
Single	263	47.4
Married	271	48.8
Divorced	21	3.8
Educational status		
Primary	83	15.0
Secondary	244	44.0
Certificate and above	228	41.1

their job. Sixty percent did not attend any kind of safety training. The majority, 83.2 and 82.0 %, complained lack of work shift and safety supervision during work, respectively. About 93.2 % used at least one kind of PPE during work. The majority, 91.8, 85.4 and 61.3 %, of them used goggle, coverall, and safety shoe, respectively. Fifty eight percent drank alcohol followed by 44.0 % smoked cigarette and 39.5 % chewed khat (Table 2).

Work-related health complaints
Two-thirds, 66.8 %, of the workers reported they experienced at least one health complaint related to their work. The most common complaints were 99.6 % vision problems, 94.2 % injuries to the body, and 54.1 % back pain (Table 3).

Participants' awareness of occupational hazards
The majority, 86.5 %, of participants were aware of occupational hazards that might occur during the welding process. The highest level of awareness was observed among participants of 94.9 % large scale industries followed by 86.2 % medium scale and 83.5 % small scale.

Factors associated with awareness of occupational hazards
Work experience, employment pattern, marital status, educational status, khat chewing, cigarette smoking, job satisfaction, safety training, supervision, work regulation, and health complaint showed significant association with awareness in the bivariate analysis. However, only work experience, job satisfaction, work regulation, marital

Table 2 Workplace and behavioral characteristics of welders at Lideta Sub-City, Addis Ababa, Ethiopia, 2015

Variables	Number	Percent
Employment pattern		
Permanent	417	75.1
Temporary	108	19.5
Work experience (in years)		
≤5	151	27.2
5–9	208	37.5
10–14	99	17.8
≥15	97	17.5
Hours worked per week		
≤40	23	4.1
>40	532	95.9
Job satisfaction		
Satisfied	400	72.1
Dissatisfied	155	27.9
Attended safety training		
Yes	220	39.6
No	335	60.4
Safety supervision		
Yes	99	17.0
No	456	82.0
Work shift		
Yes	92	16.6
No	463	83.2
Used PPE		
Yes	194	35.0
No	361	65.0
Type of PPE used		
Goggle	509	91.8
Coverall	476	85.4
Safety shoe	340	61.3
Glove	200	36.0
Respirator	110	19.8
Helmet	30	5.4
Ear plug	24	4.3
Drink alcohol		
Yes	322	58.0
No	233	42.0
Smoke cigarette		
Yes	244	44.0
No	311	56.0
Chew khat		
Yes	219	39.5
No	336	60.5

Table 3 Health complaints reported by welders at Lideta Sub-City, Addis Ababa, Ethiopia, 2015

Variables	Number	Percent
Vision problems		
Yes	553	99.6
No	2	0.4
Breathlessness		
Yes	166	29.9
No	389	70.1
Chronic cough		
Yes	12	2.2
No	543	97.8
Metallic fume fever		
Yes	20	3.6
No	535	96.4
Injuries to the body		
Yes	523	94.2
No	32	5.8
Back pain		
Yes	300	54.1
No	255	45.9
Hearing impairment		
Yes	69	12.4
No	486	87.6

status, and educational status remained significant in the multivariable logistic regression model (Table 4).

Discussion

Welding is a manufacturing industry where workers could be exposed to several hazards, like fumes and gases, dust, intense bright light, excessive noise, vibrations, electricity, intense heat, unsecured gas cylinders, awkward work postures, and fast moving machinery such as grinders. Proper awareness of these hazards is important to design safety education programs, use the different protective devices, and train in ergonomics and appropriate design of tools and machines to achieve greater efficiency of both man and machine. In this study 86.5 % of the workers were observed to be aware of the existence of different hazards related to their work. This finding is slightly different from studies reported from Nigeria (77.9–91.6 %) [5, 17]. The discrepancies between studies could be due to methodological differences, like study population, definitions of hazard awareness, methods of data collection, and workplace conditions.

This study identified important predictors influencing workers awareness of hazards related to their work. The odds of hazard awareness among employees who

Table 4 Factors associated with awareness of occupational hazards among welders in Lideta Sub-City, Addis Ababa, Ethiopia, 2015

Variables	Hazard awareness		Crude OR (95 % CI)	Adjusted OR (95 % CI)
	Yes	No		
Work experience (in years)				
<5	118	33	1.0	1.00
5–9	179	29	1.7(0.1, 3.0)	2.7(1.3, 5.6)
10–14	91	8	3.2(1.4, 7.2)	5.6(1.7, 18.8)
≥15	92	5	5.1(1.9, 13.7)	2.4(0.6, 9.9)
Work regulation				
Yes	305	25	3.5(2.1, 5.8)	2.4(1.1, 5.2)
No	175	50	1.0	1.0
Job satisfaction				
Yes	381	19	11.3(6.4, 20.0)	9.3(4.3–20.1)
No	99	56	1.0	1.0
Marital status				
Married	239	32	18.7(6.8, 51.6)	12.6(3.4, 46.6)
Single	235	28	21.0(7.5, 58.4)	11.4(3.1–41.9)
Divorced	6	15	1.0	1.0
Educational status				
Primary	62	21	1.0	1.0
Secondary	207	37	1.9(1.0, 3.5)	2.8(1.2, 6.6)
Certificate and above	211	17	4.2(2.1, 8.5)	2.7(1.1, 6.7)

had longer work experience were nearly six times higher compared to those who served for less than five years. The possible explanation for this may be that those workers who served longer could have good knowledge and skills on machines and tools in use and become familiar to the work environment. In addition to this they might be exposed to different safety training sessions that could improve their awareness.

In this and other studies workers hazard awareness was found to be significantly associated with the presence of workplace safety regulations [13]. It is a fact that proper implementation of workplace safety regulations could help to monitor workers behavior and allow them complies with the safe procedures of their jobs. This, in proper integration with other safety programs, is a good strategy to mitigate safety culture impediments and to enhance workers awareness of occupational hazards.

Another important finding of this study was that the odds of hazard awareness among employees who were satisfied in their jobs were more than nine times higher compared to those who were not. An increasing number of studies have considered job satisfaction as pervasive and influential factor in the prevention of workplace hazards [18]. This could be linked to fact that when workers were satisfied in their jobs, they could

experience meaningfulness, greater responsibility, and better use of their knowledge and skills in their jobs. Increased job satisfaction could lead to greater attention to safety motivation, knowledge, and compliance [19].

Higher odds of hazard awareness were observed among married [20] and single workers compared to those who were divorced in this study. This could be to the fact that those who were divorced could be worried with unrelated issues and might not give an attention towards their safety. This striking difference warrants further investigation on whether this group may be less attentive towards personal safety.

Workers' awareness of occupational hazards was dependent on their increased level of educational attainment. This is in agreement with study conducted in Nigeria [5]. This might be due to the fact that workers who attained a higher level of education could have the tendency to change available information into mature stage which increased their awareness of hazards.

Social desirability bias is a potential limitation in self-reported studies like this one, in that employees might report more socially acceptable responses than their actual day to day practice. As this is a cross-sectional study, the limitations that come with this type of design need to be taken into consideration when interpreting the findings.

Conclusion

This study revealed that the level of awareness of occupational hazards among welders was high.

However, this does not mean that there will be no need for further strengthening of the safety measures as significant proportions of the workers still had low awareness. Interventions to boost workers awareness of occupational hazards should focus on areas, such as provision of safety trainings, promotion of safety advocacy, and enforcement of appropriate workplace safety regulation.

Competing interests
The authors declare that they have no competing interests.

Authors' contributions
ST: Involved in write up of the research proposal, the data analyses, and wrote the manuscript, KB: Involved in write up of the research proposal, the data analyses, and wrote the manuscript, BD: Involved in write up of the research proposal, the data analyses, and wrote the manuscript, YA: Involved in write up of the research proposal, the data analyses, and wrote the manuscript. All authors read and approved the final manuscript.

Acknowledgements
The authors wish to thank the Lideta Sub-City's large, medium and small scale industry offices for logistic and administrative support, and data collectors for their support in making this study possible. They also extend their deepest gratitude to the study participants.

Author details
[1]Institute of Public Health, the University of Gondar, Gondar, Ethiopia. [2]City Government of Addis Ababa Health Bureau, Addis Ababa, Ethiopia.

References
1. Lund F, Marriott A. Occupational health and safety and the poorest: School of Development Studies, University of KwaZulu-Natal. 2011.
2. Du J, Leigh JP. Incidence of workers compensation indemnity claims across socio-demographic and job characteristics. Am J Ind Med. 2011;54(10):758–70.
3. Hamalainen P, Saarela KL, Takala J. Global trend according to estimated number of occupational accidents and fatal work-related diseases at region and country level. J Saf Res. 2009;40:125–39.
4. Bhumika TV, Thakur M, Jaswal R, Pundird P, Rajware E. Occupational injuries and personal protective equpiments adopted by welding workers: a cross sectional study in South India. GJMEDPH 2014;3(5). ISSN: 2277-9604.
5. Sabitu K, Iliyasu Z, Dauda M. Awareness of occupational hazards and utilization of safety measures among welders in Kaduna metropolis, Northern Nigeria. Ann Afr Med. 2009;8(1):46.
6. Antonini JM. Health effects of welding. Crit Rev Toxicol. 2003;33(1):61–103.
7. El-Zein M, et al. Is metal fume fever a determinant of welding related respiratory symptoms and/or increased bronchial responsiveness? A longitudinal study. Occup Environ Med. 2005;62(10):688–94.
8. El-Zein M, et al. Prevalence and association of welding related systematic and respiratory symptoms in welders. Occup Environ Med. 2003;60:655–61.
9. Holm M, Kim JL, Lilhenberg L, Storass T, Jogi R, Svanes C. Incidence and prevalence of chronic bronchitis: Impact of smoking and Welding: THE RHINE study. Int J Tuberc Lung Dis. 2012;16(4):553–7.
10. Andrea TM, Paul B, David Z, Neonila SD, Peter R, Jolanta L. Welding and lung cancer in central and Eastern Europe and the United Kingdom. Am J Epidemol. 2012;175(7):706–814.
11. Mortensen P. Fertility among danish male welders. Scand J Env Health. 1998;16(5):315–22.
12. Sellapa S, Subhadra KK, Prathyuman S, Shyn J, Vellingri B. Biomonitoring of genotoxic effects among shielded manual metal arc-welders. Asian Pacific J Cancer Prev. 2011;12(16):1041–4.
13. Kumar SG, Dharanipriya A, Kar S. Awareness of occupational injuries and Utilization of personal protective equpiments among welders in coastal South India. Inter J Occup Env Med. 2013;4(4):172–7.
14. Budhathoki SS, Singh SB, Sagtani RA, Niraula SR, Pokharel PK. Awareness of occupational hazards and use of personal protective equpiments among welders: a cross-sectional study from eastern Nepal. BMJ Open. 2014;4(6): e004646.
15. Ethiopian Central Statistical Authority. Report on large and medium scale manufacturing and electricity industries survey: Statistical Bulletin 2002. Contract No. 281; 2011.
16. Ministry of Labor and Social Affairs. Labour proclamation No.377/2003. Ministry of Labor and Social Affairs, Addis Ababa, Ethiopia; 2003.
17. Isah EC, Okojie OH. Occupational health problems of welders in Benin City, Nigeria. Braz J Med Biol Res. 2006;5:64–9.
18. Chau N, Mur JM, Benamghar L, Siegfried C, Dangelzer JL, et al. Relationships between certain individual characteristics and occupational injuries for various jobs in the construction industry: a case-control study. Am J Ind Med. 2004;45:84–92.
19. Probst TM. Layoffs and tradeoffs: production, quality, and safety demands under the threat of job loss. J Occup Health Psychol. 2002;7:211–20.
20. Okuga M, Mayega RW, Bazeyo W. Awareness of occupational hazards and use of personal protective equpiments Small-scale industrial welders in Jinja Municipality, Uganda. Afr Newsl Occup Health Safety. 2012;22:35–6.

7

The effect of effort-reward imbalance on the health of childcare workers in Hamburg

Peter Koch[1*], Jan Felix Kersten[1], Johanna Stranzinger[1] and Albert Nienhaus[1,2]

Abstract

Background: The prevalence of effort-reward imbalance (ERI) among qualified childcare workers in Germany is currently estimated at around 65%. High rates of burnout and musculoskeletal symptoms (MS) have also been reported for this group. Previous longitudinal studies show inconsistent results with regard to the association between ERI and MS. As yet, no longitudinal studies have been conducted to investigate the association between ERI and burnout or MS in childcare workers. This study aims to investigate the extent to which a relationship between ERI and MS or burnout can be observed in childcare workers in Germany on a longitudinal basis.

Methods: In 2014 childcare workers ($N = 199$, response rate: 57%) of a provider of facilities for children and youth in Hamburg were asked about stress and health effects in the workplace. Follow-up was completed one year later ($N = 106$, follow-up rate: 53%) For the baseline assessment, ERI was determined as the primary influencing factor. Data on MS was recorded using the Nordic questionnaire, and burnout using the personal burnout scale of the Copenhagen Burnout Inventory (CBI). The statistical analysis was carried out using multivariate linear and logistic regression.

Results: At baseline ERI was present in 65% of the sample population. The mean burnout score at the time of follow-up was 53.7 (SD: 20.7); the prevalence of MS was between 19% and 62%. ERI was identified as a statistically significant factor for MS, after adjusting especially for physical stress (lower back: OR 4.2; 95% CI: 1.14 to 15.50, neck: OR 4.3; 95% CI: 1.25 to 15.0, total MS: OR 4.0; 95% CI: 1.20 to 13.49). With regard to burnout, a relative increase of 10% in the ERI ratio score increased the burnout score by 1.1 points ($p = 0.034$).

Conclusions: ERI was revealed to be a major factor in relation to MS and burnout in childcare workers. Based on this observation worksite interventions on the individual and organizational level should be introduced in order to prevent ERI.

Keywords: Musculoskeletal symptoms, Burnout, Psychosocial, Nursery teacher, Occupational disease, Esteem, Work-related

Background

Current German studies report unfavourable psychosocial working conditions for childcare workers. According to these studies, the prevalence of work-related effort-reward imbalance [1] is in between 64% and 67% [2–4]. In Siegrist's effort-reward imbalance model (ERI model), the health of the employee is associated with

* Correspondence: p.koch@uke.de
[1]Centre of Excellence for Epidemiology and Health Services Research for Healthcare Professionals (CVcare), University Medical Centre Hamburg-Eppendorf, Martinistrasse 52, 20246 Hamburg, Germany
Full list of author information is available at the end of the article

performance and rewards (esteem, job security and promotion). The model is based on the assumption that there should ideally be a reciprocal relationship between efforts and socially defined rewards. If rewards are lower than efforts, a stressful situation that increases the risk of stress-related diseases occurs for the employee. Empirical evidence for this hypothesis has been found mainly for coronary heart disease, cardiovascular disease and depression [5]. A special feature of the ERI model is the inclusion of over-commitment (OVC) personality as a personal trait that represents a coping strategy in combination with high demands. OVC generates excessive commitment in conjunction with expectations of high rewards. According to Siegrist employees with OVC are also at increased risk, and in combination with ERI even higher risk, for developing stress-related diseases. Observations in German teachers found that OVC negatively affected plasma coagulation, natural killer cells and T-helper cells [6, 7]. Furthermore, depression and somatic symptoms including MS were found to be associated with the interaction of OVC and ERI in nurses [8, 9].

International studies have observed an increased risk of musculoskeletal disorders among childcare workers [10–13]. The association between the increase of MS and the factors of the ERI model has been observed in longitudinal studies of employee cohorts in different industries [14–16]. In a systematic review of all industries, however, the association between ERI and MS has been evaluated as inconsistent on the basis of cross-sectional and longitudinal studies [17]. To our knowledge, there have not yet been performed any longitudinal studies examining the association between ERI and MS in childcare workers.

Another symptom associated with stress in the workplace is burnout. Employees working in the service sector show a high risk of burnout [18]. Childcare workers as an occupational group do not represent any exception to this in international comparisons [19–23]. For childcare workers in Germany, prevalence rates of between 10% and 57% have been observed for burnout symptoms [2, 10, 24, 25]. For childcare workers and teaching staff, ERI shows a strong correlation with burnout [26]. A greater tendency towards OVC was shown to be associated with burnout in cross-sectional studies of qualified childcare workers and across industries [2, 27]. Longitudinal studies investigating the association between ERI and burnout in childcare workers have not been published yet.

We aim to address the following research questions in this study:

1. Does a longitudinal approach reveal an association between the psychosocial factors of the ERI model and MS among childcare workers?
2. Does a longitudinal approach reveal an association between the ERI ratio score and a higher risk of burnout among childcare workers?

Methods

As part of a 2014 occupational risk assessment a funding provider for children and young people comprising 26 different facilities in Hamburg carried out a stress monitoring survey of its childcare workers [2]. In this paper

the results of the follow-up investigation of this multi-centre study are presented.

In November 2014, all 400 qualified childcare workers of all different facilities were asked about health and stresses they faced at work. A total of 230 questionnaires were returned (response rate: 57%); a total of 31 participants were excluded as a result of low weekly working hours (< 10 h) and employment in domestic/janitorial services (kitchens, workshops). At the time of the baseline assessment, 199 people were therefore included into the study. After twelve months (follow up), all study participants once again received a copy of the same pseudonymised questionnaire they had completed a year before. A subgroup of participants (n = 33) took part in a parallel intervention programme looking at the effects of noise in the workplace [28]. In that study, the focus was on the question of whether the use of personal hearing protection over the observational period of one year could reduce the subjective noise exposure and the risk of burnout among childcare workers.

The pseudonymised stress monitoring questionnaire was agreed with the data safety officer of the funding provider for children and young people. Before the study started, every participant gave informed written consent for taking part in the study. All study documents, including the study protocol, were reviewed and approved by the Hamburg Medical Chamber Ethics Committee as part of an application process (reference: PV4792).

Questionnaire

In addition to demographic variables, the questionnaire also collected information on work-related stress and resources. Burnout and MS were used as outcomes.

Physical stress was recorded using selected questions from a standardised questionnaire [29]. Five different types of stress (*awkward body postures, standing, sitting, lifting heavy loads/children* and *carrying heavy loads/children*) were identified on a four-stage frequency scale. This resulted in a corresponding total score (ranging between 5 and 20). Using the median, the variable was dichotomised into the categories of low or high physical stress.

Subjective noise exposure was estimated using a questionnaire developed by the authors. Responding to 13 items on a five-stage scale resulted in a total score (ranging between 13 and 65). This was dichotomised into high and low subjective noise exposure by using the median. For more information, please see the publication of the cross-sectional study [2].

Psychosocial factors were recorded using the ERI questionnaire (23-item version) [30]. The psychosocial situation and the personality trait of *OVC* were evaluated using three scales (*effort*: six items, *reward*: eleven items and *OVC*: six items). The ERI ratio score was determined according to the definition using a formula that takes into account the different numbers of items in order to calculate the total on the *effort* scale as a ratio to the *reward* scale: Σ Effort/ΣReward*0.5454. An effort-reward imbalance was defined as an ERI ratio score of more than 1. Since this value is not a clinically valid cut-off value, ERI was also tested using the quartile thresholds as an ordinal influencing variable in the analysis. Regardless of the scale, increased *OVC* was defined for the value range in the upper tertile of the empirical distribution and treated as a dichotomous variable.

Other workplace-related characteristics were recorded using selected scales from a standardized instrument, the brief workplace analysis questionnaire (KFZA) [31]. This included both stress factors (*qualitative workload: two items, quantitative workload: two items*) and resources (*control: three items, collaboration: three items, information and employee participation: two items, completeness: two items, variety: three items*). The individual items were rated on a five-stage scale.

In addition, the respondent was asked about the occurrence of typical everyday situations in the workplace. Seven different statements, such as "I experience conflicts with parents" or "I don't get any breaks or chances to step away from work for a while" could be answered with yes or no.

Musculoskeletal symptoms were recorded using the Nordic questionnaire [32]. The prevalence of chronic pain in the shoulder, neck or lower back was defined as the presence of pain on at least eight days in the past twelve months, as well as pain within seven days of filling in the questionnaire. In addition, a comprehensive variable was derived for the presence of at least one type of chronic pain in the three body regions (MS total).

In order to evaluate *burnout* in childcare workers, the *personal burnout* sub-scale from the Copenhagen Burnout Inventory was used [33]. According to the definition, a higher risk of burnout is present with a value of ≥ 50 (range 0–100).

Statistical analysis

For paired group comparisons, the paired t-test was calculated in the case of normally distributed data; for not normally distributed data the Mann–Whitney U test was calculated. For dichotomous paired data, the McNemar test was used. For independent data, the Pearson correlation coefficient was used. In order to evaluate a difference in nominal variables, the chi-squared test was used.

Multivariate logistic regression was calculated for the first research question. Starting with a core variable set (ERI, physical stress, pain T0, participation in intervention programme), all variables with a *p*-value of <0.25 in the bivariate analysis were successively integrated into the model [34]. Physical stress was included as an

important confounder in the relationship between ERI and MS [16]. The following variables were taken into account as potentially influential variables: *work-related resources and stress (KFZA), typical everyday situations in the workplace, subjective noise exposure, physical stress, weekly working hours, type of institution, field of work, physical activity, age, BMI* and *gender*.

With regard to the second hypothesis, linear regression was used. Starting with a core variable set (ERI, burnout T0, age, participation in a prevention programme, type of institution) all other variables were included that showed a *p*-value of <0.2 in the bivariate analysis. In the second step, the stepwise backwards regression procedure was applied [34], where all variables with *p*-value of >0.1 were excluded from the model. In order to fulfil the requirements of linear regression, the ERI variable was transformed to the logarithmic scaling.

In all multivariate analyses a possible interaction between ERI and OVC was also tested. For logistic regression models a variable with four categories has been built: 1: ERI No/ OVC No, 2: ERI Yes/ OVC No, 3: ERI No/ OVC Yes, 4: ERI Yes/OVC Yes. For linear regression models a multiplicative term has been built from the continuous OVC variable and ERI ratio variable [35].

Missing values were replaced in the ERI scale (effort, reward, OVC) and in the personal burnout scale by individual mean values. If more than half of the individual items on a particular scale were missing for a participant, the entire scale value was set to a missing value.

A dropout analysis was performed using logistic regression. The statistical analysis was carried out using SPSS Statistics, version 23.

Results

At the time of the follow-up, the cohort comprises 106 employees (see Table 1) (Follow-up rate: 53%). The study participants are predominantly women (90.6%). The study participants in the follow-up are statistically significantly older than the dropouts (43 vs 37, *p* < 0.001); age was the only statistically significant variable in the dropout analysis. More than 90% have German nationality. Almost half of the participants have a BMI of ≥ 25 (47%). Overall, 51.9% of the employees report regular physical exercise. More than half (52.8%) work full time, with the majority working exclusively in child care (84.9%). Of all of the employees, 66% are from child day care centres, 21.7% work in school partnerships (caring for school-age children in schools) and the lowest proportion (11.3%) come from child and youth support facilities (youth projects and residential groups). As a result of too many missing values (> 50%), working hours are not evaluated.

Table 2 shows the influential and outcome variables at the time of baseline and follow-up. In terms of

Table 1 Description of the cohort at the time of follow up

Variable	n	Percent
Gender		
Women	96	90.6%
Men	10	9.4%
Age in years		
18–29	16	15.1%
30–39	22	20.8%
40–49	38	35.8%
50+	29	27.4%
n/a	1	0.9%
Nationality		
German	98	92.5%
Other	8	7.5%
BMI		
< 25	54	50.9%
≥ 25	50	47.1%
n/a	2	1.9%
Physical exercise		
Regular	55	51.9%
None	51	48.1%
Area of work		
Child care	90	84.9%
Management/administration	16	15.1%
Weekly working hours		
Full time	56	52.8%
Part time	50	47.2%
Institution		
Child day care centre	70	66%
School partnership	23	21.7%
Child and youth support work	12	11.3%
n/a	1	0.9%
Total	106	100%

resources, the mean values of the variables are ranging between 3.5 and 3.9 at both points in time. This corresponds to an occurrence of 70–78% in the upper end of the scale for individual resources. The mean value for *collaboration* shows a statistically significant decrease over time. Here, the mean decreases from 3.7 to 3.5 ($p = 0.006$). Among the stress factors, there are no statistically significant changes over time for any variables with the exception of ERI. The ERI ratio score increases from 1.2 to 1.3 points ($p < 0.001$), while the difference in the dichotomised ERI variable is also statistically significant (65.1% vs 87.4%, $p < 0.001$). Figure 1 shows which of the ERI sub-scales is mainly responsible for the significant increase in the ERI

ratio score. The mean of the *effort* scale remains nearly constant over time (73 vs. 72). For the three sub-scales of the reward scale, the following trends can be observed: *promotion* increases by three points over time (45 vs 48), *esteem* and *security*, however, decrease statistically significant over time. Here, the mean values decrease from 62 to 49 ($p < 0.001$) and from 67 to 31 ($p < 0.001$) respectively.

With regard to the outcome variables (Table 2), a slight increase in burnout can be observed (50.6 vs 53.7), which is only just not statistically significant ($p = 0.056$). For neck pain (32.1% vs 39.4%), shoulder pain (15.1% vs 19.2%) and MS overall (55.7% vs 62.1%), slight increases can be observed. The prevalence of lower back pain (39.6% vs 34.6%) decreases slightly over time. These differences are not statistically significant.

The results of the multivariate logistic regression of the association between ERI and MS are listed in Table 3. For the outcome of lower back pain, the odds ratio is 4.2 times higher for child care workers with an ERI of >1 (95% CI: 1.14 to 15.50). This correlation is statistically significant. For shoulder pain, an ERI of >1 reveals an increased odds ratio of 1.5 (95% CI: 0.40 to 5.58), which is not statistically significant. In addition, participants with low control show an odds ratio that is 4.5 times higher for shoulder pain (95% CI: 1.15 to 17.42), which is statistically significant. OVC was observed to have a protective effect that was not statistically significant (OR: 0.4; 95% CI: 0.09 to 1.40). With regard to neck pain, an ERI of >1 resulted in a statistically significant higher odds ratio of 4.3 (95% CI: 1.25 to 15.0). For the outcome of total MS, employees with an increased ERI ratio score were also observed to have a statistically significant increase in the odds ratio (OR: 4.0; 95% CI: 1.20 to 13.49). Child care workers who state that they have physical exercise regularly are shown to have a statistically significant protective effect with regard to MS (OR: 0.3; 95% CI: 0.10 to 0.98). Employees who state that they experience conflicts with parents have a statistically significant increase in the risk of MS (OR: 4.9; 95% CI: 1.55 to 15.75). No interaction between ERI and OVC was observed in any of the models.

With regard to burnout, it is shown that the ERI ratio score has a statistically significant influence on increasing the risk of burnout. Translated to the delogrithmed scaling, an increase in the ERI ratio score of 10% would increase the burnout value by 1.1 points (95% CI: 0.09 to 2.14) (Table 4). This increase is statistically significant ($p = 0.034$). The resource of variety is shown to be a protective factor (beta: −3.8; 95% CI: −0.8 to 0.37), but is not statistically significant. Age reduces the burnout value by 0.6 points per year (95% CI: −0.87 to −0.29), a statistically significant effect ($p < 0.001$). Participation in

Table 2 Resources and stress variables and outcomes at the time of baseline and follow-up (n = 106)

	Baseline				Follow Up				
Resources	x̄	SD	%	n	x̄	SD	%	n	p
Control (scale: 1–5)	3.7	0.9	.	.	3.6	0.9	.	.	0.228
Variety (scale: 1–5)	3.9	0.7	.	.	3.9	0.6	.	.	0.732
Completeness (scale: 1–5)	3.7	0.8	.	.	3.5	0.9	.	.	0.057
Collaboration (scale: 1–5)	3.7	0.7	.	.	3.5	0.8	.	.	0.006*
Information and employee participation (scale: 1–5)	3.8	0.7	.	.	3.7	0.8	.	.	0.120
Stress factors									
Qualitative workload (scale: 1–5)	2.4	0.8	.	.	2.4	0.8	.	.	0.901
Physical stress (scale: 5–20)	14.3	2.8	.	.	14.3	2.8	.	.	0.792
Subjective noise exposure (scale: 13–65)	39.7	10.3	.	.	40.6	10.5	.	.	0.220
ERI ratio score (scale: 0.2–5)	1.2	0.4	.	.	1.3	0.3	.	.	< 0.001**
ERI > 1, proportion (n)	.	.	65.1	69	.	.	87.4	90	< 0.001**
OVC (scale: 6–24)	15.8	3.4	.	.	15.3	3.5	.	.	0.084
Outcomes									
Burnout (scale 0–100)	50.6	19.7	.	.	53.7	20.7	.	.	0.056
Risk of burnout >50,	.	.	53.8	57	.	.	61.3	65	0.096
Neck pain	.	.	32.1	34	.	.	39.4	41	0.286
Shoulder pain	.	.	15.1	16	.	.	19.2	20	0.523
Lower back pain	.	.	39.6	42	.	.	34.6	36	0.523
MS total	.	.	55.7	59	.	.	62.1	64	0.700

x̄: mean, SD: standard deviation, *p < 0.05, **p < 0.001

the intervention programme has a slightly reductive effect on the target variable (beta: –2.4; 95% CI: –8.66 to 3.78). This effect is not statistically significant. In addition, it can also be observed that the burnout value for employees from child day care centres is 7 points higher than for employees from the two other types of institution (95% CI: 0.56 to 13.51). This increase is statistically significant (p = 0.034).

Discussion

In this longitudinal study, statistically significant associations between an increased ERI ratio score and the increase of MS were observed in childcare workers. In these analyses physical stress was included as a confounder variable. With regard to increasing the risk of burnout, ERI was also shown to be a statistically significant factor.

Effort-reward imbalance

We found a high prevalence of ERI among childcare workers (follow-up: 87.4% with ERI ratio > 1; mean ERI ratio: 1.3) in this study, compared to the cross-sectional study from the previous year with a prevalence rate of 65% and a mean ERI ratio of 1.17 [2].

Such unusually high levels of ERI are rare in literature. In an older study investigating childcare workers in 2004, the mean ERI was 0.5 [26]. More recent data assessed in 2012 showed ERI prevalence rates of between 64% and 67% for childcare workers, while for management staff rates of 87% [3, 4]. As was already discussed in the cross-sectional study [2], the increase in ERI over time could potentially be explained by

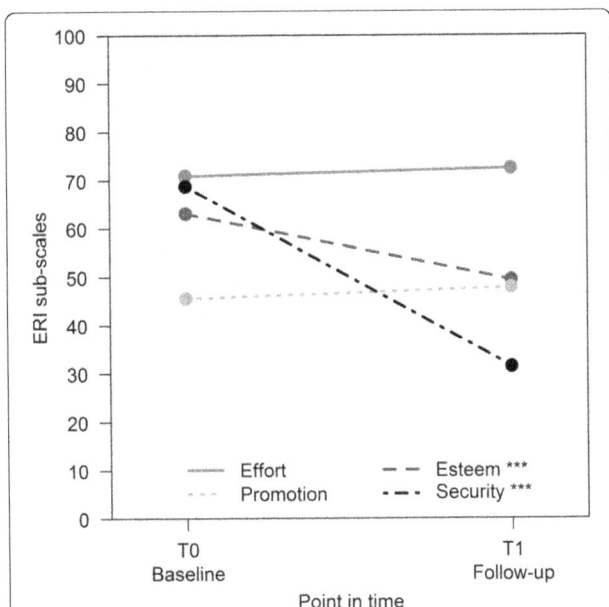

Fig. 1 Mean values for the ERI sub-scales on a standardised scale of 0 to 100 (***p < 0.001)

Table 3 Results of the multivariate logistic regressions for development of musculoskeletal symptoms (adjusted for age, MS T0)

Outcome at Follow Up:	Lower back 36 (35%)			Shoulder 20 (19%)			Neck 41 (39%)			MS total 64 (62%)		
	OR	95% CI	p	OR	95% CI	p	OR	95% CI	p	OR	95% CI	p
Influencing variables at baseline:												
ERI >1 vs ≤1	4.2*	1.14–15.50	0.031	1.5	0.40–5.58	0.547	4.3*	1.25–15.00	0.021	4.0*	1.20–13.49	0.024
Physical stress high vs low	2.8	0.94–8.10	0.064	1.1	0.33–3.69	0.876	0.9	0.33–2.61	0.891	1.2	0.37–3.87	0.758
Intervention yes vs. no	0.6	0.19–1.86	0.375	2.0	0.63–6.23	0.245	0.9	0.30–2.56	0.804	0.5	0.13–1.63	0.212
OVC 3rd tertile vs 1st + 2nd tertile	.	.	.	0.4	0.09–1.40	0.138	.	.	.	.	.	.
Control high vs low	.	.	.	4.5*	1.15–17.42	0.031	.	.	.	2.0	0.61–6.69	0.254
Physical activity yes vs no	.	.	.	.	.	.	.	.	.	0.3*	0.10–0.98	0.046
Conflicts with parents yes vs no	.	.	.	.	.	.	.	.	.	4.9*	1.55–15.75	0.007
R²	R² = 0.44			R² = 0.19			R² = 0.39			R² = 0.45		

*p < 0.05

increasing dissatisfaction with working conditions among childcare workers: since 2013, parents in Germany have had a legal right to a childcare place for infants aged 1 to <3, additionally to the existing claim for children aged 3 to 6. In recent years, this has led to larger group sizes, unfavourable staffing conditions and an increase in temporary working contracts. As a result, there was a wave of strikes instigated by childcare workers in Germany in 2015. The questionnaires were returned just a few months after the strikes had taken place. This professional-policy environment is linked with increased awareness of the lack of value accorded to this occupational group in Germany, which is made clear by the drop in the ERI sub-scale *esteem*. The decline in the *job security* sub-scale is also very clear. Paradoxically, almost all staff in the institutions had permanent contracts at the time. The decrease in the two-item *job security* sub-scale was caused in detail by the low scores for the item: "My own job is at risk". Discussion with employee representatives and the management revealed, that at the time of the follow-up the majority of employees were subject to an internal rotation process in their job. This principle meant that, at that time, employees often switched jobs within an institution or between institutions. In this context, answers to this question on the ERI questionnaire were bound to have been biased.

The prevention of ERI by using an ERI model based worksite stress management program, as demonstrated in interventional studies, is feasible and can positively influence psychosocial work environment and mental health [36, 37]. Aiming to reduce overcommitted work-related attitudes, Aust et al. conducted successfully interventions that were performed on individual and organisational levels [36]. With a participative approach Bourbonnais et al. involved employees of a hospital in formulating goals in terms of psychological demands and rewards. After 12 months a reduction of adverse psychological factors was investigated in the experimental group [37].

Musculoskeletal symptoms

We found significant associations between ERI and MS in three out of four body regions in qualified childcare workers: back, neck and combination of back, neck and shoulder (MS total). The association between ERI and lower back pain (OR: 4.2) has been observed in other longitudinal studies investigating employees of a transport company [14], employees in public administration [15] and in other cross-sectional studies investigating employees in healthcare, the wine-growing industry, the police and public transport companies [38–41].

There was a tendency towards association between ERI and the increase of shoulder pain in this study (OR: 1.5)

Table 4 Multivariate linear model for burnout (adjusted for burnout T0)

R²: 0.53	Regression coefficient	Standardised beta coefficient	95% CI	p
Increase in the ERI ratio score by 10%	1.1*	0.18	0.09–2.14	0.034
Variety (scale 1–5)	−3.8	−0.14	−8.0 – 0.37	0.074
Intervention yes vs no	−2.4	−0.06	−8.66 – 3.78	0.439
Age (per year)	−0.6*	−0.29	−0.87 – −0.29	0.001
Child day care centres yes vs other institutions	7.0*	0.16	0.56–13.51	0.034

*p < 0.05
**p < 0.001

but not to a statistically significant degree. Lower control (OR: 4.5) was revealed to be a significant influencing factor with regard to shoulder pain. Control as a psychosocial factor derives from the demand-control-support model [42], another stress model that describes the onset of work-related stress.

With regards to neck pain the ERI variable showed a significant effect (OR: 4.3). This effect was also observed in drivers and office workers as well as in cohorts of hospital staff and workers in the wine-growing industry in two longitudinal studies [14, 15] and three cross-sectional studies [38, 39, 43].

For the outcome of total MS, an increased risk was observed for participants with an ERI >1 (OR: 4.0).

Additionally, two other variables seemed to have had an influence on total MS: perceived conflicts with parents (OR: 4.9) and regular physical exercise (OR: 0.3) as a protective factor showed significant associations with the outcome. Childcare workers could be adequately supported with on-the-job training in conflict management to possibly prevent the increase of MS. Conflict management and company-facilitated sports activities for employees would not only directly influence the onset of MS, but would also indirectly affect ERI: childcare workers might perceive this as a kind of esteem for their seniority.

Indications of an interaction between ERI and OVC were not observed in relation to MS. To our knowledge, there is only one cross-sectional study where an interactive effect of this kind was documented with regard to MS in nursing staff [9].

Regarding the biological plausibility there are several explanations for the mechanism of psychosocial factors leading to MS: psychosocial stress might induce increased and prolonged muscle tension [44] and decreased blood supply in extremities [45]. It also blocks anabolic activity which is responsible for the repair of muscle tissue [46]. Another short-term stress response is muscle violation due to increased sensitivity of muscle fibres [44]. Due to these permanent short term responses the risk of chronic MS might increase over time.

Burnout
The prevalence of burnout at the time of the follow-up was higher, at 61.3% (mean: 53.7), than in the cross-sectional study one year before (56.8%, mean: 51.7) [2]. The reference data from the COPSOQ database from 2013 shows a mean burnout score for childcare workers of 48 (Additional file 1, Nuebling). The results of the linear regression showed a significant increase in burnout with an increase in ERI ratio (if the ERI ratio increases by 10%, the burnout risk increases by 1.12 points). In a longitudinal study, Spence et al. [47] also observed a significant association between ERI and

burnout in nurse managers. Other cross-sectional studies have confirmed this association in childcare workers and teaching staff [26, 48, 49]. In contrast to the cross-sectional study [2], however, the association with the ERI model component OVC could not be confirmed in the follow-up. As a personality trait, OVC is a good predictor of burnout and this has been confirmed in a range of studies [27, 50–52]. The analysis also revealed that the burnout value for employees working in child care centres was around seven points higher on average than for employees from school partnership or youth organisations. ERI and burnout prevention measures should therefore be carried out, in particular, among employees working in child care centres.

Limitations
One limitation of the study was the relatively small sample size. This resulted in wide confidence intervals and imprecise evaluations of the estimators. Furthermore, the relatively low follow-up rate resulted in a potential bias in the sample. A non-responder questionnaire was not carried out. On the basis of a dropout analysis, we attempted to identify potential selection effects and to take these into account.

Influential and outcome variables came from the same source – the presence of bias resulting from common methods, such as through social desirability, for example, could therefore not be excluded [53]. The factors of the ERI model only recorded part of the psychosocial situation in the workplace – no other psychosocial factors, such as those used in the job demand-control-support model [42], for example, were used – with the exception of control. Effects of a spill-over of psychosocial factors, but also biomechanical stress from employees' private lives, also could not be excluded since these factors were not recorded as part of the study. Furthermore, part of the sample population (31%) took part in a parallel occupational preventive programme for the reduction of subjective noise exposure [28]. Although the study did not appear to have a statistically significant intervention effect, there were indications that the intervention group showed some benefits in terms of burnout as compared with the reference group. This subgroup was tested in the analyses of MS and burnout, but this characteristic was not shown to have any statistically significant influence. Despite this, it cannot be ruled out that the intervention may have had an effect on the individual level.

Over time, this study shows high and rising rates of burnout and ERI. As mentioned above, we cannot rule out that the professional-policy environment may have resulted in a classification bias of ERI, burnout and MS at the time that the data was collected. It is highly feasible that the protest movement by childcare workers in Germany at the time that the data was collected had sensitised the study participants and affected their responses.

For the high-risk group identified in the ERI model, those who showed an increased ERI and increased OVC were not shown to have an increased health risk in our study with regard to the outcome variables tested. Taking into account the study limitations, however, childcare workers with an effort-reward imbalance at baseline were shown to have an increased health risk with regard to MS and burnout at follow up.

The small sample size of childcare workers in Hamburg may not be representative for Germany, nevertheless, in comparison to a representative study of German childcare workers [3] there were no differences with respect to age, gender and nationality.

Strengths

The main strength of this study was its longitudinal design. The analyses referred to prevalence rates at time of follow up and controlled for the outcome at baseline. The interpretation of the relation between independent and dependent variable was based on the chronology of time. Another strength, while investigating the relation between psychosocial factors and MS, was the assessment of physical stress and controlling for it in the models. By this approach we controlled a potential confounding effect of physical stress on the association of ERI and MS. Furthermore the assessment of psychosocial factors was performed with a validated instrument which was developed on the basis of a theoretical work stress model. With this approach the development of preventive measures is predetermined by the theory of the ERI model.

Conclusions

As part of an occupational risk assessment, childcare workers were identified as an occupational group with a high ERI prevalence. In this context ERI was identified as a risk factor with regard to burnout and MS as part of a longitudinal approach. Measures should be developed at company level that can help to counter the increase of an effort-reward imbalance. Since monetary changes are hard to carry out at the company level, other measures should be implemented at this level to promote the sense of reward and decrease efforts. These may include the development of a culture that values and recognises its staff, which can be initiated at the management level. There are already empirical indications about the feasibility and success of ERI model based interventions aiming at a positive psychosocial work environment.

Funding
No funding was received.

Authors' contributions
PK, performed the survey, carried out the statistical analyses and wrote the manuscript. JFK carried out statistical analyses and was critically reading the manuscript. JS read the draft critically and gave substantial comments for the improvement of the first draft. AN revised the manuscript critically for important intellectual content and gave final approval for the version to be published. All authors read and approved the final manuscript.

Competing interests
PK has no competing interest. JFK has no competing interest. JS has no competing interest. AN has no competing interest.

Author details
[1]Centre of Excellence for Epidemiology and Health Services Research for Healthcare Professionals (CVcare), University Medical Centre Hamburg-Eppendorf, Martinistrasse 52, 20246 Hamburg, Germany. [2]Health Protection Division (FBG), Institution for Statutory Accident Insurance and Prevention in the Health and Welfare Services (BGW), Pappelallee 33, 22089 Hamburg, Germany.

References
1. Siegrist J. Adverse health effects of high-effort/low-reward conditions. J Occup Health Psychol. 1996;1:27–41.
2. Koch P, Stranzinger J, Nienhaus A, Kozak A. Musculoskeletal Symptoms and Risk of Burnout in Child Care Workers - A Cross-Sectional Study. PLoS One. 2015;10:e0140980.
3. Schreyer I, Krause M, Brandl M, Nicko O. AQUA Arbeitsplatz und Qualität in Kitas Ergebnisse einer bundesweiten Befragung. München: Staatsinstitut für Frühpädagogik; 2014.
4. Viernickel S, Voss A, Mauz E, Gerstenberg F, Schumann M. STEGE - Strukturqualität und Erzieher_innengesundheit in Kindertageseinrichtungen. Wissenschaftlicher Abschlussbericht. http://www.gew.de/index.php?eID=dumpFile&t=f&f=20674&token=9d0413d1612a043e64cd74e9e71d51fccefd13ec&sdownload=. Last access 05/22/2017.
5. Siegrist J, Dragano N. Psychosoziale Belastungen und Erkrankungsrisiken im Erwerbsleben. Bundesgesundheitsblatt-Gesundheitsforschung-Gesundheitsschutz. 2008;51(3):305–12.
6. von Kanel R, Bellingrath S, Kudielka BM. Overcommitment but not effort-reward imbalance relates to stress-induced coagulation changes in teachers. Ann Behav Med. 2009;37(1):20–8.
7. Bellingrath S, Rohleder N, Kudielka BM. Healthy working school teachers with high effort–reward-imbalance and overcommitment show increased pro-inflammatory immune activity and a dampened innate immune defence. Brain Behav Immun. 2010;24(8):1332–9.
8. Jolivet A, Caroly S, Ehlinger V, Kelly-Irving M, Delpierre C, Balducci F, et al. Linking hospital workers' organisational work environment to depressive symptoms: A mediating effect of effort-reward imbalance? The ORSOSA study. Soc Sci Med. 2010;71(3):534–40.
9. Weyers S, Peter R, Boggild H, Jeppesen HJ, Siegrist J. Psychosocial work stress is associated with poor self-rated health in Danish nurses: a test of the effort-reward imbalance model. Scand J Caring Sci. 2006; 20:26–34.
10. Buch M, Frieling E. Belastungs- und Beanspruchungsoptimierung in Kindertagesstätten. Kassel: Eigenverlag Universität Kassel, Institut für Arbeitswissenschaft; 2001.
11. Grant KA, Habes DJ, Tepper AL. Work activities and musculoskeletal complaints among preschool workers. Appl Ergon. 1995;26:405–10.
12. Botzet M, Frank H. Arbeit und Gesundheit von Mitarbeiterinnen in Kindertageseinrichtungen. Regionalfallstudie in saarländischen Kindertageseinrichtungen. Landesarbeitsgemeinschaft für

Gesundheitsförderung Saarland e.V: Saarbrücken; 1998.

13. Gratz RR, Claffey A. Adult health in childcare: health status, behaviors, and concerns of teachers, directots, and family child care providers. Early Child Res Q. 1996;11:243–67.

14. Rugulies R, Krause N. Effort-reward imbalance and incidence of low back and neck injuries in San Francisco transit operators. Occup Environ Med. 2008;65:525–33.

15. Lapointe J, Dionne CE, Brisson C, Montreuil S. Effort-reward imbalance and video display unit postural risk factors interact in women on the incidence of musculoskeletal symptoms. Work. 2013;44:133–43.

16. Krause N, Burgel B, Rempel D. Effort-reward imbalance and one-year change in neck-shoulder and upper extremity pain among call center computer operators. Scand J Work Environ Health. 2010;36:42–53.

17. Koch P, Schablon A, Latza U, Nienhaus A. Musculoskeletal pain and effort-reward imbalance–a systematic review. BMC Public Health. 2014;14:37.

18. Schaufeli WB, Buunk BP. Burnout. An overview of 25 years of research and theorizing. In: Schabracq MJ, Winnubst JA, Cooper CL, editors. The handbook of work and health psychology. 2nd edn edition. New York: Wiley & Sons; 2003. p. 383–425.

19. Manlove EE. Multiple correlates of burnout in child care workers. Early Child Res Q. 1993;8:499–518.

20. Kushnir T, Milbauer V. Managing stress and burnout at work. A cognitive group intervention. Program for directors of day care centers. Pediatrics. 1994;94:1074–7.

21. Whitebook M, Howes C, Darrah R, Friedman J. Who's minding the child care workers? A look at staff burnout. Child Today. 1980;10:2–6.

22. Bertolino B, Thompson K. The residential youth care worker in action. Binghamton, New York: Hawthorn Press; 1999.

23. Snow K. Aggression: Just part of the job? The psychological impact of aggression on child and youth workers. J Child Youth Care. 1994;9:11–30.

24. Rudow B. Belastungen im Erzieher/innenberuf. Bildung Wissenschaft. 2004;6:6–11.

25. Jungbauer J, Ehlen S. Stress and Burnout Risk in Nursery School Teachers: Results from a Survey. Gesundheitswesen. 2015;77:418–23.

26. Scheuch K, Seibt R. Arbeits- und persönlichkeitsbedingte Beziehungen zu Burnout - eine kritische Betrachtung. In: Richter PG, Rau R, Mühlpfordt S, editors. Arbeit und Gesundheit. Lengerich: Pabst Science Publishers; 2007. p. 42–54.

27. Nübling M, Seidler A, Garthus-Niegel S, Latza U, Wagner M, Hegewald J, et al. The Gutenberg Health Study: measuring psychosocial factors at work and predicting health and work-related outcomes with the ERI and the COPSOQ questionnaire. BMC Public Health. 2013;13:538.

28. Koch P, Stranzinger J, Kersten JF, Nienhaus A. Use of moulded hearing protectors by child care workers - an interventional pilot study. J Occup Med Toxicol. 2016;11:50.

29. Slesina W. FEBA. Fragebogen zur subjektiven Einschätzung der Belastungen am Arbeitsplatz. http://www.rueckenkompass.de/out.php?idart=18. Last access: 05/23/2017.

30. Siegrist J, Starke D, Chandola T, Godin I, Marmot M, Niedhammer I, et al. The measurement of effort-reward imbalance at work: European comparisons. Soc Sci Med. 2004;58:1483–99.

31. Prümper J, Hartmannsgruber K, Frese M. KFZA - Kurzfragebogen zur Arbeitsanalyse. Zeitschrift für Arbeits- und Organisationspsychologie. 1995; 39:125–32.

32. Kuorinka I, Jonsson B, Kilbom A, Vinterberg H, Biering-Sorensen F, Andersson G, et al. Standardised Nordic questionnaires for the analysis of musculoskeletal symptoms. Appl Ergon. 1987;18:233–7.

33. Kristensen TS, Hannerz H, Hogh A, Borg V. The Copenhagen Psychosocial Questionnaire–a tool for the assessment of the psychosocial work environment. Scand J Work Environ Health. 2005;31:438–49.

34. Hosmer DW, Lemeshow S. Applied logistic regression. New York: Wiley & Sons; 2000.

35. Siegrist J, Li J. Associations of Extrinsic and Intrinsic Components of Work Stress with Health: A Systematic Review of Evidence on the Effort-Reward Imbalance Model. Int J Environ Res Public Health. 2016;13(4):432.

36. Aust B, Peter R, Siegrist J. Stress Management in Bus Drivers: A Pilot Study Based on the Model of Effort–Reward Imbalance. Int J Stress Manag. 1997; 4(4):297–305.

37. Bourbonnais R, Brisson C, Vinet A, Vezina M, Abdous B, Gaudet M. Effectiveness of a participative intervention on psychosocial work factors to prevent mental health problems in a hospital setting. Occup Environ Med. 2006;63(5):335–42.

38. Simon M, Tackenberg P, Nienhaus A, Estryn-Behar M, Conway PM, Hasselhorn HM. Back or neck-pain-related disability of nursing staff in hospitals, nursing homes and home care in seven countries–results from the European NEXT-Study. Int J Nurs Stud. 2008;45:24–34.

39. Bernard C, Courouve L, Bouée S, Adjémian A, Chrétien JC, Niedhammer I. Biomechanical and psychosocial work exposures and musculoskeletal symtoms among vineyard workers. J Occup Health. 2011;53:297–311.

40. von dem Knesebeck O, David K, Siegrist J. Psychosocial stress at work and musculoskeletal pain among police officers in special forces. Gesundheitswesen. 2005;67:674–9.

41. Dragano N, von dem Knesebeck O, Rodel A, Siegrist J. Psychosoziale Arbeitsbelastungen und muskulo-skeletale Beschwerden: Bedeutung für die Prävention. J Public Health. 2003;11:196–207.

42. Karasek RA. Job Demands, Job Decision Latitude, and Mental Strain: Implications for Job Redesign. Adm Sci Q. 1979;24:285–308.

43. Gillen M, Yen IH, Trupin L, Swig L, Rugulies R, Mullen K, et al. The association of socioeconomic status and psychosocial and physical workplace factors with musculoskeletal injury in hospital workers. Am J Ind Med. 2007;50:245–60.

44. Lundberg U, Dohns IE, Melin B, Sandsjö L, Palmerud G, Kadefors R, et al. Psychophysiological stress responses, muscle tension, and neck and shoulder pain among supermarket cashiers. J Occup Health Psychol. 1999;4(3):245.

45. Schleifer LM, Ley R, Spalding TW. A hyperventilation theory of job stress and musculoskeletal disorders. Am J Ind Med. 2002;41(5):420–32.

46. Theorell T, Emdad R, Arnetz B, Weingarten A. Employee Effects of an Educational Program for Managers at an Insurance Company. Psychosom Med. 2001;63:724–33.

47. Spence Laschinger HK, Finegan J. Situational and dispositional predictors of nurse manager burnout: a time-lagged analysis. J Nurs Manag. 2008;16:601–7.

48. Loerbroks A, Meng H, Chen ML, Herr R, Angerer P, Li J. Primary school teachers in China: associations of organizational justice and effort-reward imbalance with burnout and intentions to leave the profession in a cross-sectional sample. Int Arch Occup Environ Health. 2014;87:695–703.

49. Gluschkoff K, Elovainio M, Kinnunen U, Mullola S, Hintsanen M, Keltikangas-Jarvinen L, et al. Work stress, poor recovery and burnout in teachers. Occup Med (Lond). 2016;66:564–70.

50. Lau B. Effort-reward imbalance and overcommitment in employees in a Norwegian municipality: a cross sectional study. J Occup Med Toxicol. 2008;3:9.

51. Wang Y, Ramos A, Wu H, Liu L, Yang X, Wang J, et al. Relationship between occupational stress and burnout among Chinese teachers: a cross-sectional survey in Liaoning. China Int Arch Occup Environ Health. 2015;88:589–97.

52. Chou LP, Li CY, Hu SC. Job stress and burnout in hospital employees: comparisons of different medical professions in a regional hospital in Taiwan. BMJ Open. 2014;4:e004185.

53. Podsakoff PM, MacKenzie SB, Lee JY, Podsakoff NP. Common method biases in behavioral research: a critical review of the literature and recommended remedies. J Appl Psychol. 2003;88:879–903.

8

Prevalence of latent tuberculosis infection in healthcare workers at a hospital

Monica Lamberti[1*], Mariarosaria Muoio[1], Antonio Arnese[1], Sharon Borrelli[1], Teresa Di Lorenzo[1], Elpidio Maria Garzillo[1], Giuseppe Signoriello[2], Stefania De Pascalis[2], Nicola Coppola[2] and Albert Nienhaus[3]

Abstract

Background: Healthcare workers (HCWs) are at higher risk than the general population of contracting tuberculosis (TB). Moreover, although subjects with latent TB infection (LTBI) are asymptomatic and are not infectious, they may eventually develop active disease. Thus, a fundamental tool of TB control programs for HCWs is the screening and treatment of LTBI.

Methods: From January 2014 to January 2015, hospital personnel at Azienda Ospedaliera Universitaria, Naples, Italy, were screened for TB. To this end, a tuberculin skin test (TST) was administered as an initial examination, unless when contraindicated, in which case the QuantiFERON® TB-Gold (QFT) assay was performed. Moreover, QFT was carried out on all TST-positive cases to confirm the initial result.

Results: Of 628 personnel asked to participate, 28 (4.5%) denied consent, 533 were administered TST as the baseline examination, and 67 were tested only with QFT. In the TST group, 73 (13.2%) individuals were found positive, 418 (78.4%) were negative, and 42 (7.9%) were absent for the reading window; QFT confirmed the result in 39 (53.4%) TST-positive individuals. In the QFT-only group, 44 (65.7%) individuals were found positive. All TST- and/or QFT-positive subjects were referred for chest X-ray and examination by an infectious diseases specialist. None were found to have active TB, and were thus diagnosed with LTBI.

Conclusions: Although Italy is a low-incidence country regarding TB, our findings suggest that the prevalence of LTBI in HCWs may be relatively high. As a result, active screening for TB and LTBI is needed for these workers.

Keywords: Tuberculosis, Tuberculin skin test, Healthcare workers, Quantiferon test, Health surveillance, Occupational exposure

Background

Tuberculosis (TB) is a major health problem worldwide. The World Health Organization estimates that in 2013 there were 9.0 million new cases and 1.5 million TB-related deaths [1]. Compounding this problem is multidrug-resistant TB, which globally was estimated to affect 3.5% of new TB cases in 2013. Although Italy is considered a low-incidence country for TB-the number of estimated new cases in 2013 was less than 10/100,000 inhabitants [1] – the disease is still considered a risk owing to abandonment of vaccination campaigns, wide diffusion of primary and secondary immunosuppression, and influx of immigrants [2, 3].

Compared with the general population, healthcare workers (HCWs) have a higher risk of contracting a TB infection on account of increased exposure to individuals in a contagious phase of the disease, inadequate use of personal protective equipment, and their specific working conditions, such as having to carry out activities in poorly ventilated areas [4, 5]. Median annual incidences of active TB among HCWs in countries with low, intermediate, and high rates of TB are 67, 91, and 1,180 per 100,000 persons, respectively [6].

* Correspondence: monicalamberti@libero.it
[1]Department of Experimental Medicine, Section of Hygiene, Occupational Medicine and Forensic Medicine, Second University of Naples, Via dei Crecchi 16, 80133 Naples, Italy
Full list of author information is available at the end of the article

The majority of active TB cases in HCWs occur when the risk of TB infection is underestimated and control programs are lacking. Thus, improving the understanding of TB transmission and adopting effective control measures have been recommended to reduce the risk of nosocomial infection [6, 7]. In addition, a fundamental tool for TB control programs is the screening and treatment of latent TB infection (LTBI). This is strongly recommended in many countries, including Italy. Indeed, although individuals with LTBI do not show symptoms of TB and are not infectious, about 10% are at risk of developing active disease and becoming infectious during the course of their lifetime [1]. A recent review estimated the median annual risk of LTBI among HCWs to be 2.9% in countries with a low incidence of TB and 7.2% in countries with a high incidence [6].

The main purpose of the current study was therefore to evaluate the prevalence of active TB and LTBI among hospital personnel operating in a context of low endemicity, and to assess possible associations between the outcome of the screening tests and epidemiological variables.

Methods

From January 2014 to January 2015, a TB screening program was carried out at Azienda Ospedaliera Universitaria, Naples, Italy, a hospital with a risk classifiable as "low" according to CDC guidelines (i.e., <6TB patients/ year in a setting with ≥200 in-patient beds) [8]. The Italian Society of Occupational Medicine recommends to carry out a tuberculin skin test (TST) every 6 years in healthcare structures classified as "very low" risk, every 2 years in "low" risk structures, every year if the risk is "medium", and twice-yearly when the risk is "high" [9]. All hospital personnel, including physicians, surgeons, nurses, midwives, physiotherapists, laboratory technicians, radiographers, ambulance drivers, orderlies, and maintenance workers employed at the institution during the study period were asked to take part in this cross-sectional study. A pre-coded questionnaire on demographics, work (time in healthcare employment, type of job conducted, workplace frequented), and medical history (previous exposure to TB, TB vaccination status) was filled in by each participant.

The surveillance program required a TST as the baseline examination. The test was performed and assessed by trained personnel following standard procedures. In brief, 0.1 ml (2 TU) of the purified protein derivative RT23 (Statens Serum Institute, Copenhagen, Denmark) was injected intradermally on the volar side of the forearm of participants and read 48 to 72 h later. In accordance with national guidelines, a positive TST was defined as an induration measuring ≥10 mm [10–12].

Since vaccination data was either not available or incomplete for some participants, all TST-positive cases were then tested also with the QuantiFERON® TB-Gold (QFT) kit (Cellestis, Carnegie, Australia), a second-generation test based on an interferon-gamma release assay (IGRA) [13]. Participants with secondary immunodeficiency or a history of allergy were offered the opportunity to take the QFT test as their baseline examination in order to remove any possible risk of an allergic-type reaction [6]. Pregnant participants were also asked to take only this test because we wished to avoid multiple diagnostic exams in these woman, despite there being no evidence in the literature that adverse reactions to the Mantoux test can influence the course of pregnancy [6].

For the QFT test, 1 ml of whole blood was aliquoted into each of three QFT tubes, containing either TB-specific antigen (ESAT-6, CFP-10, and TB7.7), no antigen (negative control), or mitogen antigen (positive control), and incubated at 37 °C overnight before centrifugation, as recommended by the manufacturer's protocol. Interferon-gamma concentration was then measured by ELISA: a reading ≥0.35 IU/ml (TB antigens minus negative control) was considered positive [14, 15].

All TST- and/or QFT-positive cases were referred for chest radiography and carefully examined by an infectious diseases specialist. We elected to suspect active TB infection in the presence of clinical symptoms such as cough, weight loss, fever, nocturnal sweating, tiredness, and/or X-ray suggestive of TB, and to confirm the disease by the presence of TB pathogens in sputum culture; a diagnosis of LTBI was given to test-positive participants not presenting with clinical or radiographic signs of active TB [2].

This cross-sectional study was performed in compliance with the Declaration of Helsinki and current healthcare standards, according to the recommendations of the Italian Ministry of Health [11]. All participants were informed by a physician on the rationale and aims, and written informed consent was obtained. According to Italian legislation concerning guidelines on observational studies, ethical approval for conducting this study was unnecessary, so we did not require formal approval by local institutional review boards [16]. Personal information regarding the enrolled subjects was protected according to Italian law [17].

Statistical analysis of the data was performed using SPSS v.17.0 software. Continuous variables are given as mean and standard deviation, and categorical variables as absolute and relative frequencies. Differences in means were evaluated by unpaired Student t-test, and the Chi-squared test was applied to categorical variables. Odds ratio (OR), with a 95% confidence interval (CI), was estimated by a logistic regression model to evaluate the presence of LTBI, with sex, age, work seniority, and type of employment as covariates. A *p*-value of <0.05 was considered statistically significant.

Results

Six hundred twenty-eight personnel were asked to participate in the study: 28 (4.5%) denied consent and 42 (6.7%) failed to complete it (Fig. 1). The main demographic and epidemiological characteristics of the remaining participants are listed in Table 1: all were Italian; mean age was ~56 years; there was a slightly higher prevalence of males; mean time in employment was ~25 years; and almost half were nursing staff, with nursing and medical staff comprising over 93% of all personnel tested. No one reported knowledge of being exposed to TB outside the hospital and all were HIV-negative.

The baseline examination was the TST for 533 of the participants and the QFT assay for the remaining 67. Of the former, 73/533 (13.7%) were positive to the test, 418/533 (78.4) were negative, and 42/533 (7.9%) were absent during the reading window and were asked to repeat the test within 90 days. However, the evaluations of the retested participants occurred after January 2015, so this data was excluded from the current study. No adverse

loco-regional or systemic allergic reactions were encountered. All the TST-positive subjects were then given the QFT assay: a positive result was confirmed in 39/73 (53.4%) cases.

The QFT assay was administered as the baseline examination to 52 participants with a positive history of drug allergy, to 10 pregnant women, and to 5 individuals taking immunosuppressive drugs: none reported a history of positivity to TST. Of these 67, 44 (65.7%) resulted positive and 23 (34.3%) negative.

All the 83 participants found positive with QFT (i.e., the 39 individuals positive at both tests plus the 44 individuals positive at QFT as the baseline assay) were given a chest X-ray and a careful examination by an infectious diseases specialist. Clinical and radiographic signs of active TB were excluded for all, so they were diagnosed with LTBI. In addition, although the 34 TST-positive/QFT-negative participants were strongly suspected of being falsely positive to the baseline TST (they were unable to provide documented information on TB vaccination or possible contact with non-TB mycobacteria [15]), we decided to refer them to chest X-ray and specialist examination: no evidence of TB was found in any of these subjects either.

Table 2 gives the demographic characteristics of the study population stratified for the presence of LTBI

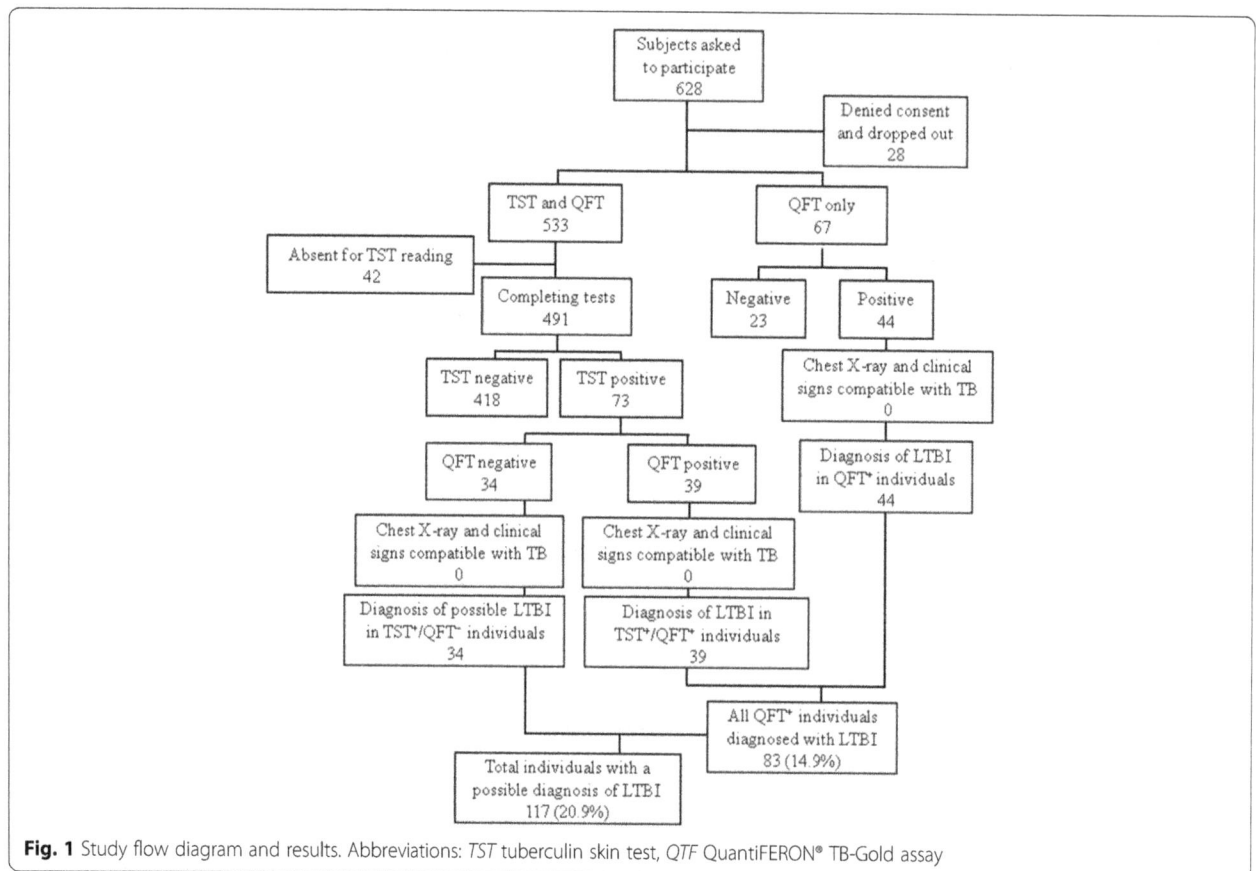

Fig. 1 Study flow diagram and results. Abbreviations: *TST* tuberculin skin test, *QTF* QuantiFERON® TB-Gold assay

Table 1 Demographic and clinical characteristics of the hospital personnel completing the study

	n (%)[a]
Subjects completing the screening[b]	558
Age, years (mean ± SD)	56.1 ± 8
Males	324 (58.2)
Work category	
• medical staff	246 (44.1)
• nursing staff	274 (49.1)
• laboratory staff	25 (4.5)
• other[c]	13 (2.3)
Workplace frequented	
• medical wards	220 (39.4)
• surgical wards	171 (30.6)
• other[d]	167 (30)
Years in employment (mean ± SD)	24.8 ± 9.8
TST as baseline examination	491 (88)
• positive	73 (14.8)
• negative	418 (85.2)
QTF as baseline examination	67 (12)
• positive	44 (65.7)
• negative	23 (34.3)
LTBI[e]	117 (20.9)
Active tuberculosis	0

Abbreviations: TST tuberculin skin test, QTF QuantiFERON® TB-Gold assay, LTBI latent tuberculosis infection
[a]values expressed as absolute frequency (percentage), unless otherwise stated
[b]28 subjects denied consent and 42 participants were absent during the TST reading window
[c]physiotherapists, orderlies, ambulance drivers, maintenance workers
[d]intensive care, clinical pathology, occupational medicine, audiology, radiology, microbiology
[e]as diagnosed for all individuals found positive at either TST or QFT

Table 2 Univariate analysis for demographic, epidemiological and occupational characteristics of the hospital personnel completing the study stratified for latent TB infection [a]

	Personnel with LTBI [b]	Personnel without LTBI[b]	p-value
n	83	475	0.47
Age, years (mean ± SD)	56.1 ± 7.2	56.1 ± 8.1	0.19
Males	45 (13.9)	279 (86.1)	0.51
Females	38 (16.2)	196 (83.8)	
Work category			
• medical staff	36 (14.6)	210 (85.4)	0.45
• nursing staff	44 (16.1)	230 (83.9)	
• laboratory staff	1 (4)	24 (96)	
• other[c]	2 (15.4)	11 (84.6)	
Workplace frequented			
• medical wards	33 (15)	187 (85)	0.35
• surgical wards	29 (17)	142 (83)	
• other[d]	21 (12.8)	146 (87.2)	
Years in employment (mean ± SD)	24.1 ± 1.0	24.9 ± 0.4	0.45

Abbreviations: LTBI latent tuberculosis infection, TST tuberculin skin test, QTF QuantiFERON® TB-Gold assay
[a]as diagnosed for TST+/QFT+ and QFT+-only participants
[b]values expressed as absolute frequency (percentage), unless otherwise stated
[c]physiotherapists, orderlies, ambulance drivers, maintenance workers
[d]intensive care, clinical pathology, occupational medicine, audiology, radiology, microbiology

as diagnosed in all QFT-positive participants. Of these personnel with LTBI, over half were nursing staff; medical staff also accounted for a large percentage of LTBI cases, whereas laboratory technicians and other categories of workers made up only a very small fraction of this group. No statistical differences were found for sex, age, work seniority, or type of employment between the participants with and without LTBI or between those taking TST or QFT as the baseline examination. This held true also when we added the data of the 34 TST-positive/QTF-negative participants (Additional file 1: Table S1). Univariate and multivariate analysis did not identify a demographic factor associated with LTBI (Tables 2 and 3, Additional file 2: Table S2).

Finally, all personnel with LTBI were referred for chemoprophylaxis. Only 6 subjects adhered to the regimen and follow-up procedure.

Discussion

Although Italy is considered a country with a low incidence of TB [1, 13], our study identified a relatively high prevalence (20.9%) of LTBI in the personnel of one hospital, confirming that the risk of TB among HCWs is higher than that observed in the general population [7]. Indeed, a recent meta-analysis reported that, globally, the risk faced by HCWs of contracting TB is consistently higher than of the general population, indicating TB as an occupational disease [7].

In the present study, no case of active TB was encountered. In other reports on HCWs conducted in Italy and other low-incidence countries, the prevalences of TB and LTBI varied depending on the country and the type of population sample studied. For example, Franchi and colleagues evaluated 1,755 HCWs in Italy in 2004, diagnosing LTBI in 6% of cases [18]; in a study conducted in France (a low-incidence country with 5.2 cases of TB per 100,000 inhabitants in 2006), 18.9% of 148 HCWs had a positive IGRA result [19]: and in a study on 134 HCWs in Spain (another low-incidence country), the pevalence of LTBI was 11.2% [20]. By contrast, a study on 2,884 hospital workers in Portugal (a high-incidence country, with 32 cases/100,000/year) reported a very high prevalence of LTBI (i.e., 29.5%) [21]. However, a

Table 3 Multivariate analysis for demographic, epidemiological and occupational characteristics of the hospital personnel completing the study stratified for LTBI[a]

Variable	OR	95% CI	p-value
Female vs Male	1.22	0.75–2.00	0.42
Age	1.02	0.98–1.07	0.35
Years of employment	0.97	0.94–1.01	0.18
Type of employment			
• nursing vs medical	1.41	0.74–2.71	0.30
• laboratory vs medical	0.34	0.04–2.73	0.31
• other[b] vs medical	1.72	0.33–8.95	0.52
Workplace			
• surgery vs medical wards	1.23	0.71–2.13	0.46
• other[c] vs medical wards	0.81	0.44–1.51	0.51

Abbreviations: LTBI latent tuberculosis infection, *OR* odds ratio, *CI* confidence interval
[a]as diagnosed for TST+/QFT+ and QFT+-only participants
[b]physiotherapists, orderlies, ambulance drivers, maintenance workers
[c]intensive care, clinical pathology, occupational medicine, audiology, radiology, microbiology

2005 meta-analysis reported that the prevalence of LTBI in HCWs ranged 5–55% in high-income countries [22].

The 20.9% prevalence of LTBI observed in our study, which represents an intermediate value compared with previous studies, can be explained, at least in part, by our HCW population's relatively high mean age and number of years in work. Indeed, the prevalences of LTBI and TB in HCWs are also dependent on the time that the workers are potentially exposed to the pathogen and, thus, on those two variables. For example, in a study on 2,028 HCWs in Germany (a low-incidence country), the prevalence of LTBI increased with the duration of employment, going from 5.4% in the subgroup with less than 5 years of employment, to 12.7% in those with more than 20 years in the healthcare sector; moreover, age was found to be the most important risk factor linked to a positive IGRA result (>55 years; OR: 14.7; 95% CI: 5.1–42.1) [23]. Both mean age and years of employment of the personnel enrolled in the present study (56.1 ± 8 and 24.8 ± 9.8 years) were higher than in the HCWs enrolled by Franchi and colleagues (39 ± 9 and 13 ± 8 years), who reported a much lower prevalence of LTBI [18]. The association between age and the prevalence of LTBI is also confirmed by data collected on healthcare students. In our recent study on undergraduate and postgraduate healthcare students in Italy (mean age: 25.8 ± 5.3 years), LTBI was diagnosed in only 35 of the 3,331 individuals tested (i.e., 1.05%) [24]. Comparable findings were reported by Durando and colleagues, who found a very low prevalence (0.5%) of LTBI in 881 Italian undergraduate students (mean age: 23.6 ± 3.1 years) [25].

Apart from age and years of employment, other factors that have been identified as associated with LTBI in HCWs are male gender, being born in a high-incidence country, prior exposure to TB, and a previous positive TST result. For example, Franchi and colleagues found that TST reactivity correlated with age (≥47 years) and the male gender [18]; Durando and colleagues reported an association with being born in a country with a high incidence of TB [25]; and a study on German HCWs identified associations with being foreign-born (OR: 1.99; 95% CI: 1.4–2.8), having TB in the individual's own history (OR: 4.96; 95% CI: 1.99–12.3), and a having a previous positive TST result (OR: 3.5; 95% CI: 2.4–4.98) [23]. However, in the present study on Italian-born HCWs of relatively high age and years of employment, we did not identify any factor associated with LTBI.

The limitations of this study are principally related to the cross-sectional design used, the lack of a control group and the relatively low number of subjects evaluated. Moreover, a single testing procedure was used, with a second test (namely an IGRA) systematically carried out only in the event of a positive TST or in subjects that did not want a skin test. In our experience, TST is safe and can be used widely (we found no instance of loco-regional or systemic allergic reactions); our decision to use IGRA as a second-level examination only in subjects found positive upon TST was aimed at optimizing costs and increasing the level of diagnostic accuracy [26]. However, both tests have their drawbacks: TST has technical limitations in that it can produce results that are hard to interpret and tends to generate a significant number of false positives [27–30]; IGRA is more specific and has a sensitivity that is at least identical to that of TST [20, 31, 32], but it is more expensive and is difficult to assess around the cut-off value. Although, the 34 TST-positive but IGRA-negative subjects in our study would normally be considered as having been infected by *M. tuberculosis*, we strongly suspected they represented false positives caused, for example, by contact with non-TB mycobacteria [15, 33]; indeed, these individuals were not able to provide us with documented data on TB vaccination. We nevertheless consider it correct to use TST as a baseline exam, especially in a country like Italy where the prevalence of BCG vaccination is low [34, 35].

Conclusions

Although Italy is considered a low-incidence country for TB, our data suggest that the prevalence of LTBI in HCWs may be high, especially in older healthcare personnel with a longer history of employment in the sector. In this epidemiological context, active screening for TB and LTBI is advised.

Acknowledgements
We thank Alessandro Izzo, Second University of Naples, for his support and assistance in data collection.

Funding
Funding Information is not available.

Authors' contributions
ML, AN, GS and NC designed the study, performed data analysis and made valuable contributions to the manuscript. AA, MM, EMG, SDP, SB, TDL were involved in data analysis and made valuable contributions to the manuscript. All authors read and approved the final manuscript.

Competing interests
All the authors of the manuscript declare that they have no conflict of interest in connection with this paper.

Author details
[1]Department of Experimental Medicine, Section of Hygiene, Occupational Medicine and Forensic Medicine, Second University of Naples, Via dei Crecchi 16, 80133 Naples, Italy. [2]Department of Mental Health and Public Medicine, Section of Infectious Diseases, Second University of Naples, Naples, Italy. [3]Institute for Health Services, Research in Dermatology and Nursing, Germany, Institution for Statutory Accident Insurance and Prevention in Healthcare and Welfare Services, University Medical Centre Hamburg-Eppendorf, Hamburg, Germany.

References
1. WHO Global Tuberculosis Report. World Health Organization. 2013. http://www.who.int/tb/publications/global_report/en/.
2. Nienhaus A, Schablon A, Preisser AM, Ringshausen FC, Diel R. Tuberculosis in healthcare workers - a narrative review from a German perspective. J Occup Med Toxicol. 2014;9:9.
3. Menzies D, Joshi R, Pai M. Risk of tuberculosis infection and disease associated with work in health care settings. Int J Tuberc Lung Dis. 2007;11:593–605.
4. Baussano I, Bugiani M, Carosso A, Mairano D, Pia Barocelli A, Tagna M, et al. Risk of tuberculin conversion among healthcare workers and the adoption of preventive measures. Occup Environ Med. 2007;64:161–6.
5. Saleiro S, Santos AR, Vidal O, Carvalho T, Torres Costa J, Agostinho MJ. Tuberculosis in hospital department health care workers. Rev Port Pneumol. 2007;13:789–99.
6. Baussano I, Nunn P, Williams B, Pivetta E, Bugiani M, Scano F. Tuberculosis among health care workers. Emerg Infect Dis. 2011;17:488–94.
7. Lamberti M, Muoio MR, Westermann C, Nienhaus A, Arnese A, Ribeiro Sobrinho AP, et al. Prevalence and associated risk factors of latent tuberculosis infection among undergraduate and postgraduate dental students: A retrospective study. Arch Environ Occup Health. 2016;28:1–7.
8. Guidelines for preventing the transmission of Mycobacterium tuberculosis in health-care settings. Department of Health and Human Services. Centers for Disease Control and Prevention. 2005. http://www.cdc.gov/tb/publications/guidelines/infectioncontrol.htm.
9. Rischio biologico per i lavoratori della sanità: linee guida per la sorveglianza sanitaria. Società Italiana di Medicina del Lavoro. 2012. http://www.aogarbagnate.lombardia.it/salviniweb/uooml/linee%20guida/Linee%20Guida%20SIMLII%20Rischio%20Biologico.pdf.
10. La tubercolosi in Italia. Ministero della Salute Ufficio V - Malattie Infettive, Direzione Generale della Prevenzione Sanitaria, Istituto Superiore di Sanità. 2008. http://www.salute.gov.it/portale/documentazione/p6_2_2_1.jsp?lingua=italiano&id=1472.
11. Duarte R, Amado J, Lucas H, Sapage JM. Portuguese Society of P. [Treatment of latent tuberculosis infection: update of guidelines, 2006]. Rev Port Pneumol. 2007;13:397–418.
12. Prevenzione della tubercolosi negli operatori sanitari e nei soggetti ad essi equiparati. Italian Ministry of Health. 2013. http://www.salute.gov.it/imgs/C_17_pubblicazioni_1901_allegato.pdf.
13. Trajman A, Steffen RE, Menzies D. Interferon-Gamma Release Assays versus Tuberculin Skin Testing for the Diagnosis of Latent Tuberculosis Infection: An Overview of the Evidence. Pulm Med. 2013;2013:601737.
14. Torres Costa J, Silva R, Sa R, Cardoso MJ, Nienhaus A. Results of five-year systematic screening for latent tuberculosis infection in healthcare workers in Portugal. J Occup Med Toxicol. 2010;5:22.
15. Salgame P, Geadas C, Collins L, Jones-Lopez E, Ellner JJ. Latent tuberculosis infection–Revisiting and revising concepts. Tuberculosis (Edinb). 2015;95:373–84.
16. Linee guida per la classificazione e conduzione degli studi osservazionali sui farmaci. Gazzetta Ufficiale 76. 2008. http://www.agenziafarmaco.gov.it/allegati/det_20marzo2008.pdf.
17. Italian Law decree n. 196, 30 June 2003 (article 24). 2003. http://www.camera.it/parlam/leggi/deleghe/03196dl.htm.
18. Franchi A, Diana O, Franco G. Job-related risk of latent tuberculosis infection in a homogeneous population of hospital workers in a low incidence area. Am J Ind Med. 2009;52:297–303.
19. Tripodi D, Brunet-Courtois B, Nael V, Audrain M, Chailleux E, Germaud P, et al. Evaluation of the tuberculin skin test and the interferon-gamma release assay for TB screening in French healthcare workers. J Occup Med Toxicol. 2009;4:30.
20. Alvarez-Leon EE, Espinosa-Vega E, Santana-Rodriguez E, Molina-Cabrillana JM, Perez-Arellano JL, Caminero JA, et al. Screening for tuberculosis infection in spanish healthcare workers: Comparison of the QuantiFERON-TB gold in-tube test with the tuberculin skin test. Infect Control Hosp Epidemiol. 2009;30:876–83.
21. Torres Costa J, Silva R, Ringshausen FC, Nienhaus A. Screening for tuberculosis and prediction of disease in Portuguese healthcare workers. J Occup Med Toxicol. 2011;6:19.
22. Seidler A, Nienhaus A, Diel R. Review of epidemiological studies on the occupational risk of tuberculosis in low-incidence areas. Respiration. 2005;72:431–46.
23. Schablon A, Harling M, Diel R, Nienhaus A. Risk of latent TB infection in individuals employed in the healthcare sector in Germany: a multicentre prevalence study. BMC Infect Dis. 2010;10:107.
24. Lamberti M, Muoio M, Monaco MG, Uccello R, Sannolo N, Mazzarella G, et al. Prevalence of latent tuberculosis infection and associated risk factors among 3,374 healthcare students in Italy. J Occup Med Toxicol. 2014;9:34.
25. Durando P, Sotgiu G, Spigno F, Piccinini M, Mazzarello G, Viscoli C, et al. Latent tuberculosis infection and associated risk factors among undergraduate healthcare students in Italy: a cross-sectional study. BMC Infect Dis. 2013;13:443.
26. Lamberti M, Uccello R, Monaco MG, Muoio M, Feola D, Sannolo N, et al. Tuberculin skin test and Quantiferon test agreement and influencing factors in tuberculosis screening of healthcare workers: a systematic review and meta-analysis. J Occup Med Toxicol. 2015;10:2.
27. Zwerling A, van den Hof S, Scholten J, Cobelens F, Menzies D, Pai M. Interferon-gamma release assays for tuberculosis screening of healthcare workers: a systematic review. Thorax. 2012;67:62–70.
28. Menzies D, Pai M, Comstock G. Meta-analysis: new tests for the diagnosis of latent tuberculosis infection: areas of uncertainty and recommendations for research. Ann Intern Med. 2007;146:340–54.
29. Menzies D. Interpretation of repeated tuberculin tests. Boosting, conversion, and reversion. Am J Respir Crit Care Med. 1999;159:15–21.
30. Ewer K, Deeks J, Alvarez L, Bryant G, Waller S, Andersen P, et al. Comparison of T-cell-based assay with tuberculin skin test for diagnosis of Mycobacterium tuberculosis infection in a school tuberculosis outbreak. Lancet. 2003;361:1168–73.
31. Pai M, Gokhale K, Joshi R, Dogra S, Kalantri S, Mendiratta DK, et al. Mycobacterium tuberculosis infection in health care workers in rural India: comparison of a whole-blood interferon gamma assay with tuberculin skin testing. JAMA. 2005;293:2746–55.
32. Kang YA, Lee HW, Yoon HI, Cho B, Han SK, Shim YS, et al. Discrepancy between the tuberculin skin test and the whole-blood interferon gamma assay for the diagnosis of latent tuberculosis infection in an intermediate tuberculosis-burden country. JAMA. 2005;293:2756–61.

33. Hermansen TS, Thomsen VO, Lillebaek T, Ravn P. Non-tuberculous mycobacteria and the performance of interferon gamma release assays in Denmark. PLoS One. 2014;9:e93986.

34. Uccello R, Monaco MG, Feola D, Garzillo EM, Muoio M, Sannolo N, et al. Managment of tuberculosis in an University of Campania. G Ital Med Lav Ergon. 2012;34:299–301.

35. Lamberti M, Uccello R, Monaco MG, Muoio M, Sannolo N, Arena P, et al. Prevalence of latent tuberculosis infection and associated risk factors among 1557 nursing students in a context of low endemicity. Open Nurs J. 2015;9:10–4.

9

Self-reported safety practices and associated factors among employees of Dashen brewery share company, Gondar

Solomon Tesfa Tezera, Daniel Haile Chercos* ⓘ and Awrajaw Dessie

Abstract

Background: According to International Labor Organization (ILO), occupational accidents and work-related diseases are the causes for millions of deaths of workers every year. In addition, many millions of workers suffer non-fatal injuries and illnesses. This research was conceived with aim to assess safety practices and associated factors among employees of Dashen brewery Share Company, Ethiopia.

Method: Institutionalbased cross-sectional study was conducted to assess the level of self-reported safety practice and associated factors from February to March 2016, among Dashen brewery workers. Stratified sampling method was employed to select 415 study participants and the data was collected by using structured interview-administer questionnaire. Observational checklist was also used to ascertain the response given by interviewee.

Results: Fourhundred 15 respondent were involved in this study. Of those individuals, almost three fourth (74.2%) of the participants were male and 43.4% of participants were single. Mean (SD) age of respondents were 28.18 (±8.67) years and half of the respondents (49.9%) were diploma holders. The finding of this study indicated that 87.2% of the respondents reported complying with good safety practice. Age, marital status, employment status, attitude, safety and health training, and management support were found to be main predictors for safety practices.

Conclusion: The level of self-reported safety practice in this study was good. Management commitment on safety and training of the employees about safety and health is very important and should be provided regularly.

Keywords: Safety practice, Prevalence, Brewery factory, Ethiopia

Background

Millions of industrial workers around the world are involved in different hazardous work-related exposures on a daily basis. Due to the presence of hazards, employees in both developed and developing countries are highly vulnerable for diverse and considerable risk of industrial accidents, diseases and death [1].

According to the International Labor Organization (ILO), an estimated 2.3 million workers die every year from occupational accidents and work-related diseases globally. The total economic loss due to this is tremendous [2]. The majority of labor force in developing countries live and work in hazardous work environment that worsens their health, social and economic condition [3].

Incidence rate of occupational injury is the highest in food and drink processing industry, which make it the most dangerous occupation, among the manufacturing industries [4]. In Bralirwa brewery industry, Republic of Rwanda,86.4%of workers suffered from work related injury annually [5]. In Durban, South Africa, about 22% of brewery industry workers were also encountered work related injury within 6 months of working period [6].

In Ethiopia, the number of industries are increasing drastically due to the country's favorable policy that supports the growth of small and large scale industries [7]. However, workers who are involved in manufacturing

* Correspondence: daniel.haile7@gmail.com
Department of Environmental and Occupational Health and Safety, Institute of Public Health, University of Gondar, P.O. Box 196, Gondar, Ethiopia

industries including brewery companies, have encountered higher level of workplace accident [8]. Though many reasons can be related to work-related injuries; majority (88%) of the injuries are caused by unsafe working practice [9].There is scant knowledge on the level of safety practice and its determinant factors among brewery workers in Ethiopia.

Brewery workers in Ethiopia have been reported to be exposed to various work hazards (excessive heat and noise levels, broken bottles, chemicals and radiation) [7]. This may end up with occupational injuries and diseases, like skin cuts and lacerations, eye injuries, respiratory problems (bronchitis and asthma), hearing impairment, skin diseases, and musculoskeletal disorder [6, 10, 11].

Methods
Aim of this study
The aim of this study was to assess the level of self-reported safety practices and associated factors among workers in Dashen Brewery Share Company.

Study design
Institution based cross-sectional study.

Study area and period
Dashen Brewery Share Company is situated in the Gondar town, approximately 750 km away from Addis Ababa, the capital city of Ethiopia. It was established in 2000 and currently has 858 employees. It has been certified with ISO 9001 quality management system (QMS) and ISO 14001 environmental management system (EMS).

The study carried out from February to March 2016; Permanent and temporary workers who engaged in production process were included in the study.

Sample size and sampling technique
The sample size was determined using the formula for a single population proportion assuming a margin of error as 5%, expected proportion of safety practice as 58% [12], 95% confidence interval and 10% of non-respondent rate to came up with a sample size of 415 respondents.

We took a list of all production process workersfrom HumanResource department and used it as sampling frame.

The following procedures were followed to identify respondents from the sampling frame;

- First, Stratified sampling was employed assuming that workers in different department would exhibit different level of safety practices. The calculated sample size was allocated to each stratum proportionally to the sample size.

- Secondly, systematic random sampling was used to select respondent from each stratumand came up with a desired sample size of 415 fromthe following; 22 respondents from Quality department, 195 from Packaging department, 107 from Engineering department, 29 from Brewing department, and 62 from Loading and unloading function.

Operational definitions

- **Safety Practice:** Respondent's score out of 20 questions was graded as Good if ≥60%; and poor <60% [13].
- **Attitude:** Attitude of the participants regarding occupational safety and health calculated from 5 point Likert scale questions.Each question had a value of 1–5 that corresponds with the scale measurement. The participants' answer graded as good attitude if the cumulative answer is ≥80% (20–25), medium attitude if 60–79% (15–19) and poor attitude if (<59%) 0–14 [14].
- **Knowledge:** Participants asked to answer 9 knowledge questions about safety and health. Graded as having "Good knowledge" if they had answered correctly (≥80%) 7–9 questions, (60–80%)5–6 as "Medium level knowledge" and (<59%) 0–4 as "Poor knowledge" [14].
- **Job satisfaction:** Whether the worker was happy or not with the job that he or she had engaged currently [15].
- **Sleep disturbance problem:** The presence of sleeping problems when the worker was at work in the factory [16].
- **Chat chewers:** Chewing chat leaves by the worker at least once per week [16].
- **Management support:** was measured by 5 point Likert scale (Strongly agree =5, Agree =4, Moderate =3, Disagree =2, and Strongly disagree =1) [17].

Data collection tools
The data was collected using interview administered questionnaire and observation checklist. The data collection were carried out by six occupational safety and health degree graduates.Two supervisorswere also involved for monitoring data collection and checking the completeness of the questionnaires.

Data quality control
Training was given for data collectors and supervisors for 3 days on procedures, techniques and ways of collecting the data. Prior to the commencement of the actual data collection process, the questionnaire was pretested on 21 (5% of sample size) Pepsi soft drink industry workers and the necessary modification was made. Reliability test was conducted and the consistence

of the research tool was ascertained (Additional file 1). Clear introduction explaining the purpose and objective of the study was provided to the respondents on the first page of the questionnaire before data collection. In addition continuous and strict supervision and on spot checking was carried out during the data collection process.

Ethical consideration
Before data collection, ethical clearance was obtained from Institutional Review Board (IRB) of University Of Gondar, College of Medicine and Health Sciences. The company manager was communicated through formal letters from University of Gondar, Institute of Public Health and permission was obtained. Written consent was sought from each respondent after explaining the purpose and objectives of the study. Confidentiality was assured for information collected from study participants.Privacy was also ensured during the interview.

Data processing and analysis
Data was entered using Epi-Info version 7, andanalyzed using SPSS statistical package for windows, version 20.0. All assumptions applied to binary logistic regression including fitness of model were checked. To determine factors associated with self-reported level of safety practice, Binary Logistic Regression model was fitted and variables with a p-value <0.2 in bivariable analysis were included in the multi-variant analysis. A p-value of less than 5% in the multi-variable analysis wasconsidered statistically significant.Crude adds (COR) ratios and adjusted Odds ratios (AOR) with 95% confidence intervalare reportedin the result.

Results
A total of 415 (100%) respondents were interviewed. Of those individuals almost three fourth 308 (74.2%) of the participants were male. The majority 250 (60.2%) respondents were aged between 14 and 29 years, with mean (±SD) age of 28.18 (±8.67) years. Nearly half of them 207 (49.9%) were diploma holders. Furthermore, 224 (54.0%) were married and more than half of respondents 255 (69.9%) were permanently employed, of which 244 (58.8%) of the respondents had worked for less than or equal to 5 years (Table 1).

The current study showed that majority 362 (87.2%) of the workers reportedhaving good level of safety practices.

This study depicted that majority of workers 357 (86%) had utilized at least one type of personal protective equipment (PPE), while were working. For those who didn't use PPE, lack of PPE 155 (37.3%) and the feeling discomfort while using PPE 65 (15.7%) were the major reasons. The adherence level of safety procedures reported by the workers and their actual performance

Table 1 Distribution of Socio-demographic characteristics of respondents, Dashen Brewery Share Company workers ($N = 415$)

Variables	Number	Percent
Age (years)		
14–29	250	60.2
30+	165	39.8
Sex		
Male	308	74.2
Female	107	25.8
Educational level		
Grade 1–8	32	7.7
Grade 9–12	116	28
Diploma	207	49.9
Degree and above	60	14.5
Marital Status		
Married	224	54
Single	180	43.4
Divorced	8	1.9
Widowed	3	0.7
Work Experience (years)		
≤ 5	244	58.8
> 5	171	41.2
Employment Status		
Temporary	125	30.1
Permanent	290	69.9
Working Department		
Quality	22	5.3
Engineering	107	25.8
Packaging	195	47
Brewing	29	7
Loading/Unloading	62	14.9

ascertained by observation showed discrepancy, but it was not statistically significant ($P = 0.082$) (Table 2).

Multivariate analysis showed that socio-demographic factors; age, marital status, and employment status were found to be the determinant factors for safety practices. Similarly factors like, attitude towards safety practice, management support and training on safety and health were found to be determinant factors for having good safety practice in the study (Table 3).

Workers aged14–29 years were 7.2 times more likely to reporthaving good safety practice than older workers[AOR; 7.2;95%; CI; (1.9–26)]. Marital status of workers was also found to be associated with safety practice. Single workers were 86% less likely to reporthaving good safety practice than married workers [AOR; 0.1; 95%; CI; (0.04–0.4)].

Table 2 Use of utilization of safety methods ascertained by self-report from interviewees and by researcher's observation in Dashen Brewery Share Company. The difference rated by observation and self-report were tested by Mann-Whitney test and the result shows the difference was not significant ($p = 0.082$)

Safety Practice	Self-reported safety practices		Observed safety practices	
	Number	Percent (%)	Number	Percent (%)
Safety shoes	349	84.1	320	77.1
High visibility vest	348	83.9	314	75.7
Overall	341	82.2	310	74.7
Goggles	324	78.1	210	50.6
Gloves	294	70.8	205	49.4
Ear plugs	299	72	179	43.1
Helmet	42	10.1	4	1
Respirator	235	56.6	0	0
Followed the correct manual lifting techniques	178	42.9	149	35.9
Followed demarcated safe walk ways	313	75.4	259	62.4

Employment status showed a statistically significant association with safety practice; in which permanent workers 5.35 times more likely to reportgood safety practice than their counterparts[AOR; 5.4; 95%; CI; (1.3–21.5)].

Workers who reported good attitude towards safety practice were 20.3 times more likely to report good safety practice than employees who reporting poor attitude [AOR; 20.3; 95%; CI; (5.8–71.1)]. The study also revealed that workers who perceived they had support by management were 11.9 times more likely to report good safety practice than workers who perceived they didn't get management support [AOR; 12.0;95%; CI; (3.4–41.9). On the other hand, those workers who attended safety and health training were 4.5 times more likely to reporthaving good safety practice than workers who didn't get safety and health training [AOR; 4.5; 95%; CI; (1.2–16.3)] (Table 3).

Discussion

The level of self-reported safety practices in Dashen Brewery was very good; in which 87.2% of the workers reported to comply with good level of safety practices. The result of this study is in agreement with the study conducted among pipeline workers in Nigeria that report 85.9% of the workers having good safety practice [13]. On the other hand, the level of self-reported safety practice was relatively good compared to other studies conducted in Ethiopia among laboratory workers 39.3% [18], in Iran among chemical industry workers 70% [19], and also in Iran among steel manufacturing workers 58.2% [20].The reason for high safety practice by workers might be related to the adoption of principles of QMS and EMS by the company. Activities undertaken to qualify for these systems might have a positive effect on safety practice of the workers. Hence, our findings

may support that implementing QMS andEMS to improvesafety and health is very crucial [21, 22].

Though not statistically significant, the discrepancy on the level of adherence to safety procedures based on self-report by the workers and actual performance ascertained by observation might be due to social desirability bias. The bias could be apparent if less robust data collection tools and techniques are used during face to face interview. Hence, adopting robust data collection tools and techniques are very important to minimize the bias [23]. In the current study, we have used pre-tested, validated and robust tools for data collection to overcome the problem.

This study found that younger workers were more likely to report good safety practices than old workers. This finding is in agreement with a study from India [24].The possible explanation could be younger workers show better motivation and information about safety and health as shown in our result. However, other studies conducted in Ethiopia found that younger workers were more likely to suffer from occupational injury thanolder workers [7, 12, 16]. In general as employees grow older, the behavior of workers improved [19, 20, 25, 26].

In our study, marital status was also significantly associated with safety practices.Married workers were more likely to report good safety practice than singles. This finding is consistent with study conducted in Komobolcha textile factory, Ethiopia [15]. One possible reason for this might be thatmarried workers wanted to take care of themselves due to their concerns for being able to provide for their partners and families [15].

Employment status was also found to be a significant predictor of safety practice; permanent workers being more likely to report good safety practice than temporary workers. This finding was consistent with another study conducted in Ethiopia [27]. The possible

Table 3 Multivariable analysis of predictors for self-reported safety practice in Dashen Brewery Share Company workers (N = 415)

Variables	Safety Practice		Crude OR (95%CI)	Adjusted OR (95%CI)
	Good n (%)	Poor n (%)		
Age (years)				
14–29	229 (91.6)	21 (8.4)	2.6 (1.5,4.7)*	7.2 (1.9,26)**
30+	133 (80.6)	32 (19.4)	1.0	1.00
Sex				
Male	274 (89)	34 (11)	1.7 (0.9,3.2)	
Female	88 (82.2)	19 (17.8)	1.0	
Educational level				
Grade 1–8	19 (59.4)	13 (40.6)	1.0	
Grade 9–12	86 (74.1)	30 (25.9)	2.0 (0.86,4.44)	
Diploma	198 (95.7)	9 (4.3)	15.0 (5.6,39.7)	
Degree and above	59 (98.3)	1 (1.7)	40.3 (4.9329)	
Marital status				
Married	212 (94.6)	12 (5.4)	1.0	1.0
Single	140 (77.8)	40 (22.2)	0.2 (0.1,0.39)*	0.1 (0.04,0.42)**
Working department				
Quality	20 (90.9)	2 (9.1)	1.0	
Engineering	102 (95.3)	5 (4.7)	2.0 (0.37,11.3)	
Packaging	176 (90.3)	19 (9.7)	0.9 (0.2,4.3)	
Brewing	26 (89.3)	3 (10.3)	0.9 (0.13,5.7)	
Loading/Unloading	38 (61.3)	24 (38.7)	0.2 (0.03,0.74)	
Employment Status				
Temporary	84 (67.2)	41 (32.8)	1.0	1.0
Permanent	278 (95.9)	12 (4.1)	11.3 (5.7,22.5)*	5.4 (1.3,21.54)**
Knowledge				
Good	285 (90.5)	30 (9.5)	4.0 (1.5,11.4)*	
Medium	63 (78.8)	17 (21.5)	1.6 (0.5,4.8)	
Poor	14 (70)	6 (30)	1.0	
Attitude				
Good	209 (96.8)	7 (3.2)	33.6 (13.9,81.8)*	20.3 (5.8,71.05)**
Medium	121 (92.4)	10 (7.6)	13.6 (6.1,30.3)*	10.7 (3.2,35.9)**
Poor	32 (47.1)	36 (52.9)	1.0	1.0
Job satisfaction				
Yes	216 (89.3)	26 (10.7)	1.5 (0.86,2.74)	
No	146 (84.4)	27 (15.6)	1.0	
Management support				
Yes	252 (96.6)	9 (3.4)	11.0 (5.3,23.7)*	12.0 (3.4,41.9)**
No	110 (71.4)	44 (28.6)	1.0	1.0
Safety and health Training				
Yes	228 (96.6)	8 (3.4)	9.6 (4.4,20.9)*	4.5 (1.2,16.3)**
No	134 (74.9)	45 (25.1)	1.0	1.0

Note: 1:0 = Reference, * Significant at P value <0.02, ** Significant at P value <0.05

explanation for this could be the difference in benefit packages, the company provides to permanent and temporary workers. Hence, temporary workers have limited access to basic safety training and use of personal protective devices. In another study conducted in Spain, the authors reasoned that job dissatisfaction and less knowledge and experience of the workplace were associated with high prevalence of occupational injury among temporary workers [28].

In the current study, attitude were associated with safety practice. This finding is in accordance corroborate with a study conducted among chemical industry workers in Iran [19]. Moreover, Another Iranian study in gas refineries reported a decrease in number of accidents with increasing safety attitudes [29]. The possible reason for this might be the existence of a direct relationship between good attitude toward safety and the actual safety practice among workers.

In this study, management support was a significant determinant factor for safety. The findings was congruent with studies conducted across the globe [30–33]. The result of this study is also in line with the view of the British Health and Safety Executive (HSE) [33]. The reason for this finding might be due to the fact that employees behave according to good safety practices when they perceive that the management value them and cares for their personal well-being.

In the present study, respondents who got safety and health training were more likely to report good safety practice than their counterparts. The result was also like the findings of a study conducted in Tendaho, Ethiopia [27]. Safety training was also indicated as important barrier for work-related injuries in different industries [10, 34]. This is based on the idea that training make employees aware of possible dangers and ways to avoid occupational injury.

Conclusion

The reported level of safety practice in this study was good. Management commitment to safety is an important factor for safety of industry workers. Training of new employees as well as temporary and permanent workers about safety and health specifically on the nature of the work place, hazard prevention and control methods is very important and should be provided regularly. Well-designed work procedures, which are fitting to the specific working conditions, should be readily available to improve adherence of hazard preventive measures, like PPE.

Acknowledgements
We would like to thank University of Gondar, College of Medicine and Health Sciences for providing ethical clearance for his study. We also like to express our gratitude forDashen Brewery Share Company management staffs and study participants.

Funding
We received logistic and financial support from University of Goondar to undertake the research project.

Authors' contributions
STH was responsible for generating the concept of this research paper, literature review and organization, preparation of draft research proposal document, organizing data collection process, and preparation of draft data analysis and interpretation. DHCparticipated in proposal research design process, data analysis, and presentation and interpretation process of result, preparation of scientific paper or the manuscript, and corresponding author of the manuscript. AD participated in proposal research design process, data analysis, and presentation and interpretation process of result, preparation of scientific paper or the manuscript, and corresponding author of the manuscript. All authors read and approved the final manuscript.

Competing interests
The authors declare that they have no competing interests.

References
1. Quartey SH, Puplampu BB. Employee health and safety practices: an exploratory and comparative study of the shipping and manufacturing industries in Ghana. Int J Business Manage. 2012;7(23):81–95.
2. ILO. Safety and health at work: a vision for sustainable prevention: XX World Congress on Safety and Health at Work: Global Forum for Prevention, 24–27 August 2014, Frankfurt, Germany. International Labour Office; 2014.
3. Jahan S, Jespersen E, Mukherjee S, Kovacevic M, Bonini A, Calderon C, Lucic S, et al. Human development report 2015: work for human development. New York: UNDP; 2015.
4. Cal/OSHA Consultation Service. Ergonomics in Action: A Guide to Best Practices for the Food-Processing Industry.Department of Industrial Relations, Research and Education Unit. California Department of Industrial Relations; 2003. p. 82.
5. Mbonigaba E. To assess the prevalence of occupational health related risks and use of safety measures among employees in Bralirwa processing industries in Rwanda. Occup Med Health Aff. 2015;
6. Chetty L. A study to determine the occupational health and safety knowledge, practices and injury patterns of workers at a specific beverage manufacturing company. Cape Town: University of Cape Town; 2006.
7. Tadesse T, Kumie A. Prevalence and factors affecting work-related injury among workers engaged in small and medium-scale Industries in Gondar wereda, north Gondar zone, Amhara regional state, Ethiopia. Ethiop J Health Dev. 2007;21(1):25.
8. Mulu G. Assessment of occupational injury and associated factors among Mugher cement factory workers. Ethiopia.AAU: Mugher; 2014.
9. Howe J. Warning: behavior-based safety can be hazardous to your Health & Safety Program. Occupational Health & Safety-Newsletter of the UAW Health & Safety Department. 1998;4:6.
10. Bankole A, Ibrahim L. Perceived influence of health education on occupational health of factory workers in Lagos state, Nigeria. British J Arts Soc Sci. 2012;8(1):57–65.
11. Tomoda S. Occupational safety and health in the food and drink industries. Geneva: International Labour Organization; 1993.
12. Berhe A, Yemane D, Gebresilassie A, Terefe W, Ingale L. Magnitude of occupational injuries and associated factors among small-scale industry Workers in Mekelle City, northern Ethiopia: Occupational Medicine & Health Affairs; 2015.
13. Adebola JO. Knowledge, attitude and compliance with occupational health and safety practices among pipeline products and marketing company (PPMC) staff in Lagos. Merit Res J Med Med Sci. 2014;2:158–73.

14. Trunong CD, Siriwnog W, Roboson MG. Knowledge, attutude, and practice on using personal protective equipment of rattan craftsmen in trade village at Kienxuong district, Thaibinh province, Vietnam. College of Public Health Sciences, Chulalongkorn University; 2008;26–38 .

15. Yessuf SS, Moges HG, Ahmed AN. Determinants of occupational injury in Kombolcha textile factory, north-East Ethiopia. Int J Occup Environ Med. 2014;5(2):84–93.

16. Aderaw Z, Engdaw D, Tadesse T. Determinants of occupational injury: a case control study among textile factory workers in Amhara regional state, Ethiopia. J Trop Med. 2011;2011. doi:10.1155/2011/657275.

17. Hosny G, Elgamal A, Mostafa M, Shalaby E-SA. The Different Perspectives of Safety Managerial Practices in Safety Certified Management System: A Case study. Organization; 2015. 7: p. 8.

18. Wondwossen K. Assessment of knowledge, attitude and practice towards occupational health and safety among medical laboratory personnel in selected governmental teaching hospitals of Ethiopia. Addis Ababa: AAU; 2015.

19. Nasab HS, Tavakoli R, Ghofranipour F, Kazemnejad A, Khavanin A. Evaluation of knowledge, attitude and behavior of workers towards occupational health and safety. Iran J Public Health. 2009;38(2):125–9.

20. Azadeh A, Mohammad FI. The evaluation of importance of safety behaviors in a steel manufacturer by entropy. J Res Health Sci. 2009;9(2):10–8.

21. Christini G, Fetsko M, Hendrickson C. Environmental management systems and ISO 14001 certification for construction firms. J Constr Eng Manag. 2004;130(3):330–6.

22. Levine DI, Toffel MW. Quality management and job quality: how the ISO 9001 standard for quality management systems affects employees and employers. Manag Sci. 2010;56(6):978–96.

23. Pannucci CJ, Wilkins EG. Identifying and avoiding bias in research. Plast Reconstr Surg. 2010;26(2):619.

24. Ghosh AK, Bhattacherjee A, Chau N. Relationships of working conditions and individual characteristics to occupational injuries: a case-control study in coal miners. J Occup Health. 2004;46(6):470–80.

25. Ibrahim M, Al Hallaq K, Enshassi A. Safety climate in construction industry the case of Gaza strip. 4th international engineering conference–towards engineering of 21st century. Gaza Strip: Islamic University in Gaza; 2012.

26. Opong-Addoh MA. Factors influencing adherence to safety protocols in Ghanaian industries: University of Ghana; 2013.

27. Yiha O, Kumie A. Assessment of occupational injuries in Tendaho agricultural d\development SC, afar regional state. Ethiop J Health Dev. 2010;24(3):167–74.

28. Benavides FG, Benach J, Muntaner C, Delclos GL, Catot N, Amable M. Associations between temporary employment and occupational injury: what are the mechanisms? Occup Environ Med. 2006;63(6):416–21.

29. Monazzam M, Soltanzadeh A. The relationship between the worker's safety attitude and the registered accidents. J Res Health Sci. 2009;9(1):17–20.

30. Michael JH, Evans DD, Jansen KJ, Haight JM. Management commitment to safety as organizational support: relationships with non-safety outcomes in wood manufacturing employees. J Saf Res. 2005;36(2):171–9.

31. Iskandar BS. Linking Management Safety Commitment and Employees' Satisfaction on Working Conditions: A Case Study in a Manufacturing Automotive Industry. 2004.

32. Garcia A, Boix P, Canosa C. Why do workers behave unsafely at work? Determinants of safe work practices in industrial workers. Occup Environ Med. 2004;61(3):239–46.

33. Executive HAS. Successful health and safety management, A.P.A.U.n.O. Unit), Editor. 2008: UK. 98.

34. Kiani F, Khodabakhsh MR, Saffarinia M. The role of attitude towards safety as a mediator of safety training effectiveness to fatalism. Health Educ Health Promot. 2014;1(2):61–75.

10

Toll-like receptor 9 partially regulates lung inflammation induced following exposure to chicken barn air

David Schneberger, Gurpreet Aulakh, Shankaramurthy Channabasappa and Baljit Singh*

Abstract

Background: Exposure to animal barn air is an occupational hazard that causes lung dysfunction in barn workers. Respiratory symptoms experienced by workers are typically associated with endotoxin and TLR4 signalling, but within these environments gram negative bacteria constitute only a portion of the total microbial population. In contrast, unmethylated DNA can be found in all bacteria, some viruses, and mold. We hypothesized that in such environments TLR9, which binds unmethylated DNA, contributes to the overall immune responses in the lung.

Methods: Using a mouse model, wild-type and TLR9$^{-/-}$ mice were exposed to chicken barn air for 1, 5, or 20 days. Blood serum and bronchiolar lavage fluid was tested against a panel of six TLR9-induced cytokines (IL-1β, IL-6, IL-10, IL-12, TNFα, and IFNγ) for changes in expression. Bronchiolar lavage fluid (BAL) was also tested for macrophage as well as monocyte migration.

Results: There were significant decreases in serum TNFα after a single day exposure in TLR9$^{-/-}$ mice. BAL concentrations of TNFα and IFNγ, as well as TNFα in serum in TLR9$^{-/-}$ mice were also reduced after barn exposure for 5 days. After 20 days of exposure IFNγ was significantly reduced in lavage of TLR9$^{-/-}$ mice. Myeloperoxidase (MPO) accumulation in the lung was reduced at 20 days of exposure in TLR9$^{-/-}$ mice, as was total lavage cell counts. However, Masson's staining revealed no apparent lung histological differences between any of the treatment groups.

Conclusions: Taken together our data show TLR9 plays a partial role in lung inflammation induced following exposure to chicken barn air potentially through binding of unmethylated DNA.

Keywords: Barn dust, TLR9, CpG DNA, Macrophages, Neutrophils, BAL

Background

Workers in high-intensity livestock operations have been recognized to be at risk for a number of chronic respiratory problems including bronchitis, rhinitis, chronic cough and phlegm, occupational asthma, and organic dust toxic syndrome to name a few [1–3]. Workers in such facilities are exposed to a wide variety of agents such as ammonia, hydrogen sulfide, dust particles, and lipopolysaccharide (LPS) [3, 4]. Even single exposure to such facilities has been shown to elevate a number of pro-inflammatory cytokines in nasal lavages and serum,

and induce lung inflammation [5–7]. The mechanisms of these complex in vivo pulmonary responses are not fully understood.

Endotoxin has been targeted as a critical component responsible for many of the lung problems seen in exposure to barn air [1, 7, 8]. More recent work however suggests that within chicken barns, endotoxin-producing gram-negative bacteria comprise only a small fraction of the bacterial species, and that these bacteria may be in the minority as far as total numbers of bacteria present [4]. In contrast, all bacteria and some viruses and mold contain unmethylated DNA in their genomes, which induces a variety of cytokines through binding the TLR9 receptor. Many of these cytokines are similar to those induced by endotoxin, which binds TLR4 [9]. Previous

* Correspondence: Baljit.singh@usask.ca
Department of Veterinary Biomedical Sciences, Western College of Veterinary Medicine, University of Saskatchewan, 52 Campus Drive, Saskatoon, SK S7N 5B4, Canada

work had shown that DNA from barn dust extracts could induce IL-10 and IL-12p40 [10], however this system exposed isolated peripheral blood mononuclear cells to purified DNA in vitro. This may not be an optimal reflection of barn and in vivo conditions, where significant production of cytokines may occur in the lung from a variety of cell types. Further, such a system does not account for effects of numerous other components in the air that may synergize with or counter responses through TLR9. Therefore, before we dissect the cellular effects in in vitro systems, we need in vivo animal model studies to understand the lung responses to chicken barn air.

Recently, we delineated expression of TLR9 in mouse and human lungs using in situ hybridization and light and electron microscope immunocytochemistry [11]. We have also reported TLR9 expression in cattle, horses, dogs and pigs that spend their lives in barns or other animal containment facilities [12, 13]. This series of studies provided the first data to show in situ expression of TLR9 in airway epithelium, alveolar septal cells and alveolar macrophages. We used this TLR9 expression data to hypothesize that TLR9 promotes in vivo lung inflammation induced by single or multiple exposures to chicken barn air. We tested this hypothesis by exposing TLR9$^{-/-}$ and wild-type mice to chicken barn air for 1, 5, or 20 days. The data show that TLR9 has a partial role in lung inflammation induced following exposure to chicken barn air.

Methods
Animals
The experimental protocols were approved by the University of Saskatchewan Committee on Animal Care Assurance and all experiments conducted according to guidelines of the Canadian Council on Animal Care. Breeding pairs of TLR9-deficient mice (C57BL/6 background) were a gift from Dr. Heather Davis and obtained from Taconic. Knockout status was confirmed by PCR on mouse lung tissue. Mice were raised at the Western College of Veterinary Medicine Animal Care Unit. C57BL/6 (wild type) mice where obtained from the Animal Resource Centre at the University of Saskatchewan.

Experimental exposure
Mice were transported in sealed cages with vents and driven to a cage-based chicken barn in the morning and placed on a shelf approximately 1.8 m (6 ft) off the ground. Mice were kept in barn for 8 h and then returned to animal care facilities at the University of Saskatchewan where they were transferred out of their cages for the evening. Each group consisted of 6 animals per group. Each exposure group was split into two to three subgroups for transport to the barn to ensure that

variation of barn or transport conditions on a single day would not account for changes seen in an exposure group. Mice were taken to the barn for 1, 5, or 20 days. The 20 day exposure animals were rested for 2 days after each cycle of 5 exposures to mimic a 5 day work week exposure. Parallel control groups of mice that were transported but not exposed to barn air were transported in separate cages along with the exposed mice.

Tissue, blood, and lavage collection
At the end of exposure time mice were euthanized (100 mg/kg ketamine + 20 mg/kg xylazine, intraperitoneal injection), and blood was collected by cardiac puncture (Sandoz, Boucherville, QC, Canada). Collection was done approximately 2 h after leaving the barn environment. Blood was separated into serum for cytokine analyses by centrifugation at 2000 g for 10 min in Vacutainer tubes (BD, Franklin Lakes, NJ). BAL fluid was collected by flushing lungs with 3 ml of cold HEPES buffer and centrifuged at 400 g for 10 min and stored at −80 °C for later use, while the cell pellet was resuspended in 100 μl HEPES and counted with a haemocytometer (Hausser Scientific, Horsham, PA). Cells were resuspended to 800 μl, counted and cytospun onto microscope slides at 1000 rpm for 10 min, and dried overnight before staining with a Hemacolor kit (EMD Chemicals, Mississauga, ON, Canada) according to manufacturer's protocol. The macrophage and neutrophil counts were converted to absolute numbers. Unfortunately, we lost some of samples from mice exposed five times to chicken barn air during processing and thus cell counts for 5 day exposure were not included in the final analysis.

Lung sections were divided in two, and one half snapfrozen in liquid nitrogen and stored at −80 °C. The other lung was fixed in 4 % paraformaldehyde overnight before dehydration and embedding in paraffin. Lung tissue sections were stained using Masson's trichrome stain as well as for hematoxylin-eosin, and mounted with cover slips.

Protein extraction
Frozen mouse lung tissue was homogenized in microcentrifuge tubes using a pestle (Bel-art, Pequannock, NJ, USA). Protein was extracted using an AllPrep DNA/RNA/Protein purification kit (Qiagen, Mississauga, ON, CA) as per manufacturer's instructions. Protein fractions were saved, quantified, and stored at −80 °C.

Dust and endotoxin measurement
Dust samples were collected from two random days of exposure on days when animals from 1,5, and 20 day animals were present in the facility. A Sensidyne constant air-flow pump (GilAir-3, Clearwater, FL) run at 2 L per

minute was used with a glass fiber filter (1.0 mm binder free type AE; SKC Inc., Eighty Four, PA). The filter was weighed prior to use. Sampling was done at the same location as animal housing in the barn facility for 8 h. Dust was resuspended in 1 ml of water and tested by Limulus Amoebocyte Lysate assay (Cambrex Bioscience, Walkersville, MD) for endotoxin. DNA purification was attempted using a QiaAmp DNA Mini Kit (Qiagen, Mississauga, ON, CA) and quantified using NanoDrop 1000 spectrophotometer (Thermo Scientific, Wilmington, DE)

Myeloperoxidase assay

Briefly, protein samples were placed on a 96-well plate at several concentrations in phosphate citrate buffer (0.2 M Na_2HPO_4 – $7H_2O$, 0.1 M citric acid, pH 5.0) in duplicate along with a recombinant standard. TMB substrate was added to all wells and developed for 2 min at room temperature before reaction was stopped with 1 M H_2SO_4 and read at a450.

Immunohistochemistry

Immunohistology was done on 5 µm thick lung tissue sections. Briefly, after de-paraffinization, rehydration, tissue peroxidase quenching (0.5 % hydrogen peroxide in methanol), and antigen unmasking with pepsin (2 mg/mL 0.01 N hydrochloric acid), the tissue sections were blocked for 1 h with 1 % BSA to block nonspecific binding. Sections were treated with F4/80 (1:75 dilution) and incubated overnight at 4 °C. The next day horseradish peroxidase-conjugated goat anti-rabbit antibody (ab6845, Abcam) was added at 1:100 dilution for 1 h at 37 °C. Color was developed using a color developing kit (Vector Laboratories, Ontario, Canada). Slides were counterstained with methyl green (Vector Laboratories) before mounting. A control was similarly run with omission of the primary antibody or the secondary antibody. We counted F4/80 positive cells in the alveolar septa of lungs to quantify number of septal macrophages. The counts were made in three fields in 4 mice randomly selected from each group in the study at 100X magnification.

Serum and BAL cytokine bio-plex enzyme linked immunosorbent assay

Cytokines IL-1β, IL-6, IL-10, IL-12, IFNγ, and TNFα were measured using bead-conjugated antibodies and recombinant standards with the Bio-Plex multiplex ELISA assay system (Bio-Rad, Mississauga ON, Canada). Assay was carried out as per manufacturer's instructions for magnetic bead ELISA and read on a Bio-Plex 200 plate reader (Bio-Rad, Mississauga ON, Canada). Lavage fluid and serum were centrifuged prior to use as described earlier.

Statistical analysis

All values given were given as mean values with error bars representing standard deviation. One-way ANOVA was preformed to determine significance between groups. Two-way ANOVA was done to assess effect of genotype versus exposure day, with p values generated by Bonferroni post-test.

Results

Dust and endotoxin measurement

Dust and endotoxin were measured in the barn over the same period of animal exposure. The average amount of respirable dust for an 8 h exposure was 1.738 µg with a standard deviation of 0.067. The levels of endotoxin measured were 3966 EU/mg of dust. These levels are less than half of those found in a comparable study [14]. Dust levels were also low in comparison. Attempts were made to purify DNA from the samples. An attempt to purify DNA from samples yielded only a single success of 1.065 µg/ml, or 0.6129 µg/µg dust, although this was near the limit of detection.

BAL total cell numbers

There were no differences in total BAL cell numbers between one day or 20 day control TLR9$^{-/-}$ and WT animals or those exposed for one day to chicken barn air (Fig. 1). The total BAL cell numbers were significantly lower in TLR9$^{-/-}$ mice compared to WT mice after 20 exposures (p ≤ 0.05).

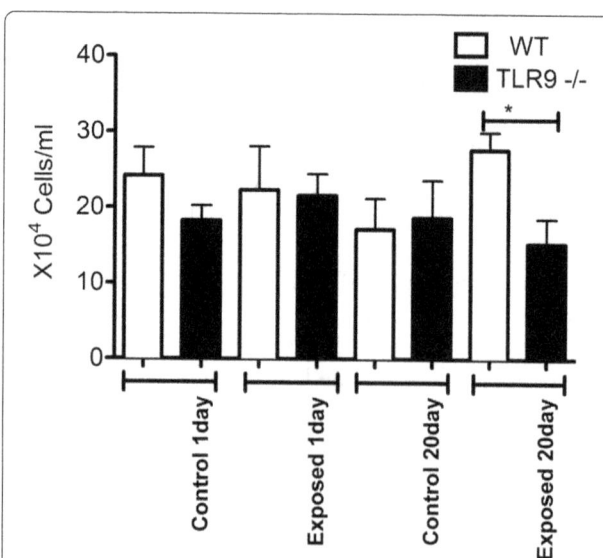

Fig. 1 BAL cell counts. BAL from exposed and unexposed WT and TLR9-deficient (TLR9-) mice (n = 6) was spun briefly at 400 g, supernatant removed, and cells resuspended to 100 µl for counting with hemocytometer. BAL cell numbers were lower in TLR9$^{-/-}$ mice compared to WT mice after 20 exposures (* = p ≤ 0.05)

Neutrophil recruitment into BAL and lung tissues

There were no effects of number of exposures and the strain on the numbers of neutrophils in BAL (Fig. 2). We used an MPO assay as a surrogate for neutrophils trapped in the lung tissues that are not amenable to lavage. MPO assay did not reveal any differences in neutrophil recruitment in lung tissues between the WT and TLR9$^{-/-}$ control mice as well as those exposed once or five times to barn air (Fig. 3). However, after 20 exposures there were reduced MPO concentrations ($p \leq 0.05$) in lung homogenates from TLR9$^{-/-}$ animals compared to similarly exposed WT mice. This reduction was not significantly lower than the unexposed control though.

Macrophage recruitment into BAL and lung tissues

In addition to neutrophils, macrophages are important players in promoting or resolving lung inflammation. There were no differences in macrophage BAL numbers from normal one day WT and TLR9$^{-/-}$ mice (Fig. 4). However, TLR9$^{-/-}$ mice had more macrophages in BAL compared to WT mice after single exposure ($p \leq 0.05$). Interestingly, the BAL macrophage numbers were lower in 20 day exposed TLR9$^{-/-}$ mice compared to 20 day wild type exposed animals ($p \leq 0.05$).

To determine the number of tissue macrophages in lavaged lungs, we stained lung sections with macrophage F4/80 antibody. Single exposure to barn air induced a significant decrease in the number of septal macrophages in TLR9$^{-/-}$ and wild-type mice compared to unexposed mice at the same time point (Fig. 5, $p \leq 0.05$ and $p \leq 0.01$). Septal macrophages were significantly

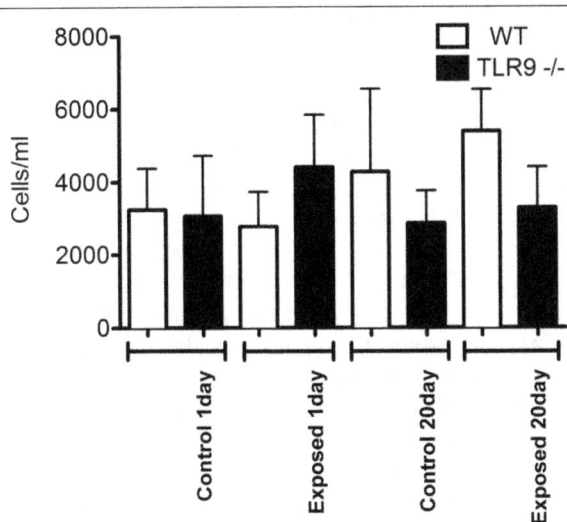

Fig. 3 Myeloperoxidase activity assay for lung neutrophil quantitation. TMB substrate was added to protein extracts of whole lung tissue from exposed and unexposed WT and TLR9-deficient (TLR9-) mice and read at a450 after 2 min ($n = 6$). Activity was assessed by comparison to a standard curve. A reduction was seen in 20 day exposed TLR9- mice compared to WT mice exposed for the same time (* = $p \leq 0.05$)

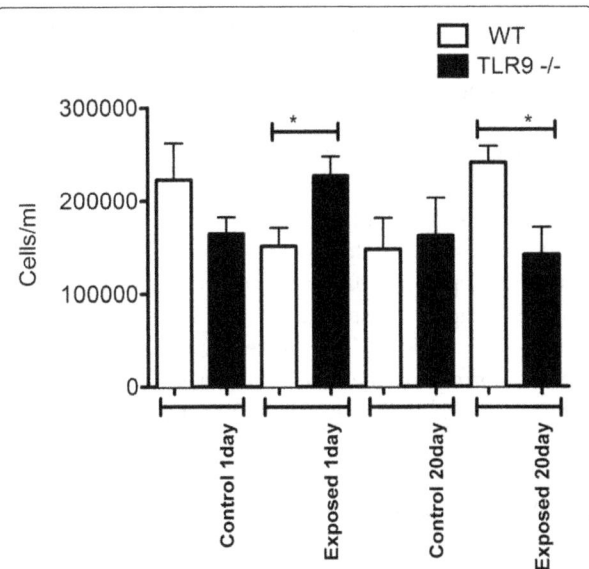

Fig. 2 Neutrophil cell counts. BAL from exposed and unexposed WT and TLR9-deficient (TLR9-) mice ($n = 6$) was spun briefly at 400 g, supernatant removed, and cells resuspended and stained with a hemacolor kit. Neutrophils were counted and numbers converted to absolute numbers. No significant differences were seen in neutrophil counts between any groups

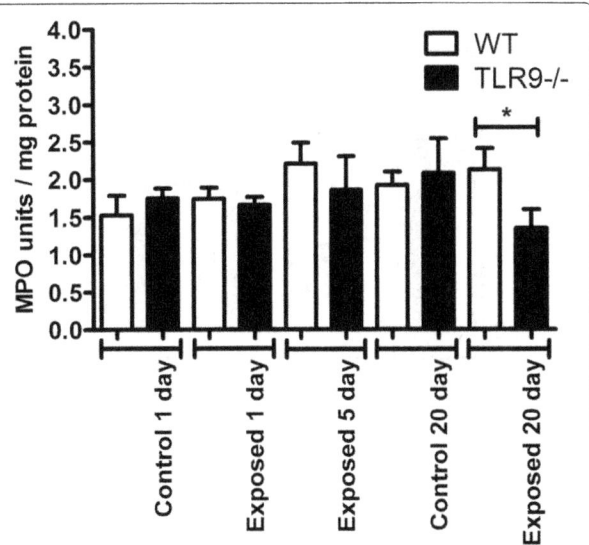

Fig. 4 Macrophage cell counts. BAL from exposed and unexposed WT and TLR9-deficient (TLR9-) mice ($n = 6$) was spun briefly at 400 g, supernatant removed, and cells resuspended and stained with a hemacolor kit. Macrophages were counted and numbers converted to absolute numbers. Macrophage numbers were higher in 1 day exposed TLR9$^{-/-}$ animals compared to WT mice (* = $p \leq 0.05$). A similar increase was seen in 20 day control TLR9$^{-/-}$ mice compared to WT mice exposed for the same time (* = $p \leq 0.05$)

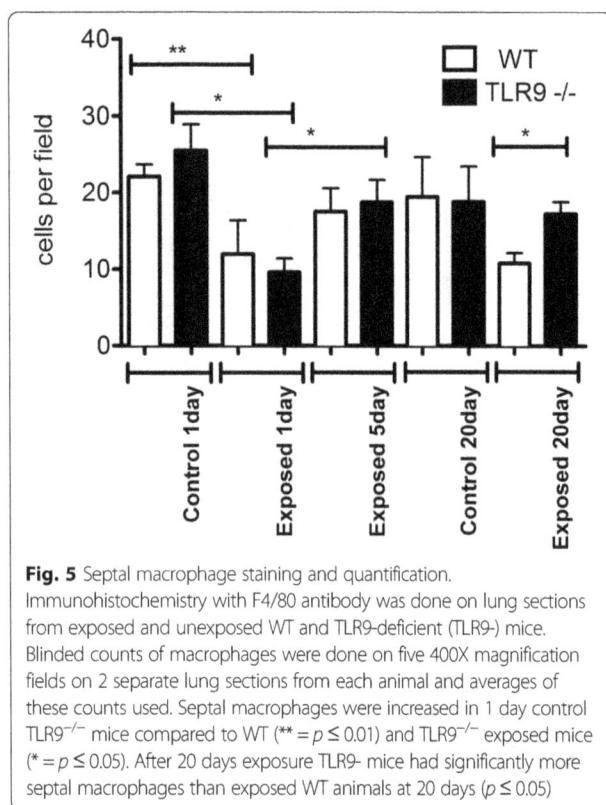

Fig. 5 Septal macrophage staining and quantification. Immunohistochemistry with F4/80 antibody was done on lung sections from exposed and unexposed WT and TLR9-deficient (TLR9-) mice. Blinded counts of macrophages were done on five 400X magnification fields on 2 separate lung sections from each animal and averages of these counts used. Septal macrophages were increased in 1 day control TLR9$^{-/-}$ mice compared to WT (** = $p \leq 0.01$) and TLR9$^{-/-}$ exposed mice (* = $p \leq 0.05$). After 20 days exposure TLR9- mice had significantly more septal macrophages than exposed WT animals at 20 days ($p \leq 0.05$)

increased in TLR9$^{-/-}$ mice after five exposures compared to a single exposure. The number of septal macrophages were significantly higher ($p \leq 0.05$) in 20 day exposed TLR9$^{-/-}$ mice compared to similarly exposed WT mice, however these values were still lower than unexposed animals. A two-way ANOVA analysis of genotype versus day of exposure failed to show any significance.

Histological assessment of lung tissues
Lung tissue sections stained with Masson's stain did not show any apparent differences in extracellular connective tissue (Fig. 6). Histologically, the lung sections from control WT and TLR9$^{-/-}$ mice appeared similar and showed normal architecture. There were no histological differences observed after 5 or 20 exposures to chicken barn air.

Expression and quantification of cytokines in lung BAL and serum
A panel of cytokines (IL-1β, IL-6, IL-10, IL-12, IFNγ, and TNFα) were examined in serum and BAL. Of these cytokines significant differences were detected for only IFNγ and TNFα in BAL (Fig. 7) and TNFα in serum (Fig. 8). We do note however that no IL-12 was detected in any samples. There were significantly lower concentrations of TNFα in BAL (Fig. 7a) from TLR9$^{-/-}$ mice compared to WT mice after five exposures barn ($p \leq 0.05$). The levels of

IFNγ in BAL (Fig. 7b) were lower in TLR9$^{-/-}$ mice compared to WT mice after five and 20 exposures to chicken barn ($p \leq 0.05$). There was significantly reduced concentrations of TNFα in serum (Fig. 8) of TLR9$^{-/-}$ mice compared to WT mice after one and five exposures to chicken barn air ($p \leq 0.05$).

Discussion
Chicken barn air has a complex biochemical and microbial composition. Inhalation of chicken barn air is therefore expected to engender a complex inflammatory response in the lungs of humans. Two major components of chicken barn air are endotoxin and unmethylated-CpG DNA. CpG originate from all bacteria, some viruses and molds, and bind to TLR9, initiating an immune response. Previous in vitro work on the effects of purified bacterial DNA on peripheral blood mononuclear cells has alluded to its role in lung immune responses [10]. To better understand the role of CpG in lung dysfunction in chicken barn workers we exposed TLR9$^{-/-}$ mice to chicken barn air for 8 h, to approximately simulate a full work day in a barn facility. The data show a partial role for TLR9, and indirectly CpG, in lung inflammation following exposure to chicken barn air.

The cell numbers in BAL are used as an indicator of lung inflammation [15]. As indicated in Materials and Methods, we unfortunately lost some of the samples from five day exposure group and omitted this group from BAL cell analyses. Our data showed no differences in total BAL cell counts between the one and 20 day control and one day exposed WT and TLR9$^{-/-}$ mice. After 20 exposures however, TLR9$^{-/-}$ mice had significantly lower total BAL cell numbers compared to WT mice. There were no effect of TLR9 on neutrophil numbers in BAL. Also, after 20 exposures, TLR9$^{-/-}$ mice showed higher numbers of septal macrophages compared to WT. Interestingly, the MPO content, indicative of neutrophils left in the lung tissues after BAL has been performed, was also lower in the knockout mice compared the WT after 20 exposures but not after one or five exposures. However, lack of perfusion of the lungs may also be responsible for some of the variation. Taken together, these cellular and histological data suggest lower lung inflammation in TLR9−/− mice compared to WT mice in longer term exposure.

The results of the current study are in contrast to the effect of pig barn air where significant increase in total neutrophil and macrophage numbers in BAL was noticed after a single exposure [16]. The reasons for the differences are not addressed by our experiments but could be related to the higher amount of endotoxin in the air in pig barn because deficiency of TLR4 resulted in significant reduction in total, neutrophil and

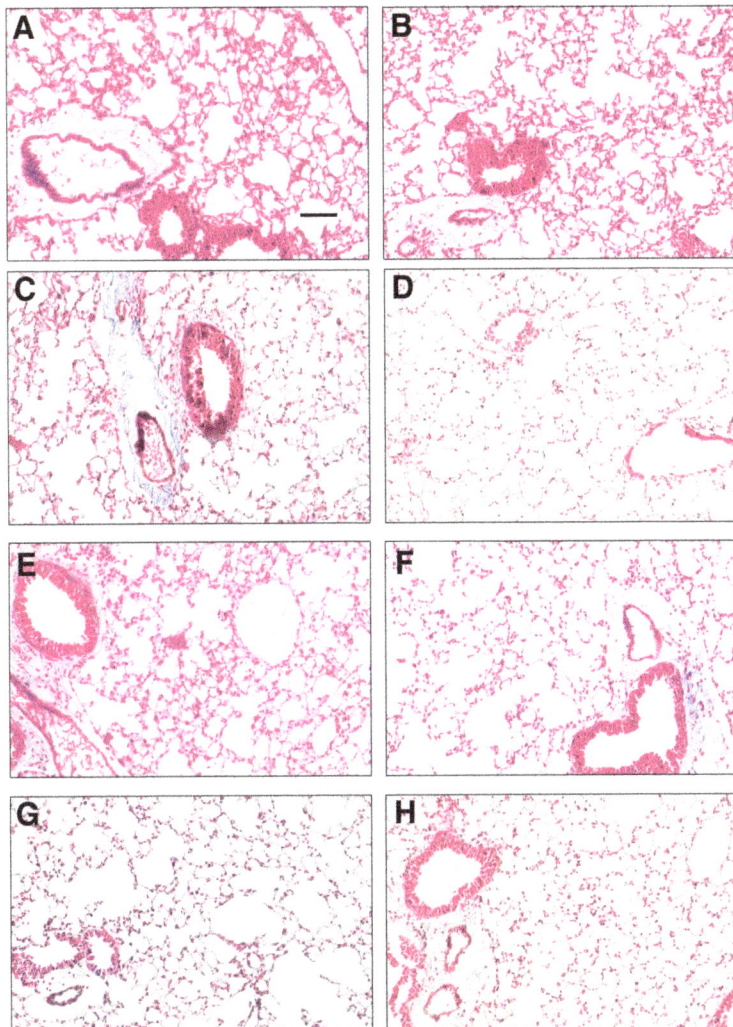

Fig. 6 Histopathology of lung samples. Histological assessment shows normal histology in unexposed WT (**a**) and unexposed mutant (**b**). One day exposed WT (**c**) and TLR9$^{-/-}$animals (**d**). WT mice exposed for five days (**e**) showed little difference to the 5 day exposed mutant mice (**f**). Lung sections from both WT (**g**) and mutant mice (**h**) exposed for 20 days showed normal histology. Bar = 100 micron

macrophage BAL numbers compared to the WT animals exposed to pig barn air [5, 7]. There are also likely differences in the total exposure doses found in each barn which could also account for these changes. Second, the differences could be related to the microbial content in chicken and pig barns as even the WT animals didn't show acute inflammation as experienced after exposure to pig barn air. The migration of inflammatory cells into alveolar spaces is regulated through development of a chemotactic gradient produced through production of chemokines such as IL-8, MIP-1 and MCP-1 by airway epithelial cells and alveolar macrophages stimulated by inhaled molecules such as endotoxins [17]. The maintenance in the number of macrophages which resolve and modulate inflammation in the BAL of TLR9$^{-/-}$ mice compared to WT mice following one exposure suggests a modulatory role for TLR9. The early increase in

macrophages without any effect on neutrophils or total cells in the BAL in TLR9$^{-/-}$ mice is interesting when combined with fewer tissue neutrophils but comparable tissue macrophages after 20 exposures to chicken barn air. Although neutrophils migrate during the early phase of acute lung inflammation, their migration may continue over a longer period of time in chronic inflammation stimulated through repeated exposures in diseases such as COPD [18, 19]. The data suggest that deficiency of TLR9 dampens lung inflammation induced by exposure to chicken barn air.

The expression of inflammation including recruitment of neutrophils and macrophages is regulated through adhesion proteins and inflammatory mediators [20, 21]. To understand the role of inflammatory mediators, we examined the expression of IL-1β, IL-6, IL-10, IL-12, IFNγ, and TNFα in BAL and serum of mice in our study.

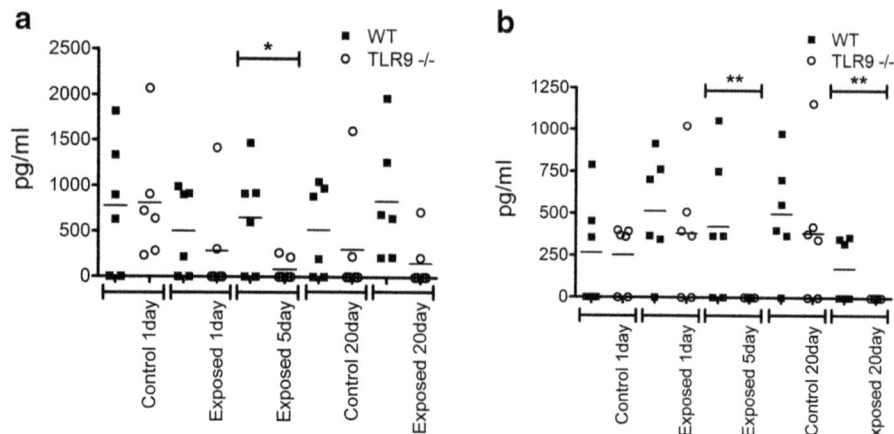

Fig. 7 Bio-plex ELISA of mouse bronchoalveolar lavage. BAL was collected by washing lungs 3 times with cold HEPES buffer from exposed and unexposed WT and TLR9$^{-/-}$ mice ($n = 6$). Samples were centrifuged briefly to remove cells and fluid decanted. ELISA was done with antibodies to IL-1β, IL-6, IL-10, IL-12, IFNγ, and TNFα. TNFα (**a**) was significantly reduced after 5 days exposure in TLR9$^{-/-}$ mice compared to WT (* = $p \leq 0.06$). IFNγ (**b**) was significantly reduced after 5 and 20 days exposure in TLR9$^{-/-}$ mice compared to WT (** = $p \leq 0.05$)

These cytokines are produced following ligation of bacterial DNA by TLR9 [22, 23]. We did not find any differences in control or exposed WT or TLR9$^{-/-}$ mice for IL-1β, IL-6, IL-10, and IL-12. This would suggest that while the barn may be an environment known to induce inflammation in the lung, changes in many individual cytokines may not be significantly elevated, or that responses are too variable. While IFNγ was reduced in BAL from TLR9$^{-/-}$ mice after 5 and 20 exposures, TNFα was reduced only after 5 exposures. The levels of IFNγ were

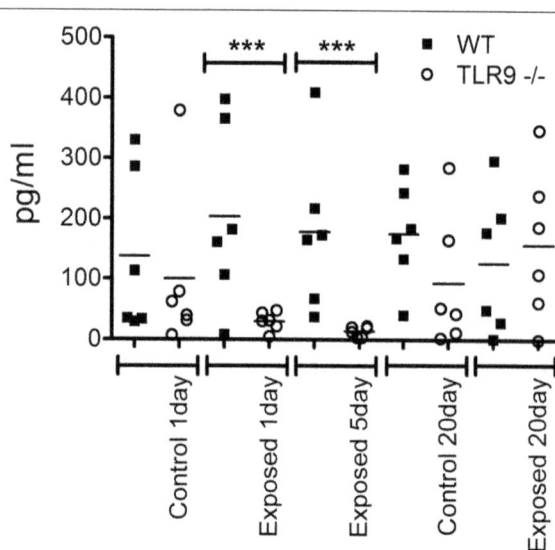

Fig. 8 Bio-plex ELISA of mouse serum. Serum was collected by collecting blood via cardiac puncture and then briefly centrifuging to remove cells from exposed and unexposed WT and TLR9$^{-/-}$ mice ($n = 6$). ELISA was done with antibodies to IL-1β, IL-6, IL-10, IL-12, IFNγ, and TNFα. IFNγ was significantly reduced after 1 and 5 days exposure in TLR9$^{-/-}$ mice compared to WT (*** = $p \leq 0.01$)

lower in the serum of TLR9$^{-/-}$ mice compared to WT mice exposed once or five times to chicken barn air. Although there were differences in IFNγ and TNFα in BAL fluid between WT and TLR9$^{-/-}$ mice after five exposures, there were no differences in the numbers of cells recruited into alveoli after one or five exposures. There were however more septal macrophages in TLR9$^{-/-}$ mice compared to WT mice following five exposures. Because macrophages play a role in resolution of inflammation [21], reduced levels of TNFα along with increased numbers of macrophages may indicate a pro-inflammatory role for TLR9 in lung inflammation induced following exposure to chicken barn air. Because TNFα promotes expression of adhesion molecules [24], reduced levels of TNFα may have also contributed to reduced migration of neutrophils in lungs of TLR9$^{-/-}$ mice compared to WT mice following 20 exposures to chicken barn air. However, there were more septal macrophages present at the same time. TNFα produced by activated airway epithelial cells and alveolar macrophages is an important regulator of lung inflammation as well [24]. Because of the role of TLR9 signaling in induction of pulmonary IFNγ expression [25], the reduced levels of IFNγ in the knockout mice is understandable. However, the effects of reduced expression of IFNγ on the inflammation phenotype in our experiments are not apparent. The role of IFNγ as a modulator of Th2 immune response is something that we need to address in future experiments. It is known that IFNγ is reduced in many cases of asthma [26] and in cases of endotoxin exposure [27]. This is typically associated with a more Th2 cytokine profile. Pig and cattle farm workers had higher incidence of asthma compared to other farm workers [28] which has been attributed to higher endotoxin levels.

The lack of pronounced differences in lung inflammation in WT mice compared to TLR9$^{-/-}$ mice may be due to impaired expression of TLR9 in murine alveolar macrophages [29]. Because alveolar macrophages play critical roles in lung inflammation induced following inhalation of microbes or their products [30–32], impaired TLR9 expression may explain lack of distinct differences in inflammation between WT and TLR9$^{-/-}$ mice. While recognition of endotoxin is still intact in both mouse strains, the differences in lung inflammation are rather subtle. This however does not inform us of the reasons for lack of differences between WT control and one or five day exposed mice. This issue needs to be addressed through comparison of lung inflammation in mice in which alveolar macrophages are depleted prior to their exposure to barn air.

One possible explanation for both BAL and septal macrophage results is that the septal macrophages exert an anti-inflammatory effect on the lung, leading to fewer BAL cells. There is evidence for this in a recent study that showed that signaling through TLR4 and TLR9 in septal macrophages induced expression of cytokines such as IL-10 and generally induced an anti-inflammatory response [33]. Yet another possibility is that migration of macrophages into the alveolar space requires a transition through the alveolar septa [34]. If this is the case then a reduction in macrophages at one time point in the septa being mirrored by an increase in the BAL could be a reflection of the increased movement of these cells into the alveolar space as appears to happen in our experiments. This however still raises the question of the reason for such an increased migration of macrophages.

The response of cellular influx in and out of the lung with TLR9 inhibition is quite intriguing and somewhat perplexing. We suspect that within the first day of exposure lack of TLR9 signaling reduces the rate of out-migration of alveolar macrophage to tissue and lymph nodes [35]. The general reduction in exposed group interstitial macrophages which are known to secrete anti-inflammatory cytokines to the same stimuli [33] suggest migration in and out of BAL may be more likely at this point.

By day 20 however TLR9-/- animals are seeing increases in these interstitial macrophage populations, suggesting a less permissive migration scenario. At this point we see this reflected in reduced total BAL cells, BAL macrophages, and tissue neutrophils. As such, we would hope to do more work on the effects of dusts and TLR9 signaling in interstitial macrophages to better determine their role in lung cellular migration.

Lung responses to bacterial DNA will depend on the amount of inhaled DNA. Attempts to purify DNA from barn dust from a previous experiment typically produced around 1 μg of DNA from a filter kept in a similar barn for 8 h (unpublished observations). Of this a portion of recovered DNA will be methylated eukaryotic DNA, further reducing the amount of stimulatory DNA. Therefore, the predicted exposure to bacterial DNA in the barn is probably quite low, certainly in comparison to what is used in in vitro trials [10]. However, as has been mentioned, dust and endotoxin levels in this facility were lower compared to a wider survey [3]. We would thus predict a greater effect of bacterial DNA in many facilities compared to what is shown here. Although some differences between WT and TLR9$^{-/-}$ mice were noticed after single exposure, the divergence in immune responses between mouse populations at 5 days or later may indicate a requirement for exposure to a sufficient dose of stimulatory DNA that the mice do not see in a single day. Indeed, as Roy and colleagues found, 10 μg of barn dust induced detectable responses [10], which would be approximately the dose encountered by the mice after 5 exposures. This accumulated effect though would have to result from continued exposure, not an accumulation of DNA within the tissue, as other studies have shown that internalized DNA is rapidly degraded [36]. What this suggests is that a low unmethylated DNA dose (perhaps 1 μg/day) may cause changes to lung cytokine secretion, especially in the context of stimulation or challenge by other pro-inflammatory molecules or organisms (in this case endotoxins and/or proteoglycans and particulate dust). Another consideration is what happens the CpG DNA in absence of TLR9 receptor? To what degree could other potential sensing mechanisms be altered by CpG DNA not binding to TLR9?

We do note that a study like this has a number of limitations that must be recognized. First, dust and barn conditions are likely to differ between specific facilities, and moreso between facilities such as swine and chicken facilities, though there is clear evidence of worker lung problems in both as discussed earlier. Second, this study was limited to infiltration of cells and cytokine expression in the lung, possibly ignoring other potential markers of lung inflammation. Even in the cases of exposure there was not a significant increase of inflammatory cells and cytokines above controls animals of the same strain, so there was not a clear indication on inflammation in mice over the course of the experiment. This having been said however, there were clear changes in cytokine expression, macrophage numbers, and MPO concentration in the lungs of mice, with most of these changes being present after a longer term exposure to barn air.

Conclusions

In conclusion, while we saw little change to BAL cell populations and cytokines in mice that had been exposed to chicken barn air for 1, 5, or 20 days, there were subtle changes in TLR9–/– animals. In TLR9–/– animals we detected changes to total BAL cells, and alveolar macrophage numbers by 1 day exposure, and still at 20 days. Septal macrophages were also increased in the TLR9–/– animals by 20 days exposure, in a pattern opposite to that seen in alveolar macrophages. There were also reductions in TNFα and IFNγ in the TLR9–/– knockout mice. These results suggest that TLR9 plays a role in the innate immune response to chicken barn air exposure that enhances indicators of inflammation (TNFα, IFNγ, MPO) at later time points (5 day or 20 day exposures). However, the full effects of TLR9 may be more complex as shown by increased BAL cell numbers and alveolar macrophages after single day exposure, and increased septal macrophages in these same animals at 20 days.

Acknowledgements

We would like to thank Amberlea Farms Ltd. of Saskatoon, SK Canada for allowing access to their facilities for this study.

Funding

The work was supported by a Discovery Grant from the Natural Sciences and Engineering Research Council of Canada to Baljit Singh. David Schneberger was supported by a PHARE Graduate Scholarship from the Canadian Institutes for Health Research and a Founding Chairs Fellowship from the Canadian Centre for Health and Safety in Agriculture, University of Saskatchewan.

Authors' contributions

DS conceived of the study, analyzed data, and carried out most of the experiments and writing of the manuscript. GA and SC assisted with carrying out of experiments. BS assisted with experiment design, writing of paper, and guidance of the project. All authors read and approved the final manuscript.

Competing interests

The authors declare they have no competing interests.

References

1. Donham KJ, Cumro D, Reynolds SJ, Merchant JA. Dose–response relationships between occupational aerosol exposures and cross-shift declines of lung function in poultry workers: recommendations for exposure limits. J Occup Environ Med. 2000;42(3):260–9.
2. Kirychuk SP, Senthilselvan A, Dosman JA, Juorio V, Feddes JJR, Willson P, et al. Respiratory symptoms and lung function in poultry confinement workers in Western Canada. Can Respir J. 2003;10(7):375–80.
3. Kirychuk SP, Dosman JA, Reynolds SJ, Willson P, Senthilselvan A, Feddes JJ, et al. Total dust and endotoxin in poultry operations: comparison between cage and floor housing and respiratory effects in workers. J Occup Environ Med. 2006;48(7):741–8.
4. Just N, Duchaine C, Singh B. An aerobiological perspective of dust in cage-housed and floor-housed poultry operations. J Occup Med Toxicol. 2009;4:13.
5. Senthilselvan A, Zhang Y, Dosman JA, Barber EM, Holfeld LE, Kirychuk SP, et al. Positive human health effects of dust suppression with canola oil in swine barns. Am J Respir Crit Care Med. 1997;156(2 Pt 1):410–7.
6. Smit LAM, Heederik D, Doekes G, Krop EJM, Rijkers GT, Wouters IM. Ex vivo cytokine release reflects sensitivity to occupational endotoxin exposure. Eur Respir J. 2009;34(4):795–802.
7. Charavaryamath C, Juneau V, Suri SS, Janardhan KS, Townsend H, Singh B. Role of toll-like receptor 4 in lung inflammation following exposure to swine barn air. Exp Lung Res. 2008;34(1):19–35.
8. Zejda JE, Barber E, Dosman JA, Olenchock SA, McDuffie HH, Rhodes C, et al. Respiratory health status in swine producers relates to endotoxin exposure in the presence of low dust levels. J Occup Med. 1994;36(1):49–56.
9. Medzhitov R, Janeway Jr C. Innate immune recognition: mechanisms and pathways. Immunol Rev. 2000;173:89–97.
10. Roy SR, Schiltz AM, Marotta A, Shen Y, Liu AH. Bacterial DNA in house and farm barn dust. J Allergy Clin Immunol. 2003;112(3):571–8.
11. Schneberger D, Caldwell S, Kanthan R, Singh B. Expression of Toll-like receptor 9 in mouse and human lungs. J Anat. 2013;222(5):495–503.
12. Schneberger D, Caldwell S, Suri SS, Singh B. Expression of toll-like receptor 9 in horse lungs. Anat Rec (Hoboken). 2009;292(7):1068–77.
13. Schneberger D, Lewis D, Caldwell S, Singh B. Expression of toll-like receptor 9 in lungs of pigs, dogs and cattle. Int J Exp Pathol. 2011;92(1):1–7.
14. Dosman JA, Fukushima Y, Senthilselvan A, Kirychuk SP, Lawson JA, Pahwa P, et al. Respiratory response to endotoxin and dust predicts evidence of inflammatory response in volunteers in a swine barn. Am J Ind Med. 2006;49(9):761–6.
15. Balbi B, Pignatti P, Corradi M, Baiardi P, Bianchi L, Brunetti G, et al. Bronchoalveolar lavage, sputum and exhaled clinically relevant inflammatory markers: Values in healthy adults. Eur Respir J. 2007;30(4):769–81.
16. Charavaryamath C, Janardhan KS, Townsend HG, Willson P, Singh B. Multiple exposures to swine barn air induce lung inflammation and airway hyper-responsiveness. Respir Res. 2005;6:50-62.
17. Tam A, Wadsworth S, Dorscheid D, Man SFP, Sin DD. The airway epithelium: More than just a structural barrier. Ther Adv Respir Dis. 2011;5(4):255–73.
18. Stockley RA. Neutrophils and the pathogenesis of COPD. Chest. 2002;121 (5 SUPPL):151S–5S.
19. Gane J, Stockley R. Mechanisms of neutrophil transmigration across the vascular endothelium in COPD. Thorax. 2012;67(6):553–61.
20. Borregaard N. Neutrophils, from Marrow to Microbes. Immunity. 2010; 33(5):657–70.
21. Murray PJ, Wynn TA. Protective and pathogenic functions of macrophage subsets. Nat Rev Immunol. 2011;11(11):723–37.
22. Parilla NW, Hughes VS, Lierl KM, Wong HR, Page K. CpG DNA modulates interleukin Iβ-induced interleukin-8 expression in human bronchial epithelial (16HBE14o-) cells. Respir Res. 2006;7:84-92.
23. Chen L, Arora M, Yarlagadda M, Oriss TB, Krishnamoorthy N, Ray A, et al. Distinct responses of lung and spleen dendritic cells to the TLR9 agonist CpG oligodeoxynucleotide. J Immunol. 2006;177(4):2373–83.
24. Lauterbach M, O'Donnell P, Asano K, Mayadas TN. Role of TNF priming and adhesion molecules in neutrophil recruitment to intravascular immune complexes. J Leukocyte Biol. 2008;83(6):1423–30.
25. Zhou R, Norton JE, Zhang N, Dean DA. Electroporation-mediated transfer of plasmids to the lung results in reduced TLR9 signaling and inflammation. Gene Ther. 2007;14(9):775–80.
26. Kumar RK, Webb DC, Herbert C, Foster PS. Interferon-γ as a possible target in chronic asthma. Inflamm Allergy Drug Targets. 2006;5(4):253–6.
27. Alexis NE, Lay JC, Almond M, Peden DB. Inhalation of low-dose endotoxin favors local TH2 response and primes airway phagocytes in vivo. J Allergy Clin Immunol. 2004;114(6):1325–31.
28. Eduard W, Douwes J, Omenaas E, Heederik D. Do farming exposures cause or prevent asthma? Results from a study of adult Norwegian farmers. Thorax. 2004;59(5):381–6.
29. Suzuki K, Suda T, Naito T, Ide K, Chida K, Nakamura H. Impaired toll-like receptor 9 expression in alveolar macrophages with no sensitivity to CpG DNA. Am J Respir Crit Care Med. 2005;171(7):707–13.

30. Palmberg L, Larsson B, Malmberg P, Larsson K. Induction of IL-8 production in human alveolar macrophages and human bronchial epithelial cells in vitro by swine dust. Thorax. 1998;53(4):260–4.

31. Koay MA, Gao X, Washington MK, Parman KS, Sadikot RT, Blackwell TS, et al. Macrophages are necessary for maximal nuclear factor-kB activation in response to endotoxin. Am J Resp Cell Mol Biol. 2002;26(5):572–8.

32. Zhao M, Fernandez LG, Doctor A, Sharma AK, Zarbock A, Tribble CG, et al. Alveolar macrophage activation is a key initiation signal for acute lung ischemia-reperfusion injury. Am J Physiol Lung Cell Mol Physiol. 2006;291(5): L1018–26.

33. Hoppstadter J, Diesel B, Zarbock R, Breinig T, Monz D, Koch M, et al. Differential cell reaction upon Toll-like receptor 4 and 9 activation in human alveolar and lung interstitial macrophages. Respir Res. 2010;11:124.

34. Landsman L, Jung S. Lung macrophages serve as obligatory intermediate between blood monocytes and alveolar macrophages. J Immunol. 2007; 179(6):3488–94.

35. Thepen T, Claassen E, Hoeben K, Breve J, Kraal G. Migration of alveolar macrophages from alveolar space to paracortical T cell area of the draining lymph node. Adv Exp Med Biol. 1993;329:305–10.

36. Kawabata K, Takakura Y, Hashida M. The fate of plasmid DNA after intravenous injection in mice: involvement of scavenger receptors in its hepatic uptake. Pharm Res. 1995;12(6):825–30.

11

Fipronil induces lung inflammation in vivo and cell death in vitro

Kaitlin Merkowsky[1], Ram S. Sethi[2], Jatinder P. S. Gill[3] and Baljit Singh[1*]

Abstract

Background: Fipronil is an insecticide that acts at the *gamma*-aminobutyric acid receptor and glutamate-gated chloride channels in the central nervous systems of target organisms. The use of fipronil is increasing across the globe. Presently, very little data exist on the potential impact of exposure to fipronil on the lungs.

Methods: We studied effects of intranasal ($N = 8$) and oral ($N = 8$) treatment with fipronil (10 mg/kg) on lungs of mice. Control mice were given groundnut oil orally ($N = 7$) or ethanol intranasally ($N = 7$) as these were the vehicles for respective treatments.

Results: Hematoxylin-eosin stained lung sections showed normal histology in the control lungs compared to the thickened alveolar septa, disruption of the airways epithelium and damage to vascular endothelium in the intranasal and the oral groups. Mice exposed to fipronil either orally or intranasally showed increased von Willebrand factor staining in the endothelium and septal capillaries. Compared to the control mice, TLR4 expression in airway epithelium was increased in mice treated intranasally but not orally with fipronil. Oral fipronil reduced TLR9 staining in the airway epithelium but intranasal exposure caused intense staining in the alveolar septa and airway epithelium. There were higher numbers of TLR4 positive cells in alveolar septa in lungs of mice treated intranasally ($P = 0.010$) compared to the respective control and orally treated mice but no significant differences between treatments for TLR9 positive stained cells ($P = 0.226$). The U937 macrophage cells exposed to fipronil at concentrations of 0.29 μm to 5.72 μm/ml over 3- or 24-hour showed significant increase in cell death at higher concentrations of fipronil ($P < 0.0001$). Western blots revealed no effect of fipronil on TLR4 ($P = 0.49$) or TLR9 ($P = 0.94$) expression on macrophage cell line.

Conclusion: While both oral or intranasal fipronil treatments induced signs of lung inflammation, the number TLR4-positive septal cells was increased only following intranasal treatment. Fipronil causes macrophage cell death without altering TLR4 and TLR9 expression in vitro.

Keywords: Macrophage, Pesticides, Lung Inflammation, TLR4, TLR9

Background

The Sumerians were probably the first to used elemental sulphur against insects and mites in 2500 BC and ancient Chinese cultures treated body lice with arsenic and mercury. While the ingenuity of these ancient cultures can be appreciated, it is unlikely arsenic would be embraced today as an effective pesticide due to its deleterious effects on human health. The most prominent example in modern times of the struggle between insect control and public health concerns is dichlorodiphenyltrichloroethane (DDT), which belongs to organochlorine group of pesticides [1], and showed unparalleled effectiveness in bringing down cases of malaria. While pesticides and insecticides are the tools to manage pests and insects, many health effects of these chemicals have also be recorded.

Fipronil ((±)-5-amino-1- (2,6-dichloro-α,α,α-trifluoro-p-tolyl)- 4-trifluoromethylsulfinylpyrazole-3-carbonitrile) belongs to the phenylpyrazole family and is extensively used around the world in various anti-flea and tick sprays and for pest control in agriculture [2]. Fipronil acts as an antagonist at GABA-gated chloride channels but has a higher affinity for these channels in insects compared to non-target organisms such as humans, making it a

* Correspondence: baljit.singh@usask.ca
[1]Department of Veterinary Biomedical Sciences, Western College of Veterinary Medicine, University of Saskatchewan, 52 Campus Drive, Saskatoon, SK S7N 5B4, Canada
Full list of author information is available at the end of the article

seemingly safer product in these regards [3–5]. Fipronil is metabolized into many metabolites including sulfone, sulphide, and desulfinyl. However, it has been demonstrated the primary metabolite of fipronil, fipronil sulfone, actually has a much greater affinity for these channels in mammals than those in insects indicating potential detrimental effects of the break-down products to non-target organisms [6]. One of the studies found that following a single oral exposure fipronil sulfone persists for much longer duration than fipronil in high fat containing tissues especially adipose tissue, adrenals and the liver which leads to bioamplification along the food chain [7, 8]. It has been shown that both sulfone and desulfinyl are potent mitochondrial uncouplers and calcium efflux inducers but may differ in their potencies [9]. Nevertheless, exposure to the parent compound is pre-requisite for the generation of fipronil metabolites. Combined subchronic exposure to fipronil and fluoride induces biochemical alterations in buffalo calves [10, 11]. Fipronil also induces oxidative stress and activation of MAPK, induction of apoptosis via caspase-9 and caspase-3, and reduction in differentiated cell numbers [12–14]. During an examination of effects of fipronil on liver p450 enzymes, it was found that fipronil is an inducer of hepatic phase I CYP enzymes that may increase potential for interactions with xenobiotics [15]. While recent studies have shown the toxic effects of fipronil on liver especially the mitochondria in liver cells [9, 16], there currently are no data on the pulmonary effects of fipronil in animals.

This study was designed to investigate the pulmonary effects of fipronil following oral or intranasal exposures through testing of hypothesis that exposure to low levels of fipronil will induce lung inflammation and cell death. The inhalation route remains a major route of exposure in developing countries where agricultural workers generally spray pesticides without appropriate personal protective gear. The oral route occurs through contamination of food and water with pesticides. We also investigated the effects of fipronil on a macrophage cell line in vitro. The data show fipronil causes cell death in vitro and induces lung inflammation following both oral and intranasal routes of administration but increases number of TLR4 cells only after intranasal treatment.

Methods
In vivo experiments
Experiment was conducted following approval from the Institutional Animal Ethics Committee (IAEC), Guru Angad Dev Veterinary and Animal Sciences University, Ludhiana. Swiss albino mice, ages 8–10 weeks, were housed in laboratory animal cages at 18–22 °C and 12:12 light–dark cycles. Mice had access to feed (Ashirwad Industries, Chandigarh, Punjab, India) and water ad libitum.

Experiment design
An initial experiment was first conducted where mice ($n = 8$) were exposed to 8 mg/kg or 2 mg/kg of fipronil via intranasal or oral routes ($n = 2$ each) or treated with respective vehicles ($n = 2$ each for ethanol for intransal and corn oil for oral route) to determine an appropriate dose of fipronil (Sigma-Aldrich S. Louis, USA; <=100 % purity). Based on the preliminary study, we decided on 8 mg/kg of fipronil as the dose for both intranasal and oral exposure routes. This dose was determined as it was 10 % of the oral LD_{50} for mice to reduce chances of acute toxicity and death and treated mice for seven days to induce sub-chronic toxic effects (http://npic.orst.edu/factsheets/fiptech.pdf).

Control mice ($N = 7$) received groundnut oil, which was used as a vehicle for treating mice ($N = 8$) orally with fipronil (8 mg/kg/day). Mice ($N = 8$) were treated intranasally with fipronil (8 mg/kg/day) in dissolved in ethanol. Control mice ($N = 7$) received intranasal treatment ethanol. Unfortunately the intranasal groups of mice experienced high mortality following anaesthesia and the ketamine/xylazine dose was adjusted daily to reduce chances of mortality in the mice.

After 7 days mice were euthanized with a lethal dose of ketamine/xylazine (0.1 µl/10 g of body weight) and cardiac puncture was done to collect blood. The trachea was isolated and a small cannula was inserted to perform lung lavage. Lungs were lavaged 3 times with 0.5 ml of phosphate buffered saline to collect broncho-alveolar lavage (BAL) fluid. The left lung was fixed in 10 % formalin overnight (24 h). Lungs were placed in filter capsules and processed by the acetone and benzene method to obtain 5 µm thick paraffin sections.

Hematoxylin and eosin staining
The paraffin sections of lungs from all groups were stained with H&E staining for routine histopathology.

Immunohistochemistry
The immunohistochemistry was performed as reported earlier (Sethi 2013). Briefly tissue sections were de-paraffinized and rehydrated. The tissue peroxidases were inactivated with 0.5 % H_2O_2 in methanol for 20 min. Pepsin (2 mg/ml in 0.01 N HCl) was used to unmask antigen-binding sites (60 min) and then 1 % bovine serum albumin (BSA) in PBS was used to prevent non-specific binding (30 min). Next the tissues were incubated overnight (16 h) at 4 °C with the following antibodies: von Willebrand Factor (1:500, DAKO A0082), Toll-Like Receptor 4 (1:25, IMG-578A, IMGENEX) and Toll-Like Receptor 9 (1:50, IMG-3051, IMGENEX) followed by appropriate secondary antibody (vWF at 1:300 and TLR at 1:100, all from DAKO). VECTOR VIP Peroxidase Substrate Kit (Vector laboratories, Burlingame,

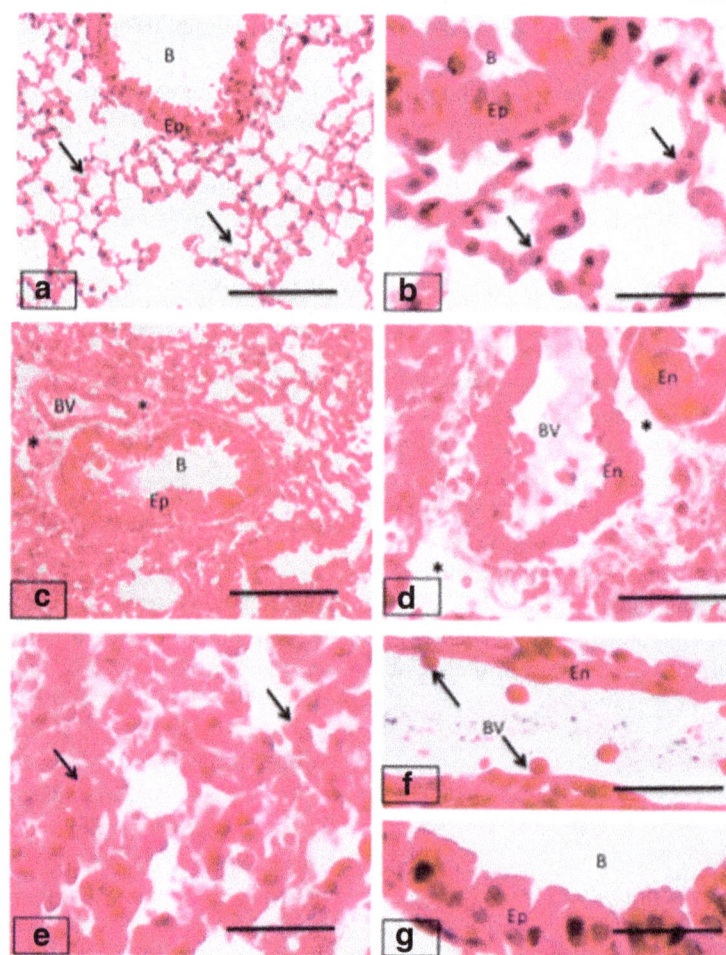

CA) was used for colour-development ed followed by counter staining with methyl green (Vector laboratories).

Grading for immunohistochemistry

Lungs sample from all the animals were used for grading of immunohistochemical staining intensity and quantification of the number of TLR4 or TLR9 positive cells in the alveolar septa (Table B). For each tissue section five random fields of vision was assessed and a score of 1–4 (1 being least intense, 4 being most intense) was assigned for each of the criteria. The cells were counted in 5 consecutive fields under 100X. The sections were graded depending on the staining intensity of vWF in the large blood vessels, or TLR4 or TLR9 in the bronchial epithelium and continuity of the airways epithelium as interrupted or intact (Table B). One individual who was blinded to what treatments of each animal performed the scoring.

In vitro experiments

U937 cell line was obtained from ATCC®. RPMI Complete Media +10 % Fetal Bovine Serum (FBS) (Gibco) was warmed to 37 °C. Aliquots of cells were thawed in a hot water bath (37 °C) and combined with 10 ml warm media in 15 ml clinical centrifuge tubes. The tubes were spun at $258\,g$ for 3 min, the supernatant was discarded and the pellet then resuspended in 10 ml media in a closed flask and incubated at 37 °C, 5 % CO_2. The cell suspension was removed from the flask and transferred to a 15 ml centrifuge tube and spun at $258\,g$ for 3 min. The supernatant was discarded and cells were resuspended in 5 ml media, split and transferred into 2 new flasks and topped with media (~15 ml). Incubation continued at 37 °C, 5 % CO_2, and this procedure was repeated every 2–3 days till the desired concentration (5×10^6 cells/ml) of cells was achieved.

Fig. 1 H&E staining of mice lungs. Lung sections from control mice (**a-b**) have normal lung histology of alveolar septa (*arrows*) and bronchiolar (B) epithelium (Ep). The oral treatment with fipronil caused lung inflammation and lung sections (**c-d**) show inflammation (*asterisks*) around bronchioles (B) and blood vessels (BV). Lung sections from mice treated intranasally with fipronil (**e-g**) show septal congestion in septa (*arrows*; **e**)), cells adhering (*arrows*) to endothelium (En; **f**) and swollen epithelium (Ep) of bronchioles (B; 1 g). Bar: 100 μm

Fipronil exposure and viability assessment

Once the cells reached a concentration of 5×10^5 cells/ml, the cells were incubated with 12 ml media + Phorbol-12-myristate-13-acetate (PMA) in 12 well plate for 48 h to differentiate into macrophages. The cells were treated with various concentrations of fipronil (0.29 μm to 5.72 μm per 1 ml) dissolved in DMSO for 3 h. Following desired incubation, 50 μl of 0.25 % Trypsin in Ethylenediaminetetra-acetic acid (EDTA) was added to each well in order to facilitate removal of the differentiated macrophages. 150 μl of the cells in media were combined with 50 μl Trypan blue to assess the viability of cells by trypan blue exclusion method.

Western blots for TLR4 and TLR9

Following a 3-hour exposure to fipronil, 50 μl of 0.25 % Trypsin in EDTA was added to each well for 5 min. Each sample was collected in 1.5 ml centrifuge tubes and spun for 10 min at 258 g. The supernatant was aspirated off and the pellet was washed with 1 ml Hanks Balanced Salt Solution (HBSS). This step was repeated twice. The supernatant was again aspirated off and one tablet of Protease inhibitor (Roche) was added to 7 ml Radioimmuno-precipitation assay (RIPA) (Sigma-Aldrich) buffer. A 300 μl of this RIPA buffer mix was added to each centrifuge tube and vortexed thoroughly. The samples were kept in a 4 °C refrigerator for 15 min and vortexed twice during this

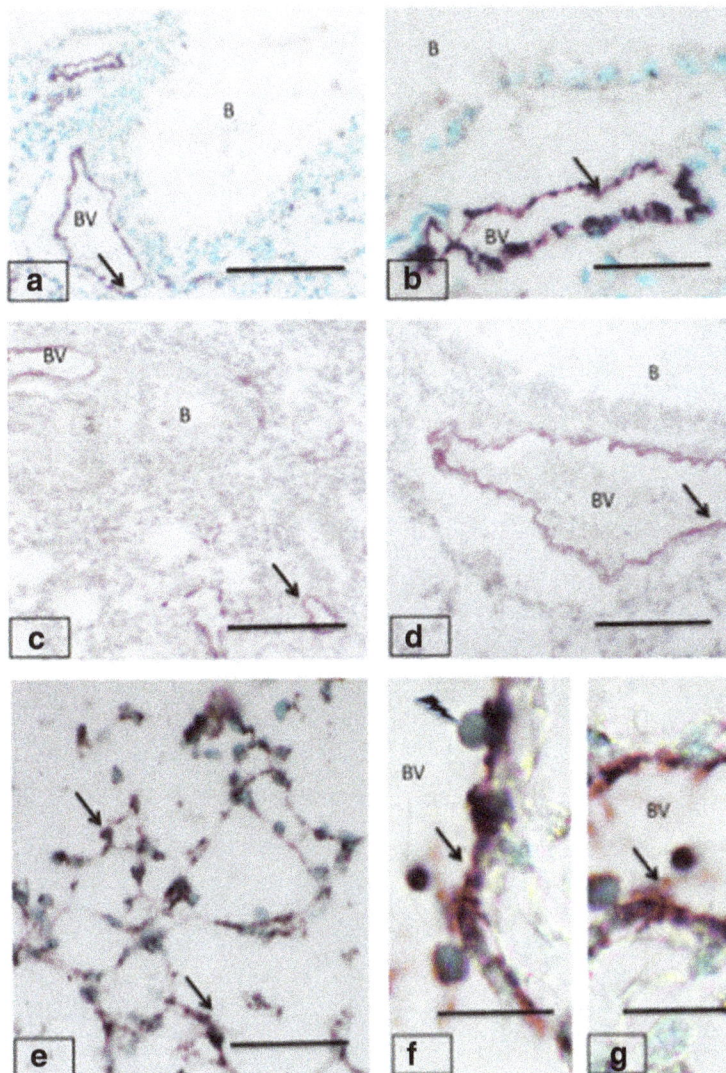

Fig. 2 von Willebrand Factor expression in mice lungs. Lungs from control groups (**a-b**) show normal vWF staining (*arrows*) in endothelium of blood vessels (BV) but not in bronchiolar (B) epithelium. The oral treatment with fipronil (**c-d**) caused inflammation but the expression of vWF (*arrows*) in blood vessels (BV) remained unchanged. The intranasal fipronil (**e-g**) showed increased expression (*arrows*) in alveolar septum (**e**), endothelium of blood vessels (**f-g**) as well as the vascular cells. Note vascular cells (*lightening arrow*) attaching to the endothelium (**f**). Bar: 100 μm

incubation. The samples were put in the centrifuge at 10,000 g for 5 min. The supernatant was then carefully removed without disturbing the pellet and stored at -45 °C until needed for future assays for up to 1 month. 25 μl of protein samples plus indicator were boiled for 5 min and then loaded into a 12 % SDS-PAGE gel. The proteins were separated via gel electrophoresis at 160 V for 45–60 min. The gel was collected and placed between 2 sponges, 4 filter papers and Immobilon – FL membrane in a western blot sandwich all previously soaked in the transfer buffer. The protein transfer was performed at 100 V for 70 min. Following transfer, the membrane was washed in 15 ml PBS and then incubated in ~15 ml blocking buffer (5 % BSA in PBS) for 1 h. Primary antibodies were mixed with the above blocking buffer with the addition

of 0.1 % Tween-20. Primary antibodies (Anti-TLR4, AF1478 R&D at 1:200 and Anti-TLR9, IMG 305A at 1:200, IMGENEX) were incubated with membranes overnight at 4 °C. Following overnight incubation membranes were washed with PBS and PBST and then incubated with secondary antibody (Goat, anti-mouse Cy5.5 or Donkey Anti-goat Cy3, both at 1:1000, AbCam) in PBS for 30 min. Washing was repeated after this step and then membranes were allowed to dry before visualization using the Typhoon 3 laser fluorescence scanner.

Statistical analyses

Statistical analysis was performed using statistical software (SPSS, IBM version 21.1 for Windows). For in vivo work a one-way analysis of variance (ANOVA) was run

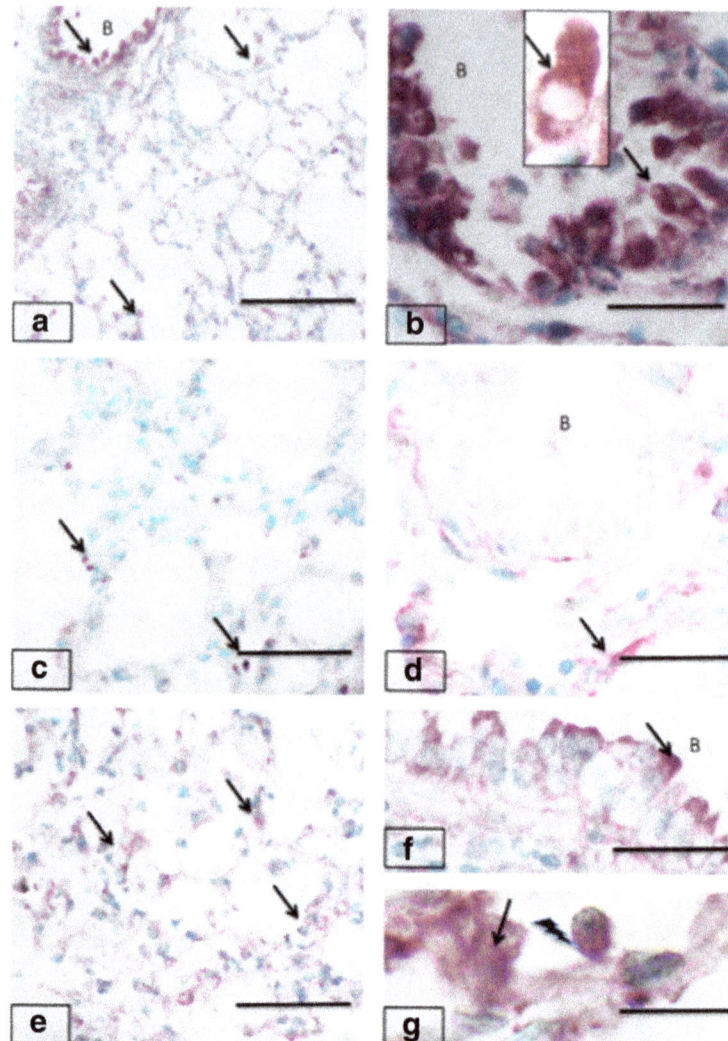

Fig. 3 Toll-like receptor 4 expression in mice lungs. Lungs from control groups (**a-b** and) show strong staining (*arrows*) in bronchiolar epithelium (B) and alveolar septum. Note rich cytoplasmic staining in bronchiolar epithelial cells (**b** and inset). The lungs sections (**c-d**) from mice treated orally with fipronil show barely minimal staining (*arrows*) in alveolar septum (**c**) while it is nearly absent in bronchiolar (B) epithelium. Lung sections from mice exposed to fipronil (**e-g**) show TLR4 staining similar (*arrows*) to the control lungs in alveolar septum (**e**) and epithelium (*arrows*) of bronchioles (B, **f**). Note TLR4 staining (3 g) in endothelium (*arrow*) and adhering cells (*lightening arrows*). Bar = 100 μm

to determine if the number of TLR4/9 positive cells present in the alveolar septa was significantly different between treatments groups. If there was a significant difference, Tukey's Multiple Comparison test was performed to see which treatments differed. For in vitro work, one-way or two-way ANOVA was run to see if there were significant difference between average cell viability. Dunnet's or Tukey's Multiple Comparison Test was ran to see the differences. Since only 2 treatments were used for western blots, Student's Independent T-test was used to determine significant differences.

Results

Hematoxylin and eosin staining

H&E stained lung sections from control group showed normal histoarchitecture of lungs except few black spots indicating some evidence of dust particles that the animals could have easily been exposed to throughout the experiment (Fig. 1a and b). Lung sections from animals in the oral fipronil group displayed an accumulation of inflammatory cells around the terminal bronchioles. There was a dilatation of perivascular spaces in lung sections from all the animals. The airway epithelial cells were enlarged and domed in mice treated intranasally with fipronil (Fig. 1c and d). The blood vessel showed a folded appearance. In comparison to the oral group, the intranasal fipronil group displayed overall normal lung architecture and the epithelium did not appear to be activated but there was an increase in accumulation of inflammatory cells in the alveolar septa and the alveoli (Fig. 1e, f and g). Many blood cells were attached to the vascular endothelium (Fig. 1f).

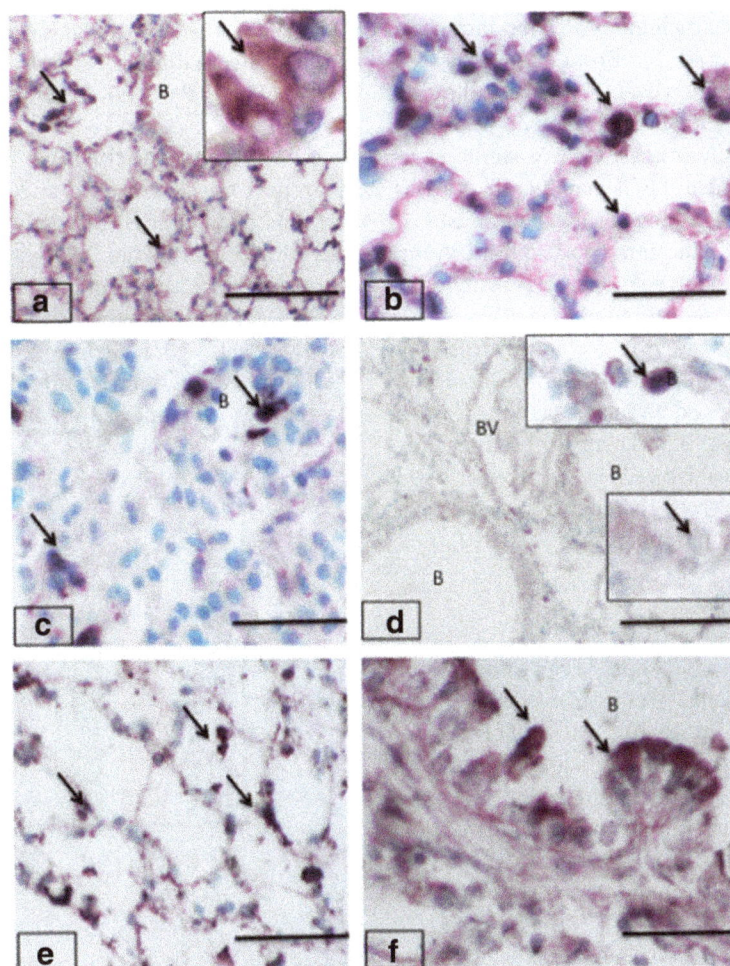

Fig. 4 Toll-like receptor 9 expression in mice lungs. Lungs sections from control groups (**a-b**) have TLR9 staining (*arrows*) in alveolar septum (**a**) and bronchiolar epithelium (**a** inset). The staining is also seen in the septal cells (*arrows*) in lung sections from control mice (**b**). The oral treatment reduced TLR9 staining in lung sections (**c-d**) and the staining (*arrows*) was observed in occasional septal cells (**c**). Bronchiolar epithelium (B; **d** and insets) showed much reduced TLR9 staining compared to the controls. Lung sections from mice treated with intranasal fipronil (**e-f**) showed intense staining (*arrows*) in alveolar septum (**e**) and bronchiolar epithelium (**f**). Bar: 100 μm

Expression of von Willebrand factor

Lung sections from control animals showed immunopositive staining for vWF in vascular endothelium that was more prominent in larger blood vessels compared to the alveolar septal capillaries (Fig. 2a and b). There was no vWF staining of the bronchiolar epithelium in lung sections from any of the treatment groups. The mice of the oral fipronil group did not have an altered expression of vWF though there was an indication of inflammation in the lung (Fig. 2c and d). An increase in vWF staining was displayed in lung sections from the intranasal fipronil group in areas such as septal capillaries and in the cells accumulated in septal areas (Fig. 2e, f and g). There was specially increased focal vWF staining in endothelial cells and the adhering blood cells (Fig. 2f).

Expression of Toll-like Receptor 4

The immunopositive TLR4 cells were observed in the cytoplasm of bronchiolar epithelium of oral and intranasal control groups (Fig. 3a and b). Bronchial associated lymphoid tissues (BALT) were present, however indicating the animals were kept in a dusty environment, as BALTs are not normally present in animals kept in sterile environments. The BALTs lacked TLR4 staining. There was reduced staining for TLR4 in lungs of mice administered fipronil orally (Fig. 3c, d). The intranasal fipronil group showed TLR4 staining in alveolar septa, bronchiolar epithelium and vascular endothelium (Fig. 3e, f, g). There reaction was more marked in the apical surface of the airway epithelium (Fig. 3f). The interface of blood cells, vascular endothelium and alveolar macrophages also showed TLR4 staining (Fig. 3g). There was significantly higher number of TLR4 positive cells in the alveolar septa in the intranasal fipronil group compared to intranasal control ($P = 0.050$) and oral fipronil group ($P = 0.010$).

Expression of Toll-like Receptor 9

TLR9 staining was observed in septa, airway epithelium and blood vessels in the lungs sectins from the oral and intranasal control groups (Fig. 4a, b). Further,, TLR9 staining assumed focal appearance in the septa but the airway epithelial staining was considerably reduced in oral fipronil group (Fig. 4c, d). There was minimal TLR9 reaction in vascular endothelium (Fig. 4d). However, TLR9 expression was intense and more prominent in the alveolar septa specially in the large cells in lungs of mice exposed intranasally to fipronil (Fig. 4e). The airway epithelium also showed intense surface staining for TLR9 while the cytoplasmic reaction was reduced in this group compared to control group (Fig. 4f). There was no significant difference for the number of TLR9 positive cells among treatment and control groups.

In vitro results

Fipronil reduces cell viability

There was a significant difference in percentage of living cells between the control and both fipronil concentrations. At 3 and 9 h the low fipronil concentration also had a significantly higher percentage of living cells than the high concentration (Fig. 5). At 24 h there was not a significant difference in the % of living cells between the low and high fipronil concentrations (Fig. 6). Further, there was no significant interaction between time vs. concentration ($F_{4,120} = 11.01$, $P = 0.115$).

Expression of TLR4 and TLR9

After the U937 cells were incubated with a high (5.72 μm) concentration of fipronil for 3 h, protein extraction was done and western blots were performed for TLR4 and TLR9 followed by densitometric quantification. Figure 7 depicts the average relative density of western blots that were performed three times. The expression of TLR4 and TLR9 did not show any significant difference between the group treated with fipronil vs. the group treated only with DMSO. TLR4 ($P = 0.49$), TLR9 ($P = 0.94$).

Discussion and conclusions

We report the first in vivo and in vitro effects on lungs and macrophage cells, respectively, of fipronil. The data show lung inflammation following both oral and intranasal treatments with fipronil and an increase in TLR4 positive cells in alveolar septa with intranasal treatment. The in vitro treatment with fipronil caused a concentration dependent reduction in the number of viable U937 macrophage cells but had no effect on the TLR4 or TLR9

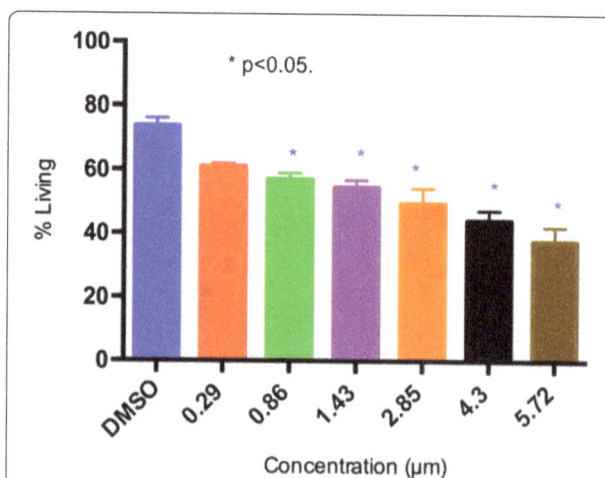

Fig. 5 Average U937 cell viability (%) is presented as a function of concentration (μm) of fipronil. Data are presented as means with error bars representing standard error of the mean. Significant results were obtained with a 1-way analysis of variance (ANOVA) and Dunnet's Multiple comparison Test ($F_{3,13} = 1.651$, $P = 0.226$). * depicts the result is significantly different from the control (DMSO). $F_{6,67} = 14.03$, $P < 0.0001$)

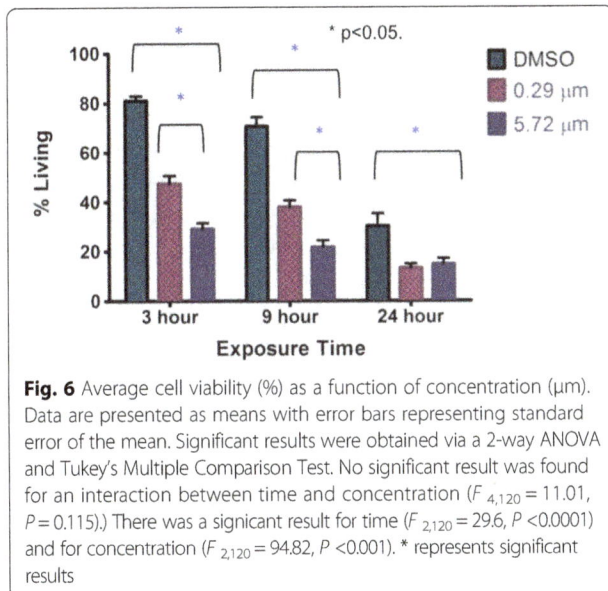

Fig. 6 Average cell viability (%) as a function of concentration (μm). Data are presented as means with error bars representing standard error of the mean. Significant results were obtained via a 2-way ANOVA and Tukey's Multiple Comparison Test. No significant result was found for an interaction between time and concentration ($F_{4,120} = 11.01$, $P = 0.115$).) There was a signicant result for time ($F_{2,120} = 29.6$, $P < 0.0001$) and for concentration ($F_{2,120} = 94.82$, $P < 0.001$). * represents significant results

expression. Taken together, these data suggest that exposure to fipronil induces lung inflammation and may increase its susceptibility for subsequent endotoxin exposure.

Because of the growing use of fipronil as a pesticide, we examined the effects of oral and intranasal exposures to fipronil on non target organs like lungs. Because this was the first study on pulmonary effects of fipronil, we chose to use fipronil and to focus on any of its metabolite such as sulfone or disulfiny in later studies. Fipronil resulted in lung inflammation in mice as evidenced by accumulation of inflammatory cells, which is considered

a hallmark of inflammation [17]. Further, In addition to the routine histology, we also used vWF as a marker of inflammation. the expression of vWF was especially upregaulated in the septal capillaries in mice treated intranasally with fipronil suggesting signs of microvascular inflammation. The expression of vWF in lungs of mice treated orally with fipronil remained changed except some apparent increase in larger pulmonary blood vessels. vWF is a resident adhesive protein in Wiebel-Palade bodies in endothelial cells, which is exocytosed along with IL-8 and P-selectin by activated endothelial cells [18, 19]. The data suggest that fipronil given orally or intranasally induced lung inflammation including that in the vasculature.

Lung inflammation is regulated through activation of innate immune system comprised of Toll-like receptors such as TLR4 and TLR9 that bind, respectively, to lipopolysaccharides and CpG molecules [20–22]. We report the first study that fipronil given orally apparently reduced the immunohistochemical expression of TLR4 and TLR9. Intranasal treatment with fipronil increased airway epithelial and vascular endothleial expression of TLR4 and TLR9. The intranasal treatment also increased the number of septal cells expressing TLR4. Previously, the herbicide paraquat given intraperitoneally increased in TLR4 mRNA in the myocardium [23]. Oral treatment with sodium methyldithiocarbamate (SMD), a commonly used pesticide in the U.S., altered expression of TLR4 and inhibited the MAP kinases, which are downstream of TLR4, to reduce the production of pro-inflammatory cytokines [24, 25]. Therefore, the observed increase in TLR4 expressing cells in the alveolar septa

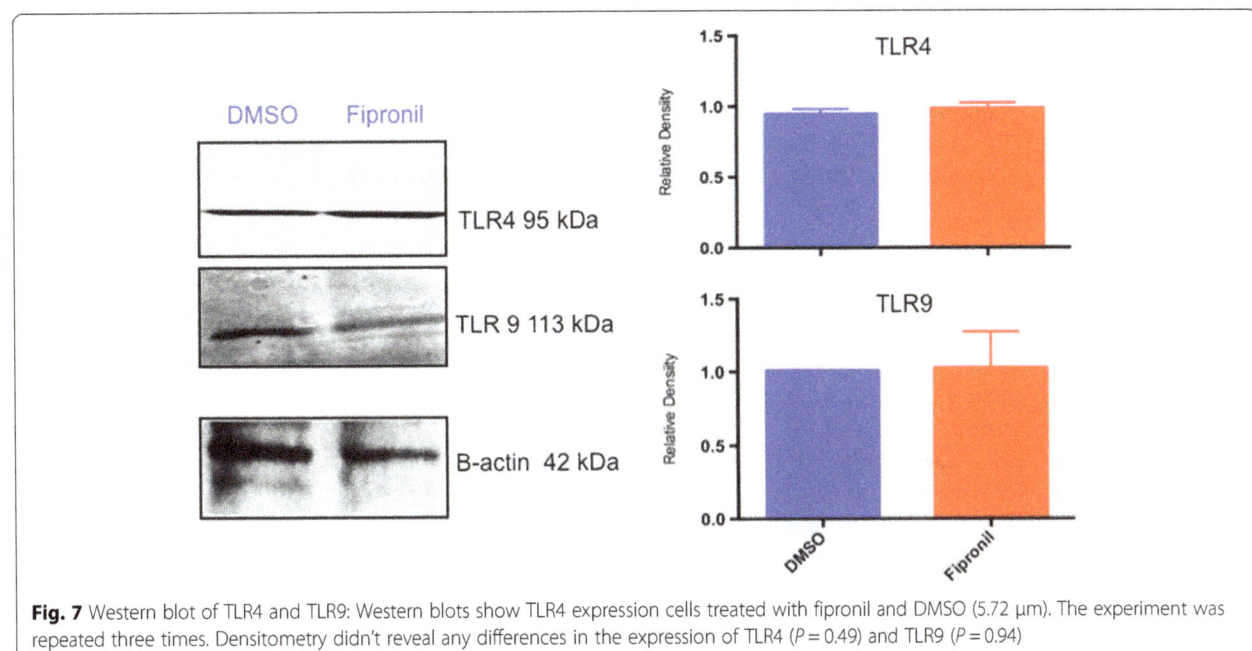

Fig. 7 Western blot of TLR4 and TLR9: Western blots show TLR4 expression cells treated with fipronil and DMSO (5.72 μm). The experiment was repeated three times. Densitometry didn't reveal any differences in the expression of TLR4 ($P = 0.49$) and TLR9 ($P = 0.94$)

would increase susceptibility of animal and humans to endotoxin exposures, which are found in higher amounts in agriculture buildings such as grain elevators and pig barns. Therefore, we need to undertake additional studies where experimental animals exposed to fipronil are challenged with LPS to understand the interactions between the two. The present studies also do not address the reasons for a significant increase in TLR4 positive cells after intranasal but not oral treatment with fipronil. One of the reasons may be the fipronil in the oral group was metabolized and a significantly lesser amount of the original chemical or the metabolite reached the lungs thus activating a fewer number of TLR4 positive cells. Possibly the passage of the chemical or its metabolite(s) through the liver may have attenuated its toxicity for the lung.

We used a macrophage cell line for in vitro studies on the effects of fipronil as many of the septal cells recruited following intranasal treatment are macrophages. Macrophages are central to lung immunity and generation of immune responses [26]. The data showed a reduction in percentages of living cells with a range of concentrations from 0.86 μmol to 5.72 μmol but not at 0.29 μmol. We used 0.29 μmol and 5.72 μmol and found that only the higher concentration caused significant reduction in cell viability at 3 and 9 h of incubation with fipronil compared to the control and the lower concentration. However, both concentrations reduced cell viability after 24 h of the exposure. Previously, chlorpyrifos, which is linked to abnormal immune responses in humans induced apoptosis in U937 cells through caspase-3 activation [27]. Our histological observations didn't reveal signs of cell necrosis/apoptosis in lungs following in vivo treatment with fipronil. The in vitro induction of cell death by fipronil may be due to more direct interaction of the pesticide with only one cell type available in the culture, and requires additional studies.

Macrophages express TLR such as TLR4 and TLR9 and use these molecules to sense microbial molecules [26, 28]. Western blot data showed lack of effect of fipronil on TLR4 and TLR9 expression in macrophage cell line. Because fipronil kills macrophages, the lack of differences in TLR4 and TLR9 expression may be due to increased expression of TLR4 and TLR9/cell to result in lack of differences between the control and the treated macrophage. This would in turn suggest that the expression of TLR4 and TLR9 on live cells may actually be increased as was the case in vivo where the number of septal cells expressing TLR4 was increased following intranasal treatment with fipronil. The preliminary immunofluorescence data on TLR4 expression showed lack of difference between control and fipronil treated cells. However, further studies are needed to clarify the issue.

We report the first in vivo and in vitro effects of fipronil on lungs and macrophage cells, respectively. The data

show lung inflammation following both oral and intranasal treatments with fipronil and an increase in TLR4 positive cells in alveolar septa with intranasal treatment. The in vitro treatment with fipronil caused a concentration dependent reduction in the number of viable U937 macrophage cells but had no effect on the TLR4 or TLR9 expression. Taken together, these data suggest that exposure to fipronil induces lung inflammation and may increase its susceptibility for subsequent endotoxin exposure.

Competing interests
The authors declare they have no competing interests.

Authors' contributions
KM conceived of the study, analyzed data, and carried out most of the experiments and writing of the manuscript. JPSG and RSS participated in the exposure experiments, data analyses and writing of manuscript. BS assisted with experiment design, writing of paper, and guidance of the project. All authors read and approved the final manuscript.

Acknowledgements
The work was supported by an International Partnership Project Grant from the University of Saskatchewan Discovery Grant and the Natural Sciences and Engineering Research Council of Canada to Baljit Singh. The work in the laboratories of Dr. JPS Gill and Dr. RS Sethi was supported through funds from the Guru Angad Dev Veterinary and Animal Sciences University, Punjab, India.

Author details
[1]Department of Veterinary Biomedical Sciences, Western College of Veterinary Medicine, University of Saskatchewan, 52 Campus Drive, Saskatoon, SK S7N 5B4, Canada. [2]School of Animal Biotechnology, Guru Angad Dev Veterinary and Animal Sciences University, Ludhiana, India. [3]School of Veterinary Public Health, Guru Angad Dev Veterinary and Animal Sciences University, Ludhiana, India.

References
1. Kannan K, Tanabe S, Giesy JP, Tatsukawa R. Organochlorine pesticides and polychlorinated biphenyls in foodstuffs from Asian and oceanic countries. Rev Environ Contam Toxicol. 1997;152:1–55.
2. Jennings KA, Canerdy TD, Keller RJ, Atieh BH, Doss RB, Gupta RC. Human exposure to fipronil from dogs treated with frontline. Vet Hum Toxicol. 2002;44(5):301–3.
3. Ratra GS, Erkkila BE, Weiss DS, Casida JE. Unique insecticide specificity of human homomeric rho 1 GABA(C) receptor. Toxicol Lett. 2002;129(1–2):47–53.
4. Ratra GS, Casida JE. GABA receptor subunit composition relative to insecticide potency and selectivity. Toxicol Lett. 2001;122(3):215–22.
5. Ratra GS, Kamita SG, Casida JE. Role of human GABA(A) receptor beta3 subunit in insecticide toxicity. Toxicol Appl Pharmacol. 2001;172(3):233–40. doi:10.1006/taap.2001.9154.
6. Zhao X, Yeh JZ, Salgado VL, Narahashi T. Sulfone metabolite of fipronil blocks gamma-aminobutyric acid- and glutamate-activated chloride channels in mammalian and insect neurons. J Pharmacol Exp Ther. 2005;314(1):363–73. doi:10.1124/jpet.104.077891.
7. Badgujar PC, Chandratre GA, Pawar NN, Telang AG, Kurade NP. Fipronil induced oxidative stress involves alterations in SOD1 and catalase gene expression in male mice liver: Protection by vitamins E and C. Environ Toxicol. 2015. doi:10.1002/tox.22125.
8. Cravedi JP, Delous G, Zalko D, Viguie C, Debrauwer L. Disposition of fipronil in rats. Chemosphere. 2013;93(10):2276–83. doi:10.1016/j.chemosphere.2013.07.083.
9. Tavares MA, Palma ID, Medeiros HC, Guelfi M, Santana AT, Mingatto FE. Comparative effects of fipronil and its metabolites sulfone and desulfinyl on the isolated rat liver mitochondria. Environ Toxicol Pharmacol. 2015;40(1):206–14. doi:10.1016/j.etap.2015.06.013.

10. Gill KK, Dumka VK. Biochemical alterations induced by oral subchronic exposure to fipronil, fluoride and their combination in buffalo calves. Environ Toxicol Pharmacol. 2013;36(3):1113–9. doi:10.1016/j.etap.2013.09.011.

11. Gill KK, Dumka VK. Antioxidant status in oral subchronic toxicity of fipronil and fluoride co-exposure in buffalo calves. Toxicol Ind Health. 2013. doi:10.1177/0748233713500376.

12. Zhang B, Xu Z, Zhang Y, Shao X, Xu X, Cheng J, et al. Fipronil induces apoptosis through caspase-dependent mitochondrial pathways in Drosophila S2 cells. Pestic Biochem Physiol. 2015;119:81–9. doi:10.1016/j.pestbp.2015.01.019.

13. Ki YW, Lee JE, Park JH, Shin IC, Koh HC. Reactive oxygen species and mitogen-activated protein kinase induce apoptotic death of SH-SY5Y cells in response to fipronil. Toxicol Lett. 2012;211(1):18–28. doi:10.1016/j.toxlet.2012.02.022.

14. Lassiter TL, MacKillop EA, Ryde IT, Seidler FJ, Slotkin TA. Is fipronil safer than chlorpyrifos? Comparative developmental neurotoxicity modeled in PC12 cells. Brain Res Bull. 2009;78(6):313–22. doi:10.1016/j.brainresbull.2008.09.020.

15. Caballero MV, Ares I, Martinez M, Martinez-Larranaga MR, Anadon A, Martinez MA. Fipronil induces CYP isoforms in rats. Food Chem Toxicol. 2015;83:215–21. doi:10.1016/j.fct.2015.06.019.

16. de Medeiros HC, Constantin J, Ishii-Iwamoto EL, Mingatto FE. Effect of fipronil on energy metabolism in the perfused rat liver. Toxicol Lett. 2015;236(1):34–42. doi:10.1016/j.toxlet.2015.04.016.

17. Williams AE, Chambers RC. The mercurial nature of neutrophils: still an enigma in ARDS? Am J Physiol Lung Cell Mol Physiol. 2014;306(3):L217–30. doi:10.1152/ajplung.00311.2013.

18. Michaux G, Cutler DF. How to roll an endothelial cigar: the biogenesis of Weibel-Palade bodies. Traffic. 2004;5(2):69–78.

19. Hannah MJ, Williams R, Kaur J, Hewlett LJ, Cutler DF. Biogenesis of Weibel-Palade bodies. SeminCell DevBiol. 2002;13:313–24.

20. Ben DF, Yu XY, Ji GY, Zheng DY, Lv KY, Ma B, et al. TLR4 mediates lung injury and inflammation in intestinal ischemia-reperfusion. J Surg Res. 2012;174(2):326–33. doi:10.1016/j.jss.2010.12.005.

21. Aharonson-Raz K, Lohmann KL, Townsend HG, Marques F, Singh B. Pulmonary intravascular macrophages as proinflammatory cells in heaves, an asthma-like equine disease. Am J Physiol Lung Cell Mol Physiol. 2012;303(3):L189–98. doi:10.1152/ajplung.00271.2011.

22. Hoppstadter J, Diesel B, Zarbock R, Breinig T, Monz D, Koch M, et al. Differential cell reaction upon Toll-like receptor 4 and 9 activation in human alveolar and lung interstitial macrophages. Respir Res. 2010;11:124. doi:10.1186/1465-9921-11-124.

23. Dong XS, Xu XY, Sun YQ, Wei L, Jiang ZH, Liu Z. Toll-like receptor 4 is involved in myocardial damage following paraquat poisoning in mice. Toxicology. 2013;312:115–22. doi:10.1016/j.tox.2013.08.009.

24. Tan W, Pruett SB. Effects of sodium methyldithiocarbamate on selected parameters of innate immunity and clearance of bacteria in a mouse model of sepsis. Life Sci. 2015;139:1–7. doi:10.1016/j.lfs.2015.08.001.

25. Pruett SB, Zheng Q, Schwab C, Fan R. Sodium methyldithiocarbamate inhibits MAP kinase activation through toll-like receptor 4, alters cytokine production by mouse peritoneal macrophages, and suppresses innate immunity. Toxicol Sci. 2005;87(1):75–85. doi:10.1093/toxsci/kfi215.

26. Schneberger D, Aharonson-Raz K, Singh B. Monocyte and macrophage heterogeneity and Toll-like receptors in the lung. Cell Tissue Res. 2011;343(1):97–106. doi:10.1007/s00441-010-1032-2.

27. Nakadai A, Li Q, Kawada T. Chlorpyrifos induces apoptosis in human monocyte cell line U937. Toxicology. 2006;224(3):202–9. doi:10.1016/j.tox.2006.04.055.

28. Schneberger D, Caldwell S, Kanthan R, Singh B. Expression of Toll-like receptor 9 in mouse and human lungs. J Anat. 2013;222(5):495–503. doi:10.1111/joa.12039.

12

Prevalence, predictors and economic burden of morbidities among waste-pickers

Praveen Chokhandre[1], Shrikant Singh[2] and Gyan Chandra Kashyap[1*]

Abstract

Background: The occupation of waste-picking characterised as 3Ds – dangerous, drudgery and demanding. In this context, the study aimed to assess occupational morbidities among the waste-pickers and attempts to identify potential individual level risk factors enhancing health risks. Additionally, economic burden of morbidities has been assessed.

Methods: The burden of the morbidities was assessed and compared with a comparison group through a cross-sectional survey. Waste-pickers ($n = 200$) and a comparison group ($n = 103$) working for at least a year were randomly selected from the communities living on the edge of the Deonar dumping site. The difference in the prevalence of morbidities was tested using the chi-square test. The effect of waste picking resulting the development of morbidities was assessed using the propensity score matching (PSM) method. A multivariate logistic regression model was employed to identify the individual risk factors. T-test has been employed in order to analyse the difference in health care expenditure between waste pickers and non-waste pickers.

Results: The prevalence of morbidities was significantly higher among the waste-pickers, particularly for injuries (75%), respiratory illness (28%), eye infection (29%), and stomach problems (32%), compared to the comparison group (17%, 15%, 18%, and 19% respectively). The results of the PSM method highlighted that waste-picking raised the risk of morbidity for injuries (62%) and respiratory illness (13%). Results of logistic regression suggest that low level of hygiene practices [household cleanliness (OR = 3.23, $p < 0.00$), non-use of soap before meals (OR = 2.65, $p < 0.05$)] and use of recyclable items as a cooking fuel (OR = 2.12, $p < 0.03$) enhanced health risks among the waste pickers when adjusted for the age, duration of work, duration of stay in community and substance use. Additionally, the high prevalence of morbidities among waste pickers resulted into higher healthcare expenditure. Findings of the study suggest that not only healthcare expenditure but persistence of illness and work days lost due to injury/illness is significantly higher among waste pickers compared to non-waste pickers.

Conclusions: The study concluded that waste-picking raised the risk of morbidities as also expenditure on healthcare. Results from the study recommend several measures to lessen the morbidities and thereby incurred healthcare expenditure.

Keywords: Injuries, Occupational morbidities, Respiratory illness, Stomach problems, Waste-pickers

Background

In the absence of any urban market-based skills, investment and social capital, which are precursors to get gainful employment, many of the migrant urban poor are forced to engage in the filthy occupation of waste picking. On the other hand, the very structure of solid waste management in the cities of developing countries offers an opportunity of survival to millions of waste-pickers [1]. In the developing countries, the rough estimate of waste-pickers was 15 million, of which around 1.5 million belonged to India [2].

The reasons for engaging in the occupation of waste-picking could range from high unemployment to a proliferating amount of solid waste and a growing global market for recycled materials. Waste-pickers work informally and earn a meagre income by collecting and

* Correspondence: statskashyap@gmail.com
[1]International Institute for Population Sciences, Govandi Station Road Donor, Mumbai 400088, India
Full list of author information is available at the end of the article

selling recyclable items out of municipal solid waste. While providing the opportunity for survival, waste-picking also has health hazards. Characterised by 3Ds – dangerous, drudgery and demanding – waste-picking leads to fatal and non-fatal morbidities. Past studies indicate that relationship exists between solid waste handling and increased health risks [3–5]. On the other hand, non-fatal morbidities are mainly musculoskeletal in nature. Past studies have revealed a significant relationship between work environment and complaints of musculoskeletal disorders. Workplace activities, such as heavy lifting, manual handling, prolonged bending and repetitive tasks, increase musculoskeletal disorders (MSDs) significantly [6–8]. A study based on waste-pickers suggest that MSDs were significantly higher for the lower back, knees, upper back, shoulders and ankles among the waste-pickers than in the comparison group [9]. In addition to the occupational health risks, their deplorable living conditions, poor hygiene practices and substance use enhance susceptibility to health risks.

In the light of the growing number of the urban poor opting for waste picking and given the nature of waste picking and the associated morbidities, limited studies have been carried out in India. Most of these studies having been done using pilot based data or non-representative samples. Further, these studies have also not taken into account the occupational and individual characteristics which too determine the health risks facing the waste pickers. Moreover, past studies have focused on morbidity prevalence among the waste pickers but have not considered the relative health risks of waste picking compared with the other occupational groups. Following to health risk, to date, hardly any study investigated the health expenditure among waste pickers. Considering this, the present study investigates the occupational health risks among the waste pickers and an attempt has been made to identify the potential risk factors which enhance their health vulnerabilities followed by economic burden of the morbidities.

Materials and methods
Design/setting
A cross-sectional study with a comparison group was conducted upon waste-pickers working at the Deonar dumping site – one of the oldest dumping sites in Asia, located in Mumbai.

Study population
Waste-pickers engaged in waste-picking at the dumping site at least for a year and aged 18 years and above were considered as cases for the study. A group of workers with similar characteristics and engaged in occupations other than waste-picking were considered as the comparison group. They were drawn randomly from in and around the communities where the waste-pickers reside.

They were mostly engaged as daily wage labourers, or in embroidery (*zari*) work and other manual occupations.

Sampling design
There are many slum communities living on the edge of the *Deonar* dumping site. Many of the waste-pickers stay in these communities. Three out of those communities were selected, using probability proportional to size (PPS) sampling. In order to ensure the effective representation of the communities, they were divided into a number of clusters having a household (HH) size ranging from a minimum of 40 to a maximum of 100 HHs. Cluster areas were identified on the basis of natural divisions of the communities. Among the total clusters, approximately 10% were selected using the PPS sampling procedure. In the next stage, mapping and listing operation was carried out in the sampled clusters, where a screener (that is age, occupation and years of working) was canvassed to find targeted participants. Through mapping and listing, we got a sampling frame for the waste-picker households and for the comparison group. Based on the sampling frame, the required number of households were selected from both the groups by using systematic random sampling.

Sample size
The total sample size for this study was determined based on the proportion of waste-pickers in the selected communities. A community based organisation reported that around 30% of the households in the study area had at least one person engaged in waste-picking. The estimated sample size was 426 households with a p value 0.30, a response rate of 0.90 with design effect of 1.20. In order to conduct case-comparison study, the total sample was divided into two equal parts. Finally, a sample of 200 waste-pickers and 200 from comparison group were interviewed (94% response rate). Further, 93 cases were dropped from the comparison group as they were housewives. The results are presented for waste pickers ($n = 200$) and comparison group ($n = 103$). The data was collected during March to July 2014.

Variables used
Response variables
The considered morbidities were based on the past studies and enquired from both the groups. The symptoms of self-reported morbidities of respiratory illness, stomach problem, eye and skin infections, and injuries while picking waste, were recorded for the study. In addition to this, other morbidities that may arise due to the waste picking occupation or due to their poor housing and living conditions were also covered including stomach problem, skin infection, typhoid, jaundice, fever, and cold and cough.

8 Medicine

Confounding factors

For the present study, age of the respondent, years of working in the occupation, weekly working hours and duration of stay in the community were considered confounding variables, whereas hygiene practices and substance use were considered as effect modifiers.

Data analysis

The data was entered in the CSPro.06 software and analysed using the STATA (Version 13.1). Descriptive statistics, such as means, percentages and 95% confidence intervals, were used to describe socio-demographic information. Differences in the prevalence of morbidities among the groups were tested using the chi-square test. Similarly, the difference in healthcare expenditure between waste-pickers and non-waste pickers has been tested using t-test.

Methods

In order to examine the impact of the waste-picking occupation on the development of the selected morbidities, the study adopted the nearest neighbourhood method of propensity score matching PSM [10, 11]. This approach gives an opportunity to assess the impact of exposure on outcomes through cross-sectional survey data [12–14]. The propensity score is estimated by logistic regression, with the dichotomous exposure/treatment variable. For instance, 1 = exposed to waste-picking occupation; 0 = unexposed to waste-picking occupation, using the associated observed demographic and occupational characteristics of the waste-pickers used as predictor variables.

In this case, the difference in the reported symptoms of the selected morbidities between the waste-pickers and the comparison group can be directly compared to show the impact of the waste-picking occupation on the waste-pickers. This is known as average exposure effect on exposed (AEEE). In order to calculate the impact of waste-picking on the occurrence of the selected morbidities, the average effects in both the groups were weighted by the proportion of the respondents in the exposed and the comparison groups, which measured the increase/decrease in the morbidities due to the waste-picking occupation. Similarly, in order to understand the individual risk factors affecting the health of the waste-pickers for selected morbidities, logistic regression analysis was employed, with adjustment of confounding factors such as age, years of working in the occupation and duration of stay in the community.

Results

Demographic and occupational profile

Table 1 suggests that the waste-pickers were comparable with the comparison group in terms of demographic and occupational characteristics. The average age of the

Table 1 Profile of study groups

Characteristic	Waste-pickers (n = 200)	Comparison group (n = 103)
Age of workers		
Below 35 years	53.0	47.6
35 & above	47.0	52.4
Mean ± SD	34.0 ± 10.2	35.5 ± 10.3
Duration of stay in the community		
Below 15 years	29.5	43.7
15 & above	70.5	56.3
Mean ± SD	18.7 ± 9.7	15.2 ± 8.8
Working years		
Below 10 yrs.	41.5	37.9
10 & above	58.5	62.1
Mean ± SD	11.2 ± 6.7	11.7 ± 7.4

waste-pickers was 34 years, similar to 36 years in case of the comparison group, with a standard deviation of 10 years each. A similar pattern was observed with regard to years of working. Marginal difference has been observed in case of average duration of stay in the community between the groups.

Prevalence of morbidities

Table 2 exhibits the prevalence of specific morbidities (during the previous six months) among the waste-pickers and the comparison group. At 75%, the prevalence of injuries was strikingly higher among the waste-pickers; whereas for the comparison group it was 17%. The injuries were mostly lacerations caused by needles or shards of glass, followed by muscle sprain. Similarly, the prevalence of respiratory symptoms was higher among the waste-pickers (28%) than the comparison group (15%). The prevalence of dyspnea and chronic cough particularly was found to be higher among the waste-pickers. Similarly, while considering eye infections, such as redness of eyes, watering of eyes or itching of eyes, the prevalence was higher among the waste-pickers (29%) than the comparison group (18%). For instance, the prevalence of eye soreness (20%) and watering of eyes (13%) was higher among the waste-pickers than the comparison group (19% & 9% respectively). Stomach problems, viz. nausea, gastroenteritis, dysentery, constipation or intestinal pain, were higher among the waste-pickers (32%) than the comparison group (19%). Episodes of gastroenteritis (20%), nausea (14%) and loose motions (14%) especially were found to be higher among the waste pickers than in the comparison group (13%, 2% and 10% respectively).

Results of PSM for the selected morbidities

The present study attempt to assess the exposure effect of the waste picking occupation on the development of

Table 2 Prevalence of morbidities among the waste pickers and the comparison group in the previous six months

	Waste pickers (n = 200)	Comparison group (n = 103)	chi2 (p-value)
Injury/Accident	75.0 [0.68 to 0.81]	16.5 [0.09 to 0.23]	(χ2 = 94.03; p = 0.000)
Fracture/contusion	3.5	2.9	(χ2 = 0.073; p = 0.786)
Muscle sprain	12.5	2.9	(χ2 = 7.451; p = 0.006)
Laceration (Needles and glass)	70.0	11.7	(χ2 = 92.58; p = 0.000)
Respiratory infection	28.0 [0.21 to 0.34]	14.6 [0.07 to 0.21]	(χ2 = 6.841; p = 0.009)
Dust allergy	12.0	2.9	(χ2 = 6.916; p = 0.009)
Dyspnea	14.5	10.7	(χ2 = 0.866; p = 0.352)
Episodes of asthma	4.0	1.9	(χ2 = 0.572; p = 0.449)
Chronic cough/Running nose	15.0	2.9	(χ2 = 10.235; p = 0.001)
Wheeze and breathlessness	7.5	2.9	(χ2 = 2.560; p = 0.110)
Eye infection	29.0 [0.22 to 0.35]	17.5 [0.10 to 0.24]	(χ2 = 4.805; p = 0.028)
Eye soreness/infection	19.5	12.6	(χ2 = 2.262; p = 0.133)
Watering of eyes	18.5	8.7	(χ2 = 5.031; p = 0.025)
Itching of eyes	8.0	1.9	(χ2 = 4.465; p = 0.035)
Stomach problem	32.0 [0.25 to 0.38]	19.4 [0.11 to 0.27]	(χ2 = 5.371; p = 0.020)
Nausea	14.0	1.9	(χ2 = 11.081; p = 0.001)
Loose motion	14.0	9.7	(χ2 = 1.141; p = 0.285)
Gastroenteritis	20.0	12.6	(χ2 = 2.564; p = 0.109)
Constipation	7.5	3.8	(χ2 = 1.512; p = 0.219)
Skin infection	6.0 [0.02 to 0.09]	2.9 [0.00 to 0.06]	(χ2 = 1.377; p = 0.241)
Typhoid/Jaundice	16.0	8.7	(χ2 = 3.064; p = 0.080)
Fever/cold & cough	34.5	34.0	(χ2 = 0.008; p = 0.928)

Values in square bracket are at 95% Confidence Interval

the selected morbidities by estimating the difference in the outcomes between the exposed group (the waste-pickers) and the matched comparison group. Analysis from Table 3 clearly highlights that episodes of injuries were 57% higher among the waste-pickers when compared with the comparison group. Similarly, self-reported symptoms of respiratory illness were found to be higher among the waste-pickers (13%) than the comparison group.

Individual risk factors for morbidities

While analysing the individual risk factors, the results of the logistic regression analysis suggest that advancing years significantly increases the likelihood of respiratory illness (OR = 1.97, p = 0.05). Similarly, those who were using wood and other recyclable items as fuel for cooking were significantly more likely to develop respiratory illness (OR = 2.12, p = 0.03) compared to those were using liquefied petroleum gases (LPG). In case of

Table 3 Average exposure effect and average exposure effect on exposed for the waste picking occupation on the selected morbidities in the previous 6 months

	Average Exposure Effect (AEE)		Average Exposure Effect on Exposed (AEEE)	
	Coef.	[95% Conf. Interval]	Coef.	[95% Conf. Interval]
Injury/Accident	0.57***	(0.463 to 0.672)	0.62***	(0.511 to 0.729)
Respiratory infection	0.13**	(0.017 to 0.233)	0.13**	(0.007 to 0.243)
Eye infection	0.04	(−0.108 to 0.194)	0.03	(−0.172 to 0.232)
Stomach problem	0.02	(−0.191 to 0.231)	0.02	(−0.265 to 0.305)
Typhoid/Jaundice[a]	0.03	(−0.112 to 0.171)	0.01	(−0.189 to 0.199)
Fever/cold & cough[a]	0.05	(−0.072 to 0.171)	0.13**	(0.003 to 0.257)

[a]Morbidities were considered for the 12 months prior to the survey
*p<0.1, **p<0.05, ***p<0.01

stomach problems, household cleaning few days a week (OR = 3.23, p = 0.00) and non-use of soap before meals (OR = 2.65, p = 0.05) emerged as significant predictors of increased risk of stomach problems (Table 4).

Economic burden of the morbidities

Along with the prevalence of morbidities among the waste-pickers, the paper attempt to assess the economic burden of the morbidities in terms of expenditure incurred on treatment, work days lost and persistence of illness among waste-pickers (Table 5). Findings suggest that the mean expenditure was significantly higher among the waste-pickers (₹1736) than the non-waste pickers (₹993). Similarly, the persistence of illness was significantly higher for the waste-pickers (31 days) than the comparison group (19 days). Further, findings suggest that the mean number of work days lost due to morbidities was significantly higher among the waste-pickers (18 days) than the comparison group (11 days). A significant difference in healthcare expenditure has been observed among the waste-pickers by the type of health-care facility. For instance, the average expenditure

Table 4 Logistic regression analysis of independent risk factors for the selected morbidities

	OR	[95% Conf. Int.]
Respiratory illness		
Age		
Below 35 years®		
35 years and above	1.97*	(0.97–3.97)
Fuel for cooking		
LPG®		
Other³	2.12**	(1.06 -4.26)
Stomach problem		
Age		
Below 35 years®		
35 years and above	1.73	(0.87–3.43)
Household cleaning		
Daily®		
Some days in a week	3.23***	(1.68–6.21)
Soap use before meals		
Yes®		
No	2.65*	(0.99–7.10)
Availability of waste-water carrying lines		
Yes®		
No	1.68	(0.87–3.21)

®Reference category; Figures are odds ratios with CI at 95%
*p < 0.1, **p < 0.05, ***p < 0.01
³Other includes wood, kerosene and material found at the dumping site and used as fuel for cooking
Model is additionally adjusted for substance use, years of working and years of stay in the communities

Table 5 Economic Burden of the morbidities among waste-pickers and non-waste pickers

	Mean (95% CI)	t-test
Health care expenditure on injuries/illness (INR Rupees)		
Waste pickers	1736 (1248–2225)	t = 1.94; p = 0.053
Non-waste pickers	993 (535–1451)	
Persistence of injury/illness (days)		
Waste pickers	31 (19–42)	t = 1.41; p = 0.078
Non-waste pickers	19 (13–25)	
Total work days lost due to injury/illness (days)		
Waste pickers	18 (15–21)	t = 2.80; p = 0.005
Non-waste pickers	11 (7–14)	
Total health care expenditure among waste pickers by type of facility (INR Rupees)		
Government	582 (364–800)	t = 2.05; p = 0.041
Private	1137 (670–1602)	

Injuries/illness comprise injuries, respiratory illness, stomach problem, eye infection, skin infection, typhoid/jaundice and fever/cold/cough

incurred at a government healthcare facility for morbidities/injuries was ₹ 582, whereas the corresponding figure for private health facility was ₹1137.

Discussion

The present study examine the prevalence of morbidities among waste-pickers by comparing with a comparison group. Results suggest that the prevalence of injuries was strikingly higher among the waste-pickers (75%) compared to the comparison group (17%). The injuries were mostly due to lacerations caused by shards of glass, followed by muscle sprain. Field insights revealed that there were frequent incidences of serious injuries and deaths occurred when waste-pickers hit by a vehicle or dozer while rushing to collect waste at the time of unloading by waste carrier vehicle. Past studies suggest there is increased risk of hepatitis B and C virus infection due to exposure to sharp instruments during waste collection [15, 16]. Similarly, exposure to fumes at the disposal sites resulted in respiratory problems. The prevalence of respiratory symptoms was found to be significantly higher among the waste-pickers (28%) compared to the comparison group (15%). Particularly, the prevalence of dyspnea (difficulty in breathing) and chronic cough were found to be higher among the waste-pickers. Field insights suggest that the majority of the waste-pickers were not using any protective clothing such as gumboot, gloves and masks, which enhanced their health vulnerabilities. The reason for not using any protective clothing could be their ignorance and poverty [17]. Stomach problems, viz. nausea, dysentery and intestinal pain, were found to be higher among the waste-pickers (32%) than the comparison group (19%). The results of logistic regression clearly highlighted that poor hygiene practices raised the risk of stomach problems. The dumping site being a breeding ground for vectors such as flies, mosquitoes and rats, a large number of diseases and infections are transmitted through these vectors due to their contact with contaminated waste material or water [18]. Results from the propensity score matching method depicted that exposure of waste-picking raised the risk of morbidities such as injuries and respiratory illness when compared to the matched comparison group. Additionally, the nature of their occupation requires the waste-pickers constant bending, which raised the risk of musculoskeletal disorders in many body parts. Waste-pickers have to climb all the way up a pile of garbage to collect waste and climb down with the pile of garbage usually with heavy bags of collected waste rested either on their back, head or shoulders. Hence carrying of heavy weights could also be a reason for the higher prevalence of MSDs among the waste-pickers. Past studies based on waste-pickers exhibit similar results particularly for injuries (82%) [17] respiratory illness (21%) [19] and stomach problems ranging from 39 to 29% [19, 20]. The results from other studies based on waste-pickers did not match with the present study due to dissimilarity in reference period for the reported morbidities.

Additionally, analysis from the study highlighted that the economic burden of the morbidities was significantly higher for the waste-pickers compared to the comparison group. This clearly implies that the economic burden of the morbidities puts them into the poverty trap. Moreover, the health of the waste-pickers is affected at two levels: one, arising out of their poverty and the conditions in which they live; and second, arising out of their exposure to disease and infection due to their occupation. Several authors have extensively recorded the work conditions of the waste-pickers and assessed how they are at the bottom of the socio-economic ladder in terms of income and respect [21–24]. These people live in unhygienic conditions, and the nature of their occupation exposes them to potentially pathogenic bio-aerosols that may lead to the spread of various diseases [25]. The abundance of fleas and offensive odours at the waste disposal sites, along with the lack of proper protective devices, makes them more susceptible to health risk. A clinical study conducted on waste-pickers in Nigeria recorded that they are potential carriers of pathogens that degrade the waste and that they serve as vehicles of transmission of pathogens that are capable of causing diseases in the body [26]. Apart from their occupational health risks, contextual factors, viz. their abysmal living environment, their health and hygiene practices, may further enhance their vulnerability to diseases. Further, several studies have also recorded the higher prevalence of substance use among the waste-pickers [20, 27, 28]. The

results of self-reported morbidities could be biased due to subjectivity in responses. Recall bias may also have affected the estimated prevalence of morbidities. Data were collected from waste-pickers who collect the waste from dumping site and not from the other type of waste-pickers who collect waste from road side or community bins and hence generalization of the results must be done with caution.

The work of the waste-pickers is not always appreciated or acknowledged, although they make a positive contribution to the society by reducing the cost of collection and transportation and by reducing the burden of the dumping site. Several studies have tried to estimate the economic contribution of the informal waste sector to the economy as it has a financial impact of several billions of US dollars every year [29]. A more detailed analysis by Medina shows that the work of the waste-pickers makes positive contributions to the society, and with support, these contributions can be even greater. Moreover, waste-picking activity reduces the cost of the proper management of waste and its collection, transportation and proper disposal. Francisco (2009) states that the work of these individuals around the world helps industries by reducing raw material imports [30]. This implies that they contribute to the conservation of natural resources and energy while reducing air and water pollution. They also reduce greenhouse gas emissions through the reuse of materials.

Suggested strategies to minimize the burden of morbidities among waste-pickers

- This study recommends both preventive and curative measures to minimize the burden of morbidities among waste-pickers.
- Health providers can play a crucial role in reducing the prevalence of morbidities through health education and by increasing the awareness of early signs and symptoms of morbidities.
- Measures should be taken to promote physical exercise as well as the use of protective equipment to reduce work-related musculoskeletal disorders.
- As waste-pickers are unorganized and earn a meagre income, the development of low cost and easy-to-use tools to minimize the occurrence of MSDs would be helpful.
- There is an urgent need of health education particularly related to health and hygiene behaviour among waste-pickers. A study conducted in Thailand exhibited that the significance of the health risk reduction behaviour model (HRRBM) decreased the healthcare costs of individuals and significantly improved knowledge, attitude and practices among the waste-pickers. The percentage of physical

symptoms was reduced due to the use of personal protective equipment (PPE) compared to the control group [25].

- Meagre income and a high prevalence of morbidities and healthcare expenditure often leads to poverty [31–33], particularly among the urban poor households [34]. Therefore, it is imperative to promote state sponsored cashless health insurance schemes like Rajiv Gandhi Jeevandayee Arogya Yojna (RGJAY) [35] and Rashtriya Swasthya Bima Yojana (RSBY) [36] among the waste-pickers.

Conclusions

Several studies including the present study have highlighted that waste-pickers are at a high risk of developing occupational morbidities particularly injuries, respiratory illness, eye infection, stomach problems, typhoid, diarrhoea, and musculoskeletal disorders. Further, individual risk factors such as poor hygiene practices, non-use of protective equipment, inhuman living conditions, and high prevalence of substance use further enhance their health vulnerabilities. This study recommends several possible strategies to abate the episodes of morbidities. Similarly, it propounds the need to promote health insurance among waste-pickers. Overall, in order for them to bargain for their rights in terms of getting a better workplace and recognition of their contribution to solid waste management, collective voices need to be built up.

Abbreviations

AEE: Average Exposure Effect; AEEE: Average Exposure Effect on Exposed; HHs: Household; HRRBM: Health Risk Reduction Behaviour Model; LPG: Liquefied Petroleum Gases; MSDs: Musculoskeletal Disorder; OR: Odds Ratio; PPE: Personal Protective Equipment; PPS: Probability Proportional to Size; PSM: Propensity Score Matching; RGJAY: Rajiv Gandhi Jeevandayee Arogya Yojna; RSBY: Rashtriya Swasthya Bima Yojana

Acknowledgements
Not applicable.

Authors' contributions
PC developed the questionnaire, collected the data, contributed in acquisition of data. SKS PC conceived and designed the experiments. PC GCK analysed the data. GCK PC wrote the manuscript. SKS critically revised the draft. All authors read and approved the final manuscript.

Funding
Not received any funding.

Authors' information
Praveen Chokhandre: PhD Student, International Institute for Population Sciences, Govandi Station Road Donor Mumbai, 400,088, India Email: praveenchokhandre@gmail.com. Shri Kant Singh: Professor, Department of Mathematical Demography & Statistics International Institute for Population Sciences, Govandi Station Road Deonar Mumbai, 400,088, India, Email: sksingh31962@gmail.com. Gyan Chandra Kashyap: PhD Student, International Institute for Population Sciences, Govandi Station Road Donor Mumbai, 400,088, India Email: statskashyap@gmail.com

Competing interests
The authors declare that they have no conflict of interest.

Author details
[1]International Institute for Population Sciences, Govandi Station Road Donor, Mumbai 400088, India. [2]Department of Mathematical Demography & Statistics, International Institute for Population Sciences, Govandi Station Road Deonar, Mumbai 400088, India.

References
1. Sebahat DT, Sertac G, Imer I, Ahmet Ragip I, Kazim G. Health and safety risks associated with waste picking. Turkish J Public Heal. 2006;4:41–4.
2. Medina M. The informal recycling sector in developing countries: organizing waste pickers to enhance their impact. Gridlines Shar Knowledge, Exp Innov public-private Partnersh Infrastruct. 2008;4:1–4.
3. Naresh K. Solid waste management : status of waste pickers and government policies. Indian Streams Res J. 2012;2:1.
4. da Silva D, Fassa M, Siqueira CE, Kriebel D. World at Work: Brazilian rag pickers. Occup Environ Med. 2005;62:736–40. doi:10.1136/oem.2005.020164.
5. Sarkar P. Solid Waste Management In Delhi – A Social Vulnerability Study. In: Bunch MJ, Suresh VM, Vasanta Kumaran T, editors. Third International Conference on Environment and Health. Chennai: Department of Geography, University of Madras and Faculty of Environmental Studies, York University; 2003. p. 451–64. http://www.yorku.ca/bunchmj/ICEH/proceedings/Sarkar_P_ICEH_papers_451to464.pdf.
6. Ijzelenberg W, Molenaar D, Burdorf A. Different risk factors for musculoskeletal complaints and musculoskeletal sickness absence. Scand J Work Environ Health. 2004;30:56–63.
7. Keyserling WM. Workplace risk factors and occupational musculoskeletal disorders, part 1: a review of biomechanical and psychophysical research on risk factors associated with low-back pain. Aihaj. 2000;61:39–50.
8. Hoozemans MJM, Kuijer PPFM, Kingma I, van Dieën JH, de Vries WHK, van der Woude LHV, et al. Mechanical loading of the low back and shoulders during pushing and pulling activities. Ergonomics. 2004;47:1–18. doi:10.1080/00140130310001593577.
9. Shrikant Singh PC. Assessing the impact of waste picking on musculoskeletal disorders among waste pickers in Mumbai, India: a cross-sectional study. BMJ Open. 2015;5:e008474.
10. Rosenbaum PR, Rubin DB. Constructing a control group using multivariate matched sampling methods that incorporate the propensity score. Am Stat. 1985;39:33–8. http://www.jstor.org/stable/2683903.
11. Stuart EA. Matching methods for causal inference: a review and a look forward. Stat Sci. 2010;25:1–21. doi:10.1214/09-STS313.
12. Rosenbaum PR, Rubin D. The central role of the propensity score in observational studies for causal effects. Biometrika. 1983;70:41–55. http://links.jstor.org/sici?sici=0006-3444(198304)70:1%3C41:TCROTP%3E2.0.CO;2-Q.
13. Rubin DB, Thomas N. Matching using estimated propensity scores: relating theory to practice. Biometrics. 1996;52:249–64.
14. Williamson E, Morley R, Lucas A, Carpenter J. Propensity scores: from naive enthusiasm to intuitive understanding. Stat Methods Med Res. 2012;21:273–93. doi:10.1177/0962280210394483.
15. Dounias G, Kypraiou E, Rachiotis G, Tsovili E, Kostopoulos S. Prevalence of hepatitis B virus markers in municipal solid waste workers in Keratsini (Greece). Occup Med (Chic III). 2005;55:60–3.

16. Tsovili E, Rachiotis G, Symvoulakis EK, Thanasias E, Giannisopoulou O, Papagiannis D, et al. Municipal waste collectors and hepatitis B and C virus infection: a cross-sectional study. Infez Med. 2014;22:271–6. http://www.ncbi. nlm.nih.gov/pubmed/25551841.

17. Syamala Devi K, Swamy AVV, Hema Krishna R. Studies on the solid waste collection by rag pickers at greater Hyderabad municipal corporation, India. Int. Res J Environ Sci. 2014;3:13–22.

18. Bhide AD, Sundaresan BB. Street cleansing and waste storage and collection in India. In: Holmes JR, editor. Managing solid waste in developing countries. USA: John Wiley & Songs Inc.; 1984. p. 149.

19. Ujawala S. The Occupational health of waste pickers in Pune: KKPKP and SWaCH members push for health rights. 2014. http://wiego.org/sites/wiego. org/files/publications/files/Samarth_OHS_Health_of_WP_in_Pune.pdf.

20. Ananthakrishnan Sneha PR. Health status and health seeking behaviour of rag pickers in the municipal dump yard in Chennai. Public Heal Res Ser. 2013;2:43–47.

21. Palnitkar S, Srinivasan V. Women Ragpickers in Bombay. Bombay; 1993.

22. Hayami Y, Dikshit AK, Mishra SN. Waste pickers and collectors in Delhi: poverty and environment in an urban informal sector. J Dev Stud. 2006;42:41–69.

23. Poornima C, Lakshmi N. Rising from the Waste—Organising Wastepickers in India, Thailand and the Philippines. In: Bangkok: Committee for Asian Women; 2009.

24. Gill K. Of poverty and plastic: scavenging and scrap trading entrepreneurs in India's urban informal economy. New Delhi: Oxford; 2012.

25. Thirarattanasunthon P, Siriwong W, Robson M, Borjan M. Health risk reduction behaviors model for scavengers exposed to solid waste in municipal dump sites in Nakhon Ratchasima Province, Thailand. Risk Manag Healthc Policy. 2012;5:97–104.

26. Wachukwu CK, Mbata CA, Nyenke CU. The health profile and impact assessment of waste scavengers (rag pickers) in Port Harcourt, Nigeria. J Appl Sci. 2010;10:1968–72.

27. Ray MR, Mukherjee G, Roychowdhury S, Lahiri T. Respiratory and general health impairments of ragpickers in India: a study in Delhi. Int Arch Occup Environ Health. 2004;77:595–8.

28. Venkateswaran S. Managing Waste – ecological, economic and social dimensions. Econ Polit Wkly. 1994;29:2907–11.

29. Medina M. The World's scavengers: salvaging for sustainable consumption and production. Lanham, MD: Alta Mira Press; 2007.

30. Salama-Younes M, Montazeri A, Ismail A, Roncin C. Factor structure and internal consistency of the 12-item general health questionnaire (GHQ-12) and the subjective vitality scale (VS), and the relationship between them: a study from France. Health Qual Life Outcomes. 2009;7:22.

31. Berman P, Ahuja R, Bhandari L. The Impoverishing Effect of Healthcare Payments in India: New Methodology and Findings. Econ Polit Wkly. 2010;xlv:65–71.

32. Krishna A. Escaping poverty and becoming poor: who gains, who loses, and why? World Dev. 2004;32:121–36.

33. Doorslaer van E, O' Donnell O, Rannan-Eliya R, Somanathan A, Adhikari SR, Akkazieva B. et al. Paying Out-of-Pocket for Health Care in Asia: Catastrophic and Poverty Impact. Rotterdam; 2005.

34. Chowdhury S. Financial burden of transient morbidity : a case study of slums in Delhi. Econ Polit Wkly. 2008;46:59–66.

35. RGJAY. Rajeev Gandhi Jeevandayee Aarogya Yojana 2008. https://www. jeevandayee.gov.in/.

36. RSBY. Rashtriya Swasthya Bima Yojna. 2008. http://www.rsby.gov.in/about_ rsby.aspx.

13

Quantification of cell-free DNA for evaluating genotoxic damage from occupational exposure to car paints

Mónica Villalba-Campos[1], Sandra Rocío Ramírez-Clavijo[1], Magda Carolina Sánchez-Corredor[1], Milena Rondón-Lagos[1], Milcíades Ibáñez-Pinilla[2], Ruth Marien Palma[3], Marcela Eugenia Varona-Uribe[2] and Lilian Chuaire-Noack[1]*

Abstract

Background: For several years, cell-free DNA has been emerging as an important biomarker for non-invasive diagnostic in a wide range of clinical conditions and diseases. The limited information available on the genotoxic effects associated with occupational exposure to car paints, as well as the fact that up-to-date there are not reports about cell-free DNA measurements for assessing this condition, led us to evaluate the DNA damage caused by the occupational exposure to organic solvents contained in car paints, through the quantification of the cell-free DNA and the comet assay, in a sample of 33 individuals taken from 10 automobile paint shops located in Bogota DC, Colombia.

Results: By applying the two methods, cell-free DNA and comet assay, we found a significant increase in the extent of DNA damage in the exposed individuals compared with the non-exposed ones within the control group.

Conclusions: Our findings provide useful information about the cell-free DNA levels in this type of exposure and can be considered as a support tool that contributes to the diagnosis of genotoxic damage in individuals occupationally exposed to car paints.

Keywords: Car painters, Organic solvents, Occupational exposure, Genotoxicity, Cell-free DNA, Comet assay

Background

The aromatic hydrocarbons used as solvents and paint removers (BTX - benzene, toluene, xylene) have been included in the list of substances to which workers in the paint industry are exposed to, according to IARC 2010 report [1]. Although most of metabolic products of these solvents, such as the S-phenyl mercapturic and trans-trans-muconic acids derived from benzene, and the hippuric acid derived from toluene are eliminated through the urine, some intermediate metabolites can interact with DNA and alter its structure, which makes benzene causes certain types of hematological disorders and cancer [2, 3] and toluene exhibits its toxic properties mainly at neuronal, urinary and reproductive level [4], among others.

In the case of individuals occupationally exposed to car paints, an increase in oxidative damage has been demonstrated [5] thus making cfDNA quantification a feasible option to assess the extent of genotoxic damage caused by the organic solvents found in these paints. In recent years, many biological biomarkers have been used to evaluate and/or quantify the different types of oxidative stress, including DNA/RNA damage, i.e., lipid peroxidation, ROS, antioxidants and protein oxidation/nitration (Table 1) [6]. To date, cfDNA has been only applied for diagnosis and prognosis of various types of pathologies or conditions (cancer, autoimmune diseases, tuberculosis, myocardial infarction, sepsis, trauma, pregnancy, among others) [7–11], considering that its usually low concentration in blood (0–100 ng/mL) [12] and other body fluids increases significantly as a result of

---
* Correspondence: lilian.chuaire@urosario.edu.co
[1]Facultad de Ciencias Naturales y Matemáticas, Universidad del Rosario, Carrera 26 63B-48, Bogotá, DC, Colombia
Full list of author information is available at the end of the article

Table 1 Biological markers of oxidative stress

Type of damage	Marker of damage
DNA/RNA Damage	8-hydroxyguanosine (8-OHG)
	Abasic (AP) sites
	BPDE DNA Adduct
	Double-strand DNA breaks
	Comet Assay (general DNA damage)
	UV DNA Damage (CPD, 6-4PP)
Lipid Peroxidation	4-Hydroxynonenal (4-HNE)
	8-iso-Prostaglandin F2alpha (8-isoprostane)
	Malondialdehyde (MDA)
	Thiobarbituric acid reacting substances (TBARS)
Reactive Oxygen Species	Universal ROS/RNS
	Hydrogen Peroxide
	Nitric Oxide
Antioxidants	Catalase
	Glutathione
	Superoxide Dismutase
	Oxygen Radical Antioxidant Capacity (ORAC)
	Hydroxyl Radical Antioxidant Capacity (HORAC)
	Total Antioxidant Capacity (TAC)
Protein Oxidation/Nitration	3-Nitrotyrosine
	Advanced Glycation End Products (AGE)
	Advanced Oxidation Protein Products (AOPP)
	BPDE Protein Adduct

cellular death associated [13]. However, cfDNA may also increase in healthy individuals [14] as a result of apoptosis or necrosis of cells of the blood or other tissues [15, 16] or as a consequence of intense exercise such as the half- or ultra-marathon running [17].

The comet assay, a biomarker of effect, has been widely used to quantify the genotoxic damage from occupational exposure, based on the appearance of nuclear fragments -product of single- and double-strand DNA breaks- and alkali- labile sites that have migrated from the nucleus and having the appearance of comet tail whose length and DNA contents may be measured and correlated with the extent of DNA damage [5, 18, 19]. Considering that occupational exposure to organic solvents, as those contained in car paints, can lead to disease and also that there is a large population of car paint workers in Colombia who, in their majority, do not observe the rules of industrial biosecurity and therefore are exposed to them, it is necessary to implement methodologies that not only allow an early identification of adverse effects caused by these genotoxic agents, but also to monitor them after the compliance with biosafety standards by owners and workers of car paint shops.

According to the above, our efforts were aimed to evaluate cfDNA concentrations in the serum of individuals occupationally exposed to the organic solvents contained in car paints and to analyze them in the light of the results of the comet assay and the levels of indoor air organic solvents, as well as of parameters such as age, time of exposure, smoking habits and alcohol intake.

Methods

Study population

This was a single blind retrospective research, which involved two cohorts. One cohort was composed by 33 male gender individuals 18–73 years old, routinely exposed to car paints, who were recruited among ten handicraft car paint shops at the "7 de agosto" neighborhood in Bogota DC, Colombia. On the other hand, 33 workers employed in a hoses factory and not occupationally exposed to organic solvents, were selected to constitute the non-exposed cohort, who were recruited in another area within the same neighborhood and with similar characteristics except for the proximity to car paint shops. This research was approved by the Ethical Committee of the Universidad del Rosario.

Selection criteria

The exposed cohort consisted of adult men being exposed to car paints for periods of at least three months. The members of the non-exposed cohort were selected using the same criteria applied for the exposed cohort except for the exposure to organic solvents and also considering that their ages were similar to the exposed group, with a maximum difference of ± 2 years.

Furthermore, we made sure that, in the case of a worker having labored in more than one shop, the biosafety conditions were similar in all the places he worked at before.

Exclusion criteria

Individuals who had suffered from hepatitis or cancer or another severe disease, or had been under chemotherapy or radiotherapy or any other recent prolonged medical treatment were excluded as well as those who provided inconsistent personal information.

Blood sampling

Two samples from peripheral blood were taken: one intended for lymphocytes isolation and further comet assay and the other for cfDNA assay. Sampling was carried out immediately after exposure at the end of the workweek. Samples to determine the cfDNA were collected in tubes with serum separator gel (BD 367988 Vacutainer® RST tubes for Rapid Obtaining Serum) and those for the comet assay in vacutainer tubes with heparin (Ref BD 367874 Vacutainer® Sodium Heparin). All samples were immediately transported to the laboratory within 10 min. The tubes for serum collection were centrifuged at 3000 RPM for 10 min and then transferred to eppendorf tubes, in order to ultra-centrifuge for 10 min at 14000 RPM twice. The supernatant was immediately frozen at –20 °C for up to three weeks. This procedure excluded the possibility that the supernatant had DNA content from blood cells. The blood samples for the comet assay were immediately processed for the isolation of lymphocytes. Samples of all individuals, exposed and non-exposed, were processed simultaneously.

Lymphocytes isolation

Lymphocytes isolation was performed by density gradients with histopaque-1077 (Sigma Aldrich, St. Louis, MO, USA) and centrifugation at 2300 rpm during 30 min. Lymphocytes pellet was re-suspended in PBS 1X (Gibco, Life Technologies, Nebraska, USA), to perform the comet assay.

Exclusion cytoxicity test

The trypan blue test (Life Technologies, Nebraska, USA) was carried out to determine that the damage to be evaluated in the cells were the result of genotoxicity and not cytotoxicity [20, 21]. The relationship between the number of live and dead lymphocytes was between 85–95 % and the volume of cell suspension used in the test was 4×10^3 lymphocytes.

Comet assay

The alkaline comet assay was performed according to the proposed Collins et al. protocol [22], using the Trevigen Comet Assay Kit (Trevigen, Gaithersburg, USA). A minimum of 100 cells per individual were analyzed by using fluorescence microscope (Nikon Instruments Inc, USA), with a magnification of 100×.

Three trials were performed. The first one was aimed to get positive controls using hydrogen peroxide (H_2O_2) as a genotoxic agent in lymphocytes; the second was conducted to evaluate cell damage due to occupational exposure to organic solvents at the car paint shops in exposed individuals and, third, to evaluate cell damage in non-exposed individuals. All assays were performed in duplicate.

The comets were classified through the Comet Score publisher program, in five categories or levels of damage according to the percentage of DNA in the tail, as follows: 0: no damage (<5 %), 1: low damage (6–25 %), 2: moderate damage (26–50 %), 3: high damage (51–75 %) and 4: severe damage (>76 %) [19, 22, 23].

In each of the sampled individuals, all types of comet were considered. For this analysis, the type of comet more often observed (mode) in each sample was used, as indicated by Moro et al. [5] and Rombaldi et al. [24].

Cell-free DNA

cfDNA was determined in the serum collected from each blood sample, following the proposed Goldshtein et al. [25] protocol. SYBR® Gold Nucleic Acid Gel Stain 10000× (Invitrogen GmbH, Karlsruhe, Germany) was used and two dilutions were made for this purpose: first, 1:1000 in pure dimethyl sulfoxide (DMS) (Sigma-Aldrich) and second, 1:8 in PBS (1×).

As concentration control, a calibration curve was constructed with known concentrations of salmon sperm DNA. Fluorescence was measured in the fluorometer (Tecan, Männedorf, Switzerland). The wavelength excitation was recorded at 485 nm and the emission wavelength at 535 nm by using data analysis software, Magellan v7.1 (Tecan Genius). These results were then confirmed by spectrophotometry (Thermo Scientific NanoDrop 2000 Series 3248, MA, USA).

cfDNA concentrations in the serum samples were calculated from the interpolation of the data obtained from the calibration curve of DNA standards. To confirm the specificity of the assay and to eliminate the possible influence of serum in the results, 10 samples of the extracted serum were randomly selected and incubated with DNAse I (500 U/mL) (Thermo Scientific, USA) at 37 °C for 5 h and used as negative control. Values of fluorescence thus obtained were then subtracted from those corresponding to the serum samples which in turn had previously been incubated with SYBR® Gold Nucleic Acid Gel Stain 10000× (Invitrogen GmbH, Karlsruhe, Germany).

The cfDNA concentrations obtained were classified into three categories or levels, according to the following reference values: low: 0–580 ng/mL; medium: 581–2500 ng/mL; high: >2500 ng/mL [25].

Determination of benzene, toluene and xylene (BTX) in air samples

Prior establishment of the risks map within the workshops, stationary air sampling was carried out through active sampling tubes, placed at 1,5 meter height and in the middle of the hall, with the aspiration flow fixed at 0,2 liters/minute, according to the "National Institute for Occupational Safety and Health" (NIOSH) analytical method 1500 for aromatic hydrocarbons [26] and then quantitative determination of BTX was performed. The reference Threshold Limit Values were those indicated by the American Industrial Hygienists Conference (ACGIH) [27].

Statistical analysis

The results were analyzed using the SPSS v22.0 (Statistical Package to Social Scientific) program. Homogeneity of variances was evaluated by the Levene's test and normality by the Shapiro-Wilk and the Lilliefors corrected Kolmogorov-Smirnov tests.

With the purpose to reduce the effect of age as a possible confounding factor, we paired 1:1 by age the exposed and the non-exposed individuals. The asymptotic or exact McNemar's test (binomial, expected values < 5) for paired samples was used to evaluate significant differences in tabaquism and alcohol intake.

The nonparametric Wilcoxon exact test for two related samples was performed to search possible significant differences in the frequencies of the type of comets as well as in cfDNA concentrations between the two cohorts. To compare the frequencies of the higher categories of comets between the two groups, an exact McNemar's test was applied. In addition, we used Spearman rank correlation to test the correlation between cfDNA concentrations and type of comets, and between exposure time and extent of DNA damage (assessed by comet assay and cfDNA) as well. To compare the extent of genotoxic damage among the visited workshops, the exact Kruskal-Wallis test was applied, excluding from analysis those having one worker exposed. Furthermore, we evaluated possible significant differences in the extent of DNA damage related to exposure time, and also BTX concentrations among car paint shops, applying the exact Kruskal-Wallis test. P-value less than 5 % ($p < 0,05^*$) and 1 % ($p < 0,01^{**}$) was considered as statistically significant.

Results

The exposed and non-exposed cohorts were comparable from a statistical point of view, which was the result of an experimental design consisting in a pairing 1:1 by age and also whereas no significant differences were found in smoking habits or alcohol intake ($p = 0,687$ and $p = 0,219$ respectively, exact McNemar's test for paired samples) (Table 2).

Comet assay and cfDNA

Similarly to that happened with the positive controls (Fig. 1a), 66,7 % of the group exposed to solvents showed type 3 and 4 comets (Table 3), in which over 50 % of total DNA was fragmented and located outside the nucleus (Fig. 1b), versus the non-exposed group, in which 82 % had type 1 comets with less than 15 % of the DNA outside the nucleus (Fig. 1c), which means that exposure to solvents has a statistically significant genotoxic effect over the exposed individuals ($p < 0,001$, Wilcoxon exact one-sided test). Frequencies of comets 3 and 4 in the exposed (66,7 %) were significantly higher than in the non-exposed ones (9,1 %) ($p < 0,001$, Exact McNemar's test).

In addition, workers employed in the #4 and #9 car paint shops had significantly higher genotoxic damage, evaluated by comet assay, compared to the other workshops ($p = 0,025$, Exact Kruskal-Wallis Test) (Additional file 1: Table S1). Having compared BTX concentrations between workshops and taking into account that It was not possible to measure them in the workshop #10, we found significant differences ($p < 0,001$, Exact Kruskal-Wallis Test). Thus, while benzene levels in workshops 1, 2, 4 and 7, and toluene levels in workshops 2, 4 and 9 were significantly higher, in turn, the distribution of the toluene levels was higher in workshops 2 and 4, followed by 7 and 9. Once compared the extent of genotoxic damage, assessed by comet assay, and the exposure time between workshops, we did not find significant differences ($p = 0,456$, Exact Kruskal-Wallis Test) (Additional file 1: Table S1).

With respect to the cfDNA quantification, its concentrations in the exposed were significantly higher than in the non-exposed individuals ($p < 0,001$, Wilcoxon exact one-sided test) (Table 4). After having rated each individual concentration (exposed and non-exposed) as low, medium or high, according to the reference values and the percentage of subjects in each category (Table 5), we found significantly higher cfDNA levels in the exposed cohort ($p = 0,016$, Wilcoxon exact one-sided test). Moreover, a significant positive correlation between the alcohol intake time of exposed individuals and the cfDNA concentration was established ($r = 0,346$, $p = 0,033$, Spearman Rank Correlation) and also with the extent of DNA damage evaluated by the type of comet ($r = 0,310$, $p = 0,047$, Spearman rank correlation). However, there was no correlation between cfDNA concentration and type of comet ($r = 0,084$, $p = 0,641$, Spearman rank correlation). In turn, a significant positive correlation between the alcohol intake time and the cfDNA concentration in non-exposed individuals was found, but not so with the alcohol intake time and the extent of DNA damage assessed by type of comet ($r = -0,085$, $p = 0,687$, Spearman rank correlation). Similarly to that happened in the exposed individuals, there was no correlation between cfDNA concentration and type of comet in the non-exposed ($r = 0,081$, $p = 0,655$, Spearman rank correlation). On the other hand, there were no significant differences in the extent of genotoxic damage assessed by cfDNA concentration or their corresponding ranges between the

Table 2 Epidemiologic characterization of the cohorts

Characteristics	Exposed (N = 33)	Non-exposed (N = 33)	Significance
Ages (mean ± SD)	46,18 ± 14.59	46,18 ± 14.68	1,000
Time of exposure in months (mean ± SD)	234,33 ± 141,38 (median = 212,00)		
Smokers	5 (15,2 %)	7 (21,2 %)	0,687 (e)
Alcohol intake	32 (97,0 %)	28 (84,8 %)	0,219 (e)

SD standard deviation

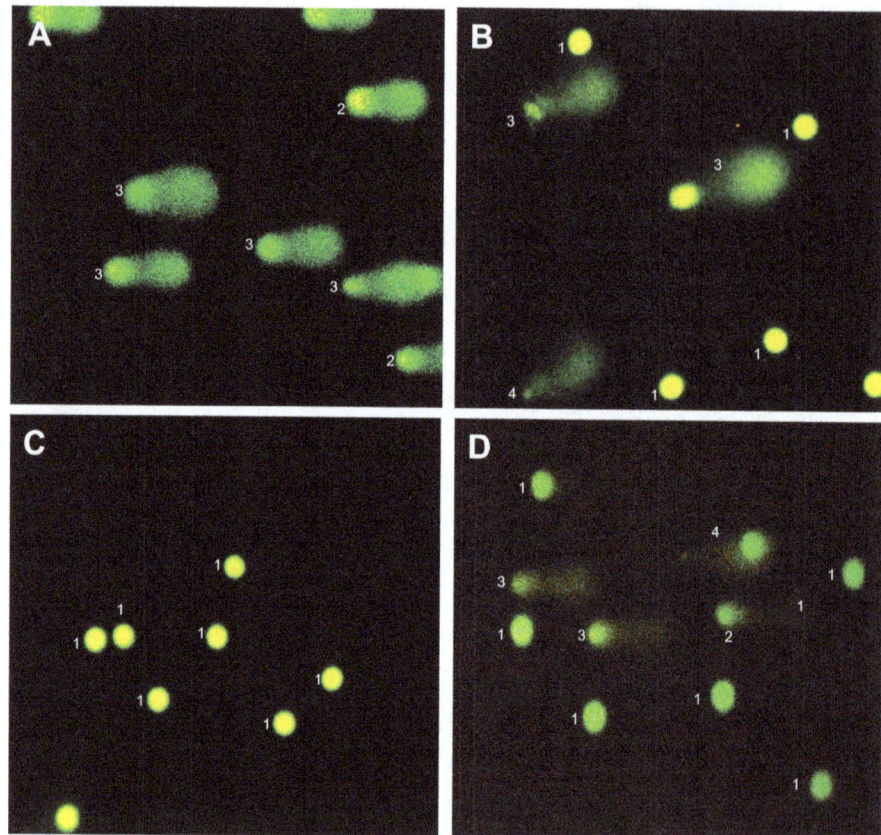

Fig. 1 Types of comet obtained from the alkaline comet assay. **a** Positive control. Predominance of type 3 is observed, which means that over 50 % of the DNA has migrated from the core. Magnification: 10×. **b** Exposed individual who had comets type 1, 3, and 4, although type 3 was the predominant after making the total count. Magnification: 10×. **c** Non-exposed individual. The observable comets correspond entirely to type 1, where less than 25 % of the DNA has migrated. Magnification: 10×. **d** In this exposed individual, comets type 1, 2, 3 and 4 are observable, being type 4 the predominant after making the total count. Magnification: 10×

car paint shops ($p = 0,297$, Exact Kruskal-Wallis Test) (Additional file 1: Table S1).

Association between DNA damage and exposure time

There was a moderate significant positive relationship between the extent of DNA damage represented by comets 3 and 4 and the exposure time to indoor airborne solvent vapors ($r = 0,317$, $p = 0,047$). Similar results were found between cfDNA concentrations and the exposure time ($r = 0,28$, $p = 0,053$, Spearman rank correlation) (Fig. 2).

It is important to mention that, in the car paint shops, the procedures used in the task of preparing mixtures for paints and applying to vehicles tend to be traditional and therefore have not changed significantly in the last 20 years. Consequently, no one had made any effort to applying any biosafety protocol in these places, so that compliance with personal protective devices was very poor. These are noteworthy facts, since the painters had

Table 3 Distribution of comets in the exposed and the non-exposed cohorts

Type of comets	Exposed % (N)	Non-exposed % (N)
0	0	0
1	21,2 (7)*	81,8 (27)*
2	12,1 (4)	9,1 (3)
3	45,5 (15)**	9,1 (3) **
4	21,2 (7)	0

**$p < 0,01$, *$p < 0,05$

Table 4 cfDNA concentrations (ng/mL) in the exposed and the non-exposed cohorts

	Exposed	Non-exposed
Mean	2398,90	1301,83
Minimum value	63	0
Maximal value	5159	3957
Standard deviation	1513,28	1276,32
Median	1991,00	994,00
N	33	33

Table 5 cfDNA levels in the exposed and the non-exposed cohorts

cfDNA levels (ng/mL)	Exposed % (N)	Non-exposed % (N)
Low (0–580)[a]	9,1 (3)	30,3 (10)
Medium (581–2500)[a]	57,6 (19)	51,5 (17)
High (>2500)[a]	33,3 (11)	18,2 (6)

[a]Reference values

been successively employed in various workshops in the same sector, which had similar features to those of their current workplace. In spite of BTX concentrations in the indoor air of the car paint shops were determined (Additional file 1: Table S1), we could not standardize the working time and daily exposure to these solvents because they varied according to workload, thus making impossible to assess the exposure of a typical handicraft car painter based on existing data, as those reported from car painting workshops belonging to the formal industrial sector, in which rights, schedules and biosafety regulations are abided and respected.

Discussion

The vast majority of paint shops of motor vehicles in Bogotá and other cities in Colombia lack adequate ventilation and personal protective equipment. For this reason painters are permanently exposed to organic solvents during all the operations involved, such as sanding of the surface, cleansing, masking, varnish preparation and spraying, activities that entail serious risks, because of their mutagenic and carcinogenic properties.

Various methods are used to date to evaluate cell damage caused by exposure to these xenobiotic agents, such as the cytogenetic and the micronucleus assays. In view of that these techniques are wasteful because of its costs and long-term analysis, in this research we conducted a new field trial evaluation of genotoxicity, based on the quantification of cfDNA in serum. This method is advantageous, not only because of its minimally invasive characteristics but also due to cfDNA stability in serum and to its easy accessibility. In addition, we used the comet assay as an alternative method for evaluating the extent of DNA damage.

Our results showed significant differences in the frequency of higher categories of comets ($p < 0,001$) and in cfDNA concentrations ($p < 0,001$) in the exposed cohort, in comparison with those observed in non-exposed (control group) (Tables 3 and 4). However, although there was a significant statistical difference in the mean of cfDNA between individuals exposed and non-exposed, these concentrations grouped into ranges or levels did not appear to be as discriminatory, it is also true the fact that in our research we tried where possible to minimize the influence of confounding factors between the two groups, such as age, degree of physical activity associated with the occupation as well as exercise habits, alcohol intake and smoking.

Although the exposed and non-exposed distribution of cfDNA concentrations in the medium level (581–2500 ng/mL) was very similar between, significant differences were observed in the distribution of the high (>2500 ng/mL) cfDNA level (Table 4), where the

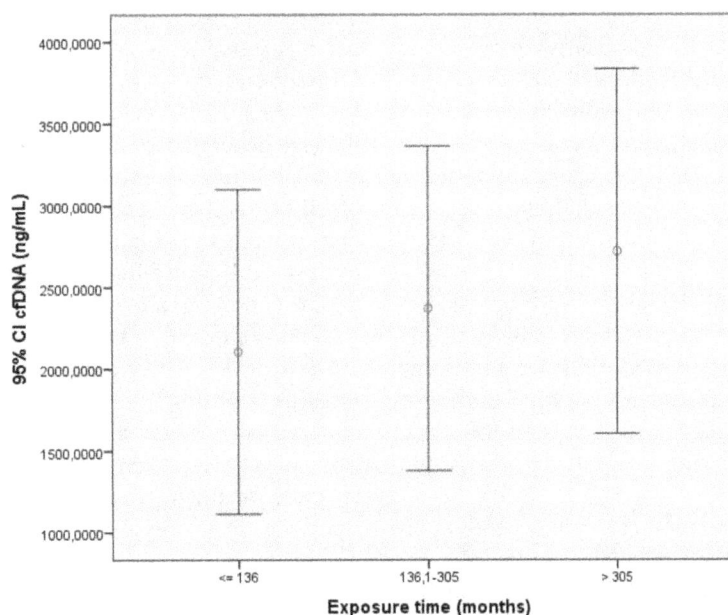

Fig. 2 Mean and 95 % confidence interval of cfDNA concentrations by range of exposure time in the exposed cohort. Exposure time to airborne solvent vapors significantly increased the extent of DNA damage assessed by cfDNA concentration ($r = 0,28$, $p = 0,053$, Spearman rank correlation)

number of exposed was greater than the non-exposed. In the low (0–580 ng/ml) cfDNA level, there was a significant statistical difference in favor of the non-exposed individuals, which were in a greater number than the exposed, fact that can be explained when considering that individuals belonging to the control group were not exposed to organic solvents and in consequence a less extent of DNA damage could be reasonable to wait.

The wide interindividual variability in cfDNA values observed in both groups (exposed and non-exposed) (Table 4), might be explained by differences in the extent of tissue damage - which may vary according to age, exposure time, workload or BTX levels at workshops – but also by differences in the oxidative metabolism of genotoxic agents, which could affect cfDNA concentrations. In the case of car painters, the exposure to those agents was obvious while in the control group, one could think in other environmental genotoxic agents e.g. carbon dioxide, alcohol, or those contained in certain products used for home cleansing. These results are in agreement with previous studies where wide variability in the mean of cfDNA concentrations was also observed [7, 28, 29]. It should be noted also that the kinetics of genotoxic damage-related cfDNA release into the bloodstream and its subsequent clearance have not yet elucidated [30] thus making the cfDNA, as rightly Danese et al. said, a "hard to read" analyte [31].

In addition, it is noteworthy that though a significant Spearman coefficient of correlation between the cfDNA content and the DNA damage (assessed by comet assay) was not observed, both parameters reflect the extent of the genotoxic damage from exposure to solvents. This finding could be explained by an adaptive response of the organism addressed to the effective cfDNA elimination from blood but also to a survival mechanism of cells with damaged DNA [32]. In fact, it has been recently reported an enhancement of DNA damage in lymphocytes along with a cfDNA content reduction, in human occupational exposure to low-dose gamma-neutron and tritium β-radiation [32].

On the other hand, occupational exposure time to organic solvents in car paint shops significantly increased the risk of genetic damage (Fig. 2), thus accomplishing the Bradford-Hill dose-response relationship criteria for causality, which means there is a valid causal connection between exposure time to airborne solvent vapors and extent of DNA damage [33].

Although cfDNA concentration can vary depending on multiple factors, including degree of exercise, the increase that has been observed after exhaustive exercise such as marathon disappears within two hours after the race [17, 34]. Consequently, activities conducted during the day could not be associated with increased concentrations of cfDNA, taking into account that the occupational-associated degree of physical activity in the two groups, exposed and non-exposed, was similar. Thus, the control group was composed of workers of a hoses factory, occupation that demands similar physical effort to that of workers in the car paint shops. In addition, none of them, exposed or non-exposed, reported exercising regularly or other possible sources of cfDNA (e.g. infection, trauma, inflammatory disease or cancer).

Considering our results together with the understanding that apoptotic and necrotic cells are the main source of cfDNA and also that its concentration increases due to an augmented vulnerability of damaged cells to cell death [35], it is possible to assume that the cfDNA is a product of cellular DNA damage. Consequently, determination of cfDNA could be taken into account along with other biomarkers, in order to support the diagnostic of genotoxicity in individuals occupationally exposed to organic solvents in car paint shops, for which this could be a useful tool, just as it has been for patients suffering from inflammatory or infectious processes, autoimmune diseases and cancer, among others [28].

The increase in DNA damage in the exposed cohort can be explained based on the oxidative metabolism of BTX, wherein the intermediate metabolites may give rise to reactive oxygen species (ROS) which, in turn, oxidize the DNA. Furthermore, these metabolites can produce DNA adducts, generating DNA modifications, such as alkali-labile sites, single-stranded breaks (SSB) or double strand breaks (DSB) [19].

Despite of the cfDNA test has been commonly used to evaluate the progression of neoplastic disease [10, 36] and also to study its relationship with apoptosis [37], using techniques such as PCR, UV-visible spectrophotometry and the newly discovered fluorometric, so far there are no reports of its application in assessing the damage generated by the organic solvents that are used to manufacture car paintings. While clinical significance of cfDNA has not been fully elucidated, the results of our research are of interest, because they allowed establishing significant differences between the cfDNA levels in the serum of individuals occupationally exposed to solvents compared to the non-exposed ones.

The high frequency of DNA damage observed in this research indicates an urgent need to implement methodologies that not only allow an early identification of adverse effects caused by these genotoxic agents, but also to monitor them after the compliance with biosafety standards by owners and workers of car paint shops.

Conclusions

Our results showed that car painters had a significant increase in the cfDNA circulating in the serum, which is an evidence of genetic damage caused by occupational exposure to organic solvents, regardless that the corresponding levels in air were or not within the allowable limits, results that should be analyzed by the appropriate control agencies in order to redefining the permissible concentrations of solvents in air. In the light of the IARC reports classifying work vehicle painting as a carcinogenic industrial process, it is clear that occupational exposure to organic solvents contained therein constitutes a public health problem in Colombia, which reiterates the need to continuously monitor them and monitor adherence to relevant biosecurity rules, as well. The feasibility of making the cfDNA test in serum as a part of the job entrance examinations and monitoring of workers in the researched labor sector could be one of the most important potential applications of the findings of our research in the field of occupational health.

Additional file

Additional file 1: Table S1. cfDNA concentrations and type of comet in the exposed individuals - grouped by car paint shops - and BTX concentrations in the indoor air. Table S2. Socio-demographic data of the exposed cohort. Table S3. Socio-demographic data of the non-exposed cohort. Table S4. Exposed cohort. cfDNA and total count and types of comet. Table S5. Non-exposed cohort. cfDNA and total count and types of comet. Table S6. Air borne solvents concentrations in workshops. Table S7. Exposed cohort. Comet score data. Table S8. Non-exposed cohort. Comet score data.

Acknowledgements
We thank the Universidad del Rosario, Bogotá DC, Colombia, and the National Institute of Health of Colombia for their help and financial support.

Funding
This work was funded by Universidad del Rosario, Bogotá DC, Colombia.

Authors' contributions
All authors made substantial contributions to the conception and design, analysis and interpretation of data, and critical review of the manuscript. MVC performed the experiments. LCN and MCSC conceived the study, analyzed and interpreted the data and wrote the manuscript. SRRC and MRL coordinated the data acquisition and analysis and participated to the manuscript writing. MIP performed the statistical analysis and participated to the manuscript writing. RMP and MEVU participated to interpretation of data and critically reviewed the manuscript. All authors read and approved the final manuscript.

Competing interests
The authors declared that they have no competing interests.

Author details
[1]Facultad de Ciencias Naturales y Matemáticas, Universidad del Rosario, Carrera 26 63B-48, Bogotá, DC, Colombia. [2]Escuela de Medicina y Ciencias de la Salud, Universidad del Rosario, Bogotá, DC, Colombia. [3]Instituto Nacional de Salud, Bogotá, DC, Colombia.

References

1. WHO-IARC. Painting, Firefighting, and Shifwork/IARC Monographs on the Evaluation of the Carcinogenic Risks of Chemicals to Humans. Occupational exposure as a painter. 2010. https://monographs.iarc.fr/ENG/Monographs/vol98/mono98.pdf. Accessed 01 Sept 2015.
2. Lan Q, Zhang L, Li G, Vermeulen R, Weinberg RS, Dosemeci M, et al. Hematotoxicity in workers exposed to low levels of benzene. Science. 2004;306(5702):1774–6. doi:10.1126/science.1102443.
3. WHO-IARC. A review of human carcinogens. Part F: Chemical agents and related occupations/IARC Working group on the evaluation of carcinogenic risks to humans. 2012. http://monographs.iarc.fr/ENG/Monographs/vol100F/mono100F.pdf. Accessed 01 Sept 2015.
4. Velandia-Neira E. Velocidad de conducción nerviosa en trabajadores que manejan solventes orgánicos. Salud Trabajo y Ambiente. 2004;11(40):12–7. http://koha.ccs.org.co/. Accessed 01 Sept 2015.
5. Moro AM, Brucker N, Charao M, Bulcao R, Freitas F, Baierle M, et al. Evaluation of genotoxicity and oxidative damage in painters exposed to low levels of toluene. Mutat Res. 2012;746(1):42–8. doi:10.1016/j.mrgentox.2012.02.007.
6. Ho E, Karimi Galougahi K, Liu CC, Bhindi R, Figtree GA. Biological markers of oxidative stress: Applications to cardiovascular research and practice. Redox Biol. 2013;1:483–91. doi:10.1016/j.redox.2013.07.006.
7. Czeiger D, Shaked G, Eini H, Vered I, Belochitski O, Avriel A, et al. Measurement of circulating cell-free DNA levels by a new simple fluorescent test in patients with primary colorectal cancer. Am J Clin Pathol. 2011;135(2):264–70. doi:10.1309/AJCP4RK2IHVKTTZV.
8. Rodriguez-Arnaiz R. Las toxinas ambientales y la genetica. In: Las toxinas ambientales y sus efectos genéticos. Fondo de Cultura Económica, México DF, México. 1995. http://www.biblioises.com.ar/. Accessed 19 Feb 2015.
9. Roth C, Pantel K, Muller V, Rack B, Kasimir-Bauer S, Janni W, et al. Apoptosis-related deregulation of proteolytic activities and high serum levels of circulating nucleosomes and DNA in blood correlate with breast cancer progression. BMC Cancer. 2011;11:4. doi:10.1186/1471-2407-11-4.
10. Schwarzenbach H, Hoon DS, Pantel K. Cell-free nucleic acids as biomarkers in cancer patients. Nat Rev Cancer. 2011;11(6):426–37. doi:10.1038/nrc3066.
11. Stroun M, Maurice P, Vasioukhin V, Lyautey J, Lederrey C, Lefort F, et al. The origin and mechanism of circulating DNA. Ann N Y Acad Sci. 2000;906:161–8.
12. Parekh H, Dashora P, Acharya A, Vaniawala S, Bapat A, Mukhopadhyaya P. Suspended in blood and circulating within, cell free (cf) DNA connects with a vast range of adverse human health conditions including cancer: A review. Res J Pharm, Biol Chem Sci. 2015;6(2):13.
13. Anker P, Stroun M. Circulating DNA in plasma or serum. Medicina. 2000;60(5 Pt 2):699–702.
14. Breitbach S, Tug S, Simon P. Circulating cell-free DNA: an up-coming molecular marker in exercise physiology. Sports Med. 2012;42(7):565–86. doi:10.2165/11631380-000000000-00000.
15. van der Vaart M, Pretorius PJ. Circulating DNA. Its origin and fluctuation. Ann N Y Acad Sci. 2008;1137:18–26. doi:10.1196/annals.1448.022.
16. Jahr S, Hentze H, Englisch S, Hardt D, Fackelmayer FO, Hesch RD, et al. DNA fragments in the blood plasma of cancer patients: quantitations and evidence for their origin from apoptotic and necrotic cells. Cancer Res. 2001;61(4):1659–65.
17. Atamaniuk J, Stuhlmeier KM, Vidotto C, Tschan H, Dossenbach-Glaninger A, Mueller MM. Effects of ultra-marathon on circulating DNA and mRNA expression of pro- and anti-apoptotic genes in mononuclear cells. Eur J Appl Physiol. 2008;104(4):711–7. doi:10.1007/s00421-008-0827-2.
18. de Oliveira HM, Dagostim GP, da Silva AM, Tavares P, da Rosa LA, de Andrade VM. Occupational risk assessment of paint industry workers. Indian J Occup Environ Med. 2011;15(2):52–8. doi:10.4103/0019-5278.90374.
19. Swanepoel A. Evaluation of DNA damage and DNA repair by the comet assay in workers exposed to organic solvents: North-West University; 2004. http://dspace.nwu.ac.za/handle/10394/1482. Accessed 01 Sept 2015.
20. Fenech M, Holland N, Chang WP, Zeiger E, Bonassi S. The HUman MicroNucleus Project–An international collaborative study on the use of the micronucleus technique for measuring DNA damage in humans. Mutat Res. 1999;428(1-2):271–83.
21. Pitarque M, Vaglenov A, Nosko M, Hirvonen A, Norppa H, Creus A, et al. Evaluation of DNA damage by the Comet assay in shoe workers exposed to toluene and other organic solvents. Mutat Res. 1999;441(1):115–27.

22. Collins AR, Dusinska M, Horska A. Detection of alkylation damage in human lymphocyte DNA with the comet assay. Acta Biochim Pol. 2001;48(3):611–4.

23. Moller P, Knudsen LE, Loft S, Wallin H. The comet assay as a rapid test in biomonitoring occupational exposure to DNA-damaging agents and effect of confounding factors. Cancer Epidemiol Biomarkers Prev. 2000;9(10):1005–15.

24. Rombaldi F, Cassini C, Salvador M, Saffi J, Erdtmann B. Occupational risk assessment of genotoxicity and oxidative stress in workers handling anti-neoplastic drugs during a working week. Mutagenesis. 2009;24(2):143–8. doi:10.1093/mutage/gen060.

25. Goldshtein H, Hausmann MJ, Douvdevani A. A rapid direct fluorescent assay for cell-free DNA quantification in biological fluids. Ann Clin Biochem. 2009; 46(Pt 6):488–94. doi:10.1258/acb.2009.009002.

26. (NIOSH) TNIfOSaH. CDC Centers for Disease Control and Prevention. CDC. 2015. http://www.cdc.gov/niosh/docs/2003-154/pdfs/1500.pdf. Accessed 07 April 2015.

27. ACGIH. Industrial Hygiene, Environmental, Occupational Health & Safety Resource. ACGIH. 2015. http://www.acgih.org/. Accessed 01 Feb 2016.

28. Gormally E, Caboux E, Vineis P, Hainaut P. Circulating free DNA in plasma or serum as biomarker of carcinogenesis: practical aspects and biological significance. Mutat Res. 2007;635(2-3):105–17. doi:10.1016/j.mrrev.2006.11.002.

29. Salazar-Jordán H, García-Robayo DA, Amaya J, Castillo M, Briceño I, Aristizábal F. Cuantificación de ADN libre en plasma sanguíneo de voluntarios sanos en una población bogotana. NOVA. 2009;7(12):63.

30. Al-Humood S, Zueriq R, Al-Faris L, Marouf R, Al-Mulla F. Circulating cell-free DNA in sickle cell disease: is it a potentially useful biomarker? Arch Pathol Lab Med. 2014;138(5):678–83. doi:10.5858/arpa.2012-0725-OA.

31. Danese E, Minicozzi AM, Benati M, Montagnana M, Paviati E, Salvagno GL, et al. Comparison of genetic and epigenetic alterations of primary tumors and matched plasma samples in patients with colorectal cancer. PLoS One. 2015;10(5):e0126417. doi:10.1371/journal.pone.0126417.

32. Korzeneva IB, Kostuyk SV, Ershova LS, Osipov AN, Zhuravleva VF, Pankratova GV, et al. Human circulating plasma DNA significantly decreases while lymphocyte DNA damage increases under chronic occupational exposure to low-dose gamma-neutron and tritium beta-radiation. Mutat Res. 2015;779:1–15. doi:10.1016/j.mrfmmm.2015.05.004.

33. Hill AB. The environment and disease: association or causation? Proc R Soc Med. 1965;58:295–300.

34. Atamaniuk J, Vidotto C, Tschan H, Bachl N, Stuhlmeier KM, Muller MM. Increased concentrations of cell-free plasma DNA after exhaustive exercise. Clin Chem. 2004;50(9):1668–70. doi:10.1373/clinchem.2004.034553.

35. Pollack M, Leeuwenburgh C. Apoptosis and aging: role of the mitochondria. J Gerontol A Biol Sci Med Sci. 2001;56(11):B475–82.

36. Garcia-Olmo DC, Picazo MG, Toboso I, Asensio AI, Garcia-Olmo D. Quantitation of cell-free DNA and RNA in plasma during tumor progression in rats. Mol Cancer. 2013;12:8. doi:10.1186/1476-4598-12-8.

37. Kaminski BC, Grabenbauer GG, Sprung CN, Sauer R, Distel LV. Inter-relation of apoptosis and DNA double-strand breaks in patients with multiple primary cancers. Eur J Cancer Prev. 2006;15(3):274–82. doi:10.1097/01.cej.0000199502.23195.29.

Occupational injuries among building construction workers in Addis Ababa

Sebsibe Tadesse[1*] and Dagnachew Israel[2]

Abstract

Background: Occupational injuries can pose direct costs, like suffering, loss of employment, disability and loss of productivity, and indirect costs on families and society. However, there is a dearth of studies clarifying the situation in most of Subsaharan African countries, like Ethiopia. The present study determined the prevalence of injury and associated factors among building construction employees in Addis Ababa, Ethiopia.

Methods: An institutional-based cross-sectional study was conducted among building construction employees in Addis Ababa, Ethiopia from February to April 2015. Multi-stages sampling followed by simple random sampling techniques was used to select the study participants. The sample size of the study was 544. A pre-tested and structured questionnaire was used to collect data. Multivariable analyses were employed to see the effect of explanatory variables on injury.

Results: The prevalence of injury among building construction employees was reported to be 38.3 % [95 % CI: (33.9, 42.7)] in the past 1 year. Use of personal protective equipments, work experience, khat chewing were factors significantly associated with injury.

Conclusion: This is among the few studies describing construction health and safety in Ethiopia. In this study a relatively higher prevalence of injury was reported among building construction employees compared to other studies. If urgent interventions are not in place, the absence from work, loss of productivity and work-related illnesses, disabilities and fatalities will continue to be a major challenge of the construction industry in the future. Therefore, programs to mitigate the burden borne by construction-related injuries should focus on areas, such as provision of safety trainings, promoting use of PPE and monitoring substance abuse in workplace.

Keywords: Construction industry, Occupational injuries, Workers, Workplace safety

Background

The World Health Organization defines occupational injury as an epidemic problem in the field of public health in developing countries [1, 2]. The human suffering caused by the injuries is hurtful to the employee, the employer and society [3–5]. According to the International Labor Organization there are 270 million occupational accidents causing 2 million deaths annually [6]. In the United States the cost of occupational injuries was $177.2 billion, and 35 million working days were lost annually [3]. The construction industry is responsible for more than half of all occupational injuries and deaths worldwide [7]. It is widely recognized as having high accident rates which result in absence from work, loss of productivity, permanent disabilities and even fatalities [8]. The estimated direct and indirect costs of fatal and nonfatal construction injuries totaled about $13 billion annually. The medical expenses of nonfatal injuries alone cost more than $1.36 billion annually [9].

Construction is a sector that has very specific hazards, like work at heights, work with power tools, more than one trade and more than one employer/contractor working on a single site with lack of coordination, working in the outdoor elements, work with power tools, contractual work as opposed to permanent employment, lack of

* Correspondence: sbsbtadesse90@gmail.com
[1]Institute of Public Health, the University of Gondar, Gondar, Ethiopia
Full list of author information is available at the end of the article

standards or regulations among workers in terms of expertise in their trade and training standards, less regulation and enforcement than other sectors. Studies reveal that there are various factors that are significantly associated with occupational injury. These factors include lack of health and safety programs, young workers, male sex [10], lack of formal education [11], smoking [12], sleeping problems [13], lack of physical exercise [14], frequent alcohol consumption [12], extended work hours [15], night work [15], physically demanding work [16], low job experience [15], and non-use of personal protective equipment [17].

The impact of occupational health and safety hazards faced by construction workers in developing countries is 10 to 20 times higher than those in industrial countries [18]. In Ethiopia information regarding construction injuries is rare, and very limited attempts have been made to investigate the prevalence and associated factors [19]. This paper presents the findings of a study which investigated prevalence and factors associated with occupational injuries among building construction workers in Addis Ababa, Ethiopia. The information could help in designing appropriate preventive and control strategies.

Methods
Study design, area and period
A construction site-based cross-sectional study was conducted to assess prevalence and factors associated with occupational injuries among building construction workers in Addis Abba, the capital city of Ethiopia from February to April 2015.

Participants
All employees who were directly involved in the process of construction in the last 1 year were included in the study until the required sample size was obtained. Workers who were absent from work for any reason during the time of data collection were excluded from the study.

Survey tool
A pre-tested and structured interview questionnaire was used to collect the data. The questionnaire contained detailed information on socio-demographic, behavioral and environmental factors that could have association with injuries. The respondents were asked the question stated as, "Have you ever had any physical injury resulting from an accident in the course of construction work in the past 1 year?" to determine prevalence of injury. A generic job satisfaction scale was used to assess workers status of job satisfaction. The respondents were also asked a close ended question to determine the main causes of injuries as perceived by them: "What are the main causes of injury at this workplace? 1. Lack of awareness 2. Poor working conditions 3. Lack of PPE 4. Others".

Sample size calculation
Epi info version 7 was used to determine the sample size of 544 by taking 6999 total population of construction workers, 38.7 % expected proportion of injury [19], 5 % confidence limit, 95 % confidence level, 5 % non-response rate, 1.5 design effect.

Sampling procedure
The multi-stage sampling technique was used to select the study participants. In the first stage, 4 condominium construction sites were randomly selected by the lottery method from 8 sites in the Addis Ababa city administration. In the second stage, the total of 544 samples was proportionally allocated to each selected sites (i.e. 82 to site 1 (N1 = 546), 128 to site 2 (N2 = 840), 148 to site 3 (N3 = 970), and 186 to site 4 (N4 = 1227)). The participants were drawn from the site's list of workers using simple random sampling. Three trained degree holders participated in the data collection processes.

Data quality control
The training of data collectors and supervisors emphasized issues such as the data collection instrument, field methods, inclusion–exclusion criteria and record keeping. The investigators coordinated the interview process, and spot-checked and reviewed the completed questionnaire on a daily basis to ensure the completeness and consistency of the data collected. The interview questionnaire was pre-tested on 20 respondents in order to identify potential problem areas, unanticipated interpretations and cultural objections to any of the questions. Based on the pre-test results, the questionnaire was adjusted contextually.

Data management and statistical analyses
Data entered and cleaned using Epi info version 7 statistical software were analyzed on SPSS version 20. Frequency distribution, mean, standard deviation and percentage, were employed for most variables. All independent variables were fitted separately into a bivariate logistic model to evaluate the degree of association with injuries. Then, variables with a p-value < 0.20 were exported to multivariable logistic regression model to control confounders. The odds ratio (OR) with a 95 % confidence interval (CI) was used to test the statistical significance of variables. Only statistically significant variables were presented.

Operational definitions

Occupational injury

Any physical injury resulting from an accident in the course of construction work in the past 1 year prior to this study.

Job satisfaction

The employee was considered as satisfied with job when his/her sum of generic job satisfaction scale score was 32 or above [20].

Personal Protective Equipment (PPE)

Utilization of specialized clothing or equipment worn by employees for protection against health and safety hazards. Workers were classified as *those who used PPE* when they were observed wearing the PPE that were necessary to be worn during a particular activity.

Permanent employee

Any contract of employment between employee and employer concluded for an indefinite period [21].

Temporary employee

Any employment contract between employee and employer made for defined period [21].

Cigarette smoker

An employee who was smoking one cigarette a day for at least 1 year [22].

Alcohol drinker

An employee who drinks at least five drinks per week for men and two drinks per week for women for at least 1 year [22].

Khat chewer

An employee chewing khat (a mild psychoactive substance) three times a week for at least 1 year [22].

Ethical considerations

The study protocol was reviewed and approved by the Institutional Review Board of the University of Gondar via the Institute of Public Health. Permission was obtained from city government of Addis Ababa Social Affair Office prior to data collection. Study participants were interviewed after informed written consent was obtained. They were also informed that their participation was voluntary and that they could withdraw from the interview at any time without consequences. The participants were assured that their responses would be treated confidentially through the use of strict coding measures. Finally, safety education was given to workers who reported injuries. They were told to avoid unsafe acts, to use PPE and to follow safety rules.

Results

Socio-demographic characteristics

A total of 504 employees completed the questionnaire making response rate 92.6 %, of whom 62.9 % were males. The majority, 89.5 %, of the employees belonged to the age group of 18–35 years. Half, 50.4 %, attended secondary and higher education. Regarding religion 72.4 % of the employees were Christian. The single were 58.3 %. The majority, 80.2 %, had a monthly salary of Birr 1000–3000 (Table 1).

Workplace and behavioral characteristics

Three-fourths, 75.8 %, of the participants were temporary employees. The majority, 84.7 %, served for less than 2 years. Regarding hours spent on work 91.9 % of the employees had worked for ≤8 h per day. More than three-fourths, 77.8 %, of them were satisfied with their job. The majority, 76.6 %, did not use PPE. Eighty four percent did not attend any kind of workplace safety training. The majority, 59.1, 73.4 and 91.3 %, of the employees didn't drink alcohol, chew khat and smoke cigarette, respectively (Table 2).

Table 1 Socio-demographic characteristics of building construction employees in Addis Ababa, Ethiopia, 2015

Variables	Number	Percent
Sex		
Male	317	62.9
Female	187	37.1
Age (in years)		
18–35	451	89.5
>35	53	10.5
Marital Status		
Single	294	58.3
Married	176	34.9
Widowed/divorced	34	6.8
Educational status		
Illiterate	30	6.0
Primary	220	43.6
Secondary and above	254	50.4
Religion		
Christian	365	72.4
Muslim	137	27.2
Other	2	0.4
Monthly salary (in US $)		
50–150	404	80.2
>150	100	19.8

Table 2 Workplace and behavioral characteristics of building construction employees in Addis Ababa, Ethiopia, 2015

Variables	Number	Percent
Employment pattern		
Permanent	122	24.2
Temporary	382	75.8
Work experience (in years)		
≤ 2	427	84.7
> 2	77	15.3
Working hours per day		
≤ 8	463	91.9
> 8	41	8.1
Job satisfaction		
Satisfied	392	77.8
Dissatisfied	112	22.2
Safety training		
Yes	82	16.3
No	422	83.7
Use PPE		
Yes	118	23.4
No	386	76.6
Drink alcohol		
Yes	206	40.9
No	298	59.1
Smoke cigarette		
Yes	44	8.7
No	460	91.3
Chew khat		
Yes	134	26.6
No	370	73.4

Prevalence of Injury

The prevalence of injury among building construction employees was reported to be 38.3 % [95 % CI: (33.9, 42.7)] in the past 1 year, of whom 62.2 % were males. The majority, 79.3 and 83.9 %, served for less or equal to 2 years and did not use PPE, respectively. The common types of injuries were 66.3 % cutting and 28.5 % falling. Nearly half, 46.6 %, of the incidents were leg injuries followed by 43.5 % finger/hand. The major cause of injuries was lack of safety awareness, 46.7 % (Fig. 1).

Factors associated with injury

Table 3 presents factors which remained statistically significant in the bivariate and multivariable logistic regression analyses. In this study the independent predictors of injury on the multivariable analysis include use of PPE [AOR: 0.4, 95 % CI: (0.2, 0.7)], work experience [AOR: 0.4, 95 % CI: (0.2, 0.7)], khat chewing [AOR: 2.6, 95 % CI: (1.6, 4.2)] (Table 3).

Discussion

Industrial safety and health problems are becoming major challenges in Ethiopia because of low occupational hazards awareness, lack of workplace safety and health policy, and inefficient safety management systems. Due to these factors employers, workers and the government are incurring measurable and immeasurable costs. Injuries remain the major occupational health problem among construction employees [8, 9]. In this study the prevalence of injury among the employees was 38.3 % [95 % CI: (33.9, 42.7)]. This finding is in line with a study from Ethiopia (38.7 %) [19], and higher than that of studies from Egypt (18.4 %) [23] and India (22.9 %) [24]. The discrepancy could be due to methodological differences, like study populations, methods of data collection and workplace conditions, like employees' level

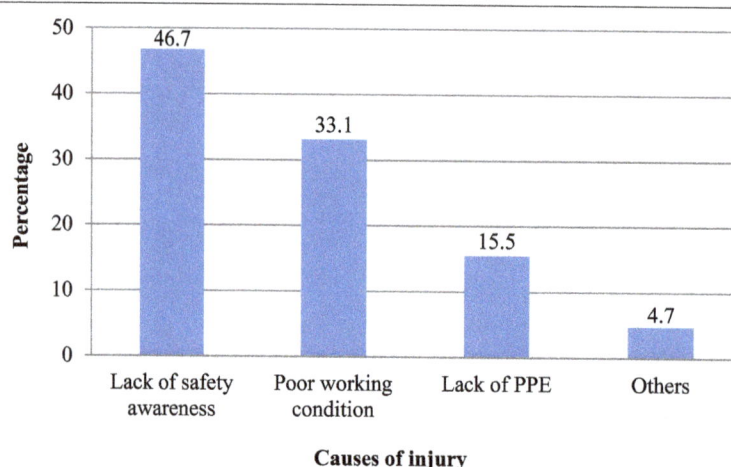

Fig. 1 Causes of injuries reported by employees

Table 3 Factors associated with injuries among building construction employees in Addis Ababa, Ethiopia, 2015

Variables	Injuries		Crude OR (95 % CI)	Adjusted[a] OR (95 % CI)
	Yes	No		
Use PPE				
Yes	31	91	0.5 (0.3, 0.7)	0.4 (0.2, 0.7)
No	162	220	1	1
Work experience (in years)				
≤ 2	153	274	0.5 (0.3, 0.8)	0.4 (0.2, 0.7)
> 2	40	37	1	1
Chew khat				
Yes	70	64	2.2 (1.5, 3.3)	2.6 (1.6, 4.2)
No	123	247	1	1

[a] The multivariable model was adjusted for age, sex, educational status, marital status, employment pattern, monthly income, cigarette smoking, alcohol drinking, job satisfaction, working hours per day and safety training

of awareness of hazard control and disease prevention and accessibility of workplace safety services. Emphasis on preventive measures, such as short and long-term training as well as encouragement to use safety tools can effectively decrease the prevalence of occupational injuries [7].

This study identified important predictors influencing the occurrence of occupational injury. The odds of injuries among employees who used PPE were 60 % less compared to those who did not. Use of PPE is one of the important measures to safeguard workers from exposure to occupational hazards, especially in developing countries where conventional occupational safety control measures remain a challenge to implement [25–27]. PPE is the lowest measure in the hierarchy of hazard control that works because it depends on workers' behavior [28]. Engineering controls, substitution and administrative controls are more effective methods that do not depend on workers' behavior. In this study more than three-fourths of the employees did not use PPE during work. This may signify that there was poor provision of PPE from employers, and lack of awareness about its importance by the workers. As a recommendation, it is imperative that safety programs need to pay more attention to provision and use of PPE.

Another important finding of this study was that the odds of injuries among employees who served for less or equal to 2 years were 60 % less compared to those who served for more than 2 years. The possible explanation for this may be that those employees who served for greater than 2 years could be accustomed to the work environment and developed false consciousness of safety which drive them not to comply with safety precautions including proper use of PPE. It might also be due to the fact that the lack of safety awareness programs in the workplaces, poor working conditions and lack of PPE,

which were described in this study, could influence employees' experience of injuries during their longer stays. Finally, there could be a healthy worker effect, since absent workers were not included in the study and may have left this workforce due to injury.

The odds of injuries among employees who chewed khat were about three times more compared to those who did not. This might be due to the fact that abuse of mind altering substances, like khat is likely to cause a change in the behavior and impair workers concentration and performance. A high blood level of such substances while at work will endanger both safety and efficiency, and be the cause of increased likelihood of mistakes, poor decision making and errors in judgment. As the result of this fact the industries' safety policy should consider control of substance abuse at workplace.

There are several limitations of this study that should be noted. Social desirability bias is a potential limitation in self-reported studies like this one, in that employees might report more socially acceptable responses than their actual day to day practice. In this study occupational injury is defined as any physical injury resulting from an accident in the course of construction work in the past 1 year prior to this study. Therefore, further studies need to be conducted to explain the nature of injury by its severity. As this is a cross-sectional study, the cause-effect relationship is not established between the different independent variables and injury. Moreover, injury status of the 40 workers who were selected but did not complete the questionnaire was not known. The prevalence is likely to be higher with the exclusion of injured workers –"healthy worker effect".

Conclusions

This is among the few studies describing construction health and safety in Ethiopia. In this study a relatively higher prevalence of injury was reported among building construction employees compared to other studies. If urgent interventions are not in place, the absence from work, loss of productivity and work-related illnesses, disabilities and fatalities will continue to be a major challenge of the construction industry in the future. Therefore, programs to mitigate the burden borne by construction-related injuries should focus on areas, such as provision of safety trainings, promoting use of PPE and monitoring substance abuse in workplace.

Competing interests
The authors declare that they have no competing interests.

Authors' contributions
ST Involved in write up of the research proposal, the data analyses and wrote the manuscript, DI Involved in write up of the research proposal, the data analyses and wrote the manuscript. Both authors read and approved the final manuscript.

Acknowledgments

The authors wish to thank the city government of Addis Ababa Social Affair Office for logistic and administrative support, and data collectors for their support in making this study possible. They also extend their deepest gratitude to the study participants.

Author details

[1]Institute of Public Health, the University of Gondar, Gondar, Ethiopia. [2]City Government of Addis Ababa Health Bureau, Addis Ababa, Ethiopia.

References

1. Karvonen M. Epidemiology in the context of occupational health. In: Karvonen M and Mikheev MI. Epidemiology of Occupational Health. WHO. Copenhagen; WHO Regional Office Office for Europe: 1986. 1–15.
2. Hamalainen P. The effect of globalization on occupational accidents. Saf Sci. 2009;47(6):733–42.
3. Larsson TJ, Field B. The distribution of occupational injury risks in the Victorian construction industry. Saf Sci. 2002;40(5):43911.
4. Lowery JT, Glazner J, Borgerding JA, Bondy J, Lezotte DC, Kreiss K. Analysis of construction injury burden by type of work. Am J Ind Med. 2000; 37(4):390–9.
5. Moradinazar M, Kurd N, Farhadi R, Amee V, Najafi F. Epidemiology of Work-Related Injuries Among Construction Workers of Ilam (Western Iran) During 2006 – 2009. Iran Red Crescent Med J. 2013;15(10):e8011.
6. International Labor Organization. Work-related fatalities reach 2 million annually 2002. Available from: http://www.nieuwsbank.nl/en/2002/05/24/K016.htm. Accessed March 20 2015.
7. Lopez-valcarcel A. Occupational safety and health in the construction work. Afr Newsl Occup Health Safety. 2001;11:4–7.
8. Eid AH, Sewefy AZ. Health Hazards and safety. J Egypt Med Assoc. 2009; 51(3):757.
9. CPWR. The center for construction research and training. Construction chart book. 4th ed. USA: CPWR; 2008.
10. Zewdie A. Determinants of occupational injury: a case control study among textile factory workers in Amhara regional state, Ethiopia. J Trop Med. 2009; 201:1–8.
11. Kunar BM, Bhattacherjee A, Chau N. Relationships of job hazards, lack of knowledge, alcohol use, health status and risk taking behavior to work injury of coal miners: a case-control study in India. J Occup Health. 2008;50: 236–44.
12. Bhattacherjee A, Chau N, Sierra CO, Legras B, Benamghar L. Relationships of job and some individual characteristics to occupational injuries in employed people: a community-based study. J Occup Health. 2003;45:382–91.
13. Salminen S, Oksanen T, Vahtera J, Sallinen M, Harma M. Sleep disturbances as a predictor of occupational injuries among public sector workers. J Sleep Res. 2010;19:207–13.
14. Gauchard GC, Chau N, Touron C, Benamghar L, Dehaene D. Individual characteristics in occupational accidents due to imbalance: a casecontrol study of the employees of a railway company. Occup Environ Med. 2003;60:330–5.
15. Dembe AE, Erickson JB, Delbos RG, Banks SM. The impact of overtime and long work hours on occupational injuries and illnesses: new evidence from the United States. Occup Environ Med. 2005;62:588–97.
16. Smith PM, Mustard C. Examining the associations between physical work demands and work injury rates between men and women in Ontario, 1990–2000. Occup Environ Med. 2004;61:750–6.
17. Kumar SG, Rathnakar U, Harsha KH. Epidemiology of accidents in tile factories of mangalore city in karnataka. Indian J Community Med. 2010;35:78–81.
18. Dong X. Long work hours, work scheduling and work-related injuries among construction workers in the United States. Scand J Work Environ Health. 2005;31:329–35.
19. Molla M, Alemu K, Kebede G, Rai H, Worku W. Occupational injuries among building construction workers in Gondar City, Ethiopia. Occup Med Health Aff. 2013;1:125.
20. Scott Macdonald MP. The Generic Job Satisfaction Scale: Scale Development and Its Correlates. 1997.
21. Ministry of Labor and Social Affairs. Labour proclamation No.377/2003. Addis Ababa: Ministry of Labor and Social Affairs; 2003.
22. Melchior M, Niedhammer I, Berkman LF, Goldberg M. Do psychosocial work factors and social relations exert independent effects on sickness absence? A six year prospective study of the GAZEL (France) cohort. J Epidemiol Community Health. 2003;57:285–93.
23. Alazab RM. Work-related diseases and occupational injuries among workers in the construction industry. Afr Newsl Occup Health Safety. 2004;14:37–42.
24. Shah CK, Mehta H. Study of injuries among construction workers in Ahmedabad City, Gujarat. Indian J Practicing Doctor. 2009;5:1–5.
25. Malik N, Mean AA, Pasha TS, Akhtar S, Ali T. Role of hazard control measures in occupational health and safety in the textile industry of Pakistan. Pak J Agric Sci. 2010;47(1):72–6.
26. Kamal A, Sayed M, Massoud A. Usage of personal protective devices among Egyptian industrial workers. Am J Ind Med. 2007;13(6):706–16.
27. Akintayo WL. Knowledge, attitude and practice on the use of personal protective equipment by traditional resist Fabrics workers in Abeokuta, Nigeria. Kuwait Rev Chapter Arab J Bus Manag Rev. 2013;2(7):31–3.
28. Jaiswal A. Case-control study among carpet thread factory workers in Uttar Pradesh, India: Occupational injury and its deteriorating factors. Glob J Hum Soc Sci Hist Anthr. 2012;12(10). ISSN: 2249–460x.

15

Effect of low-level CO_2 on innate inflammatory protein response to organic dust from swine confinement barns

David Schneberger[2], Jane M. DeVasure[2], Kristina L. Bailey[1,2], Debra J. Romberger[1,2] and Todd A. Wyatt[1,2,3]*

Abstract

Background: Organic hog barn dust (HDE) exposure induces lung inflammation and long-term decreases in lung function in agricultural workers. While concentrations of common gasses in confined animal facilities are well characterized, few studies have been done addressing if exposure to elevated barn gasses impacts the lung immune response to organic dusts. Given the well documented effects of hypercapnia at much higher levels we hypothesized that CO_2 at 8 h exposure limit levels (5000 ppm) could alter innate immune responses to HDE.

Methods: Using a mouse model, C57BL/6 mice were nasally instilled with defined barn dust extracts and then housed in an exposure box maintained at one of several CO_2 levels for six hours. Bronchiolar lavage (BAL) was tested for several cytokines while lung tissue was saved for mRNA purification and immunohistochemistry.

Results: Exposure to elevated CO_2 significantly increased the expression of pro-inflammatory markers, IL-6 and KC, in BAL fluid as compared to dust exposure alone. Expression of other pro-inflammatory markers, such as ICAM-1 and matrix metalloproteinase-9 (MMP-9), were also tested and showed similar increased expression upon HDE + CO_2 exposure. A chemokine array analysis of BAL fluid revealed that MIP-1γ (CCL9) shows a similar increased response to HDE + CO_2. Further testing showed CCL9 was significantly elevated by barn dust and further enhanced by CO_2 co-exposure in a dose-dependent manner that was noticeable at the protein and mRNA levels. In all cases, except for ICAM-1, increases in tested markers in the presence of elevated CO_2 were only significant in the presence of HDE as well.

Conclusions: We show that even at mandated safe exposure limits, CO_2 is capable of enhancing multiple markers of inflammation in response to HDE.

Keywords: Carbon dioxide, Hypercapnia, Barn dust

Background

Concentrated animal feeding operations (CAFOs) are a common feature of agriculture in developed countries. Exposure to the organic dusts within these facilities has been shown to cause a number of short and long-term problems for exposed workers. These problems include, but are not limited to, increased risk for asthma and COPD [1–3], chronic bronchitis [4], and a general decease in lung function over time exposed [5].

The immune response to organic barn dusts is mediated primarily by the innate immune system. Previous work identifies endotoxin and peptidoglycans as key components of the dust that trigger innate immune responses in humans, cell cultures, and mouse models [6–9]. These bacterial components act through the TLR4 and TLR2 receptors, respectively [10, 11], and it has been shown that one or both of these receptors may be critical to the immune response generated to these dusts [10–12], though it is doubtful that these components are the only causes of this inflammation.

Response to hog barn dust extracts (HDE) typically involves expression of pro-inflammatory cytokines and chemokines such as TNF-α [8, 13], IL-6 [13–15], and IL-8 (KC in mice) [13–16]. This increased cytokine

* Correspondence: twyatt@unmc.edu
[1]Research Service, Veterans Administration Nebraska Western Iowa Health Care System, Omaha, NE 68105, USA
[2]Pulmonary, Critical Care, Sleep & Allergy Division, Department of Internal Medicine, University of Nebraska Medical Center, 985910 The Nebraska Medical Center, Omaha, NE 68198-5910, USA
Full list of author information is available at the end of the article

expression, particularly through IL-8, results in increased infiltration of cells, particularly neutrophils, into the lung [9, 16]. Other changes to the lung will occur such as increased edema, and prolonged exposure can lead to lymphoid aggregate formation [9]. A host of other chemokines will also likely be induced in this response, but IL-6 and KC are the most often characterized markers of this inflammation.

HDE exposure does not occur in isolation of gasses in the barn air, and three gasses, in particular, are commonly recognized as being elevated in most CAFO operations: ammonia (NH_3), hydrogen sulfide (H_2S), and carbon dioxide (CO_2). Ammonia has potential negative effects on lung function and health of workers and animals in the CAFO environment [17, 18] though little is known. H_2S is recognized as a serious potential health hazard in CAFO operations, usually involving waste management and removal. H_2S in these workplace exposures is both an irritant and an asphyxiant, and if levels are high and sustained, fatal.

CO_2, on the other hand, may be elevated as high as 5000 ppm in some facilities [19], but perceived effects are often mild and do not include irritation [20]. As such, it is often not considered a potential problem in the barn environment and has thus received little to no study. Studies with cell cultures and animal models have yielded mixed results as to the pro- or anti-inflammatory nature of hypercapnia [21–23]. In almost every case, the levels used in these studies far exceed CO_2 levels that may be encountered in a workplace environment. We hypothesized that the combination of CO_2 gas exposure enhances the inflammatory response to HDE exposure.

Given that elevation of other gasses in this environment showed potential to enhance lung inflammatory symptoms [18], that CO_2 could alter response to dust extract exposures in bronchial epithelial cells [24] and that levels as low as 1000 ppm were capable of inducing changes in cognitive function [25], we hypothesized that the elevation of CO_2 gas exposure may enhance the inflammatory response to HDE exposure. We therefore looked to see if there was any effect of CO_2 on HDE exposure at the Occupational Safety and Health Administration (OSHA) 8 h workplace permissible exposure limit of 5000 ppm. Using a mouse model system of HDE exposure, we show that even at this workplace allowable limit there were significant changes to IL-6, KC, and CCL9. Further examination of CCL9 showed that the chemokine was induced by HDE, and increased in a dose-specific manner to co-exposure with elevated CO_2 at the mRNA and protein levels. As CCL9 is suggested to potentially have an effect on MMP-9, we tested and found a similar pattern in relation to MMP-9 mRNA expression. Another potential marker of enhanced inflammation in the lung, ICAM-1, may be increased or decreased during hypercapnia [26, 27]. Thus, we tested for ICAM-1 expression in mice and found a similar increase in response to HDE plus CO_2 in lung and trachea.

We therefore show that 8 h CO_2 permissible exposure levels can enhance the stimulated expression of several cytokines, chemokines, and pro-inflammatory markers in the lung in response to organic barn dusts.

Methods

Hog barn dust extracts

HDE extracts were prepared from settled dust samples combined from two separate swine confinement facilities and have been characterized as to content of protein, endotoxin, and muramic acid [28]. The bacterial composition has also been characterized [29]. Dust extracts were prepared as previously described [15]. Dust (1 g) was mixed with 10 ml HBSS without calcium and incubated for 1 h at room temperature before centrifugation for 10 min, with media being decanted and sterile-filtered for use, for a final concentration of approximately 0.105 g/ml dust. No stability problems are noted in such extracts for at least a year or more after storage. Extracts were used at a concentration of 12.5% v/v or about 0.005 g/ml dust and prepared no earlier than 2 weeks before use.

Animals

All procedures were approved by the Institutional Animal Care and Use Committee of the University of Nebraska Medical Center (protocol number 04-059-08). Female, 6–8-week-old C57BL/6 mice (Charles River, Wilmington, MA) were acclimated for one week after arrival. The animals were group-housed, and their diet consisted of commercial rodent chow and water *ad libitum*. Animals were assigned randomly to each treatment group: saline, saline + hypercapnia, HDE instillation (12.5%), or HDE instillation + hypercapnia. All mice (8 per group) were instilled nasally one time [11] with 40 μl of treatment. Mice were treated for 6 h in an exposure chamber, with controlled fresh air ventilation and a fan to circulate air within the box. Mice exposed to elevated CO_2 were given CO_2 in the same box. Levels of CO_2 were assayed using a CO_2 monitor (Extech CO210, Extech, Nashua, NH) and the chamber was manually ventilated to maintain levels for normal CO_2 (400 ppm), and hypercapnia (5000 or 7500 ppm). All treatment groups were split over two separate occasions, separated by no more than two weeks (4 animals/group/occasion; $n = 8$).

Sacrifice of animals was done within 1 min of withdrawal from exposure chamber, and staged so that BAL and lung excision did not exceed 30 min after completion of treatment.

Serum collection

Blood was taken from animals at time of sacrifice by cardiac puncture in serum collection tubes (Microtainer, Becton Dickson, Franklin Lakes, NJ) using an 18-gauge needle (Becton Dickson). Samples were centrifuged 10 min at 7000 × g and serum stored at -80 °C until used for ELISA. Blood was not taken from the 7500 ppm CO_2 exposed group by mistake.

Bronchoalveolar lavage (BAL) collection

Lungs were lavaged as detailed previously [9]. Briefly, lungs were washed three times with 1 ml sterile saline each time. BAL fluid was centrifuged 1750 × g for 10 min and supernatant samples stored at -80 °C until used. Cells were resuspended in 1 ml PBS, counted, and 1.5 × 10^3 cells adhered to glass slides via cytospin. Cells were stained using a Diff-Quik kit (Siemens Healthcare Diagnostics, Newark, DE) and cover slips mounted. A differential count of at least 200 cells was made based on morphometric criteria and expressed as absolute cell numbers (mean +/- SEM).

Lung collection

After BAL collection, lungs were excised from animals. The left lung was tied off at the primary bronchus and removed, flash frozen in liquid nitrogen and stored at -80 °C for mRNA collection. A cannula was inserted in the trachea of the remaining lung and cinched with a suture. Lungs were hung in a bath of 10% formalin fixative as 0.8 ml of this fixative was allowed to enter the lungs via the cannula for 24 h under a pressure of 15 cm H_2O. The fixed lung was then embedded in paraffin for later immunohistochemical staining.

Tracheal cell collection

A separate exposure was done with 10 mice/group at normal CO_2 (400 ppm), and hypercapnic (7500 ppm) CO_2 levels. The trachea was saved from each animal, opened, and the internal surface scraped gently with a cell scraper into cell lysis buffer (Qiagen, Chatsworth CA) and processed for RNA as per whole lung tissue (described below). Cell lysate samples were pooled from 2 mice to yield enough mRNA for testing.

ELISAs

Cytokine and chemokine quantitation of BAL fluid was done by enzyme linked immunoabsorbant assay kits to IL-6, KC, and CCL9 (R&D Systems, Minneapolis, MN) according to manufacturer's instructions. Broad spectrum testing of BAL fluid for chemokine expression was accomplished using a dot blot array kit (ARY020, R&D Systems, Minneapolis, MN).

Wet/Dry ratio

Four additional mice per group were exposed as described previously and lungs removed after treatment. Lungs were weighed at time of removal and then dried overnight in a drying oven at 60 °C and visually checked for dryness at the end of this time before being re-weighed. Ratio was calculated of wet to dry weight.

RNA purification and RT-PCR analysis

RNA was purified from lung tissue samples using a Qiagen spin miniprep kit according to manufacturer's instructions, including additional DNAse digestion (Qiagen, Chatsworth CA). Initial homogenization of tissue was done in 350 µl of lysis buffer from the miniprep kit with 2.0 mm stainless steel beads (Next Advance, Averill Park, NY) and placed in a Bullet Blender Storm 24 magnetic bead beater (Next Advance, Averill Park, NY) for 3 m at 4 °C. RNA was quantified by NanoDrop ND-1000 (Thermo Scientific, Wilmington, DE).

cDNA synthesis was performed using the Taqman reverse transcription kit (Applied Biosystems, Branchburg, NJ) with 200 ng of template mRNA. cDNA synthesis (RT-PCR) reactions contained the following reagents: 1X TaqMan RT buffer, 5.5 nM $MgCl_2$, 500 µM of each dNTP, 2.5 µM random hexamers, 0.4 U/µl RNase inhibitor, and 1.25 U/µl MultiScribe reverse transcriptase as per kit instructions (Applied Biosystems, Branchburg, NJ). Samples were incubated at 25 °C for 10 min, then 48 °C for 30 min, and 95 °C from 5 min in a thermocycler (MJ Mini; Bio-Rad, Hercules, CA).

RT-PCR was performed using probes to CCL9 (Life Technologies, Mm00441260), MMP-9 (Mm00600163), and ICAM-1 (Mm00516023). Ribosomal RNA was used as an endogenous control. PCR was conducted using an ABI PRISM 7500 Sequence Detection System (Applied Biosystems). Reactions were carried out for 2 min at 50 °C, 10 min at 95 °C, followed by 40 cycles at 95 °C for 15 s and 60 °C for 1 min each. All reactions were carried out in duplicate. For relative comparison of targets to the ribosomal RNA endogenous control, we analyzed cycle threshold (CT) value of real-time PCR data with the ΔΔCt method.

ICAM-1 tissue staining

ICAM-1 staining was localized in lung tissue as previously reported [9]. Briefly, tissue was blocked overnight at 4 °C, with primary antibody added at 1:75 (rat anti-mouse ICAM-1; Rockland Immunochemicals, Gilbertsville, PA) and incubated for 1 h at room temperature, followed by secondary antibody (rat anti-CD54, 1:300; Biolegend, San Diego, CA) for 2 h.

Statistical analysis

All data was analyzed using GraphPad Prism (Graph-Pad Software, San Diego, CA). Error bars represent the mean +/- SEM. Statistical significance was determined using ANOVA with follow-up Bonferroni test, with $p \leq 0.05$ confidence interval being considered significant.

Results

BAL cell numbers are unaffected by hypercapnia

Counts of cells harvested from BAL of mouse lungs showed that nasal instillation of barn dust induced an increase in total cell numbers in the lung (Fig. 1a), and a shift in the population from predominantly macrophages to predominantly neutrophils (Fig. 1b), as has been seen in previous studies [9, 24]. Additional exposure to elevated CO_2 conditions induced no discernable changes in either number or type of cells present in the alveolar space, both in saline as well as barn dust exposed animals, even when CO_2 was increased to 7500 ppm.

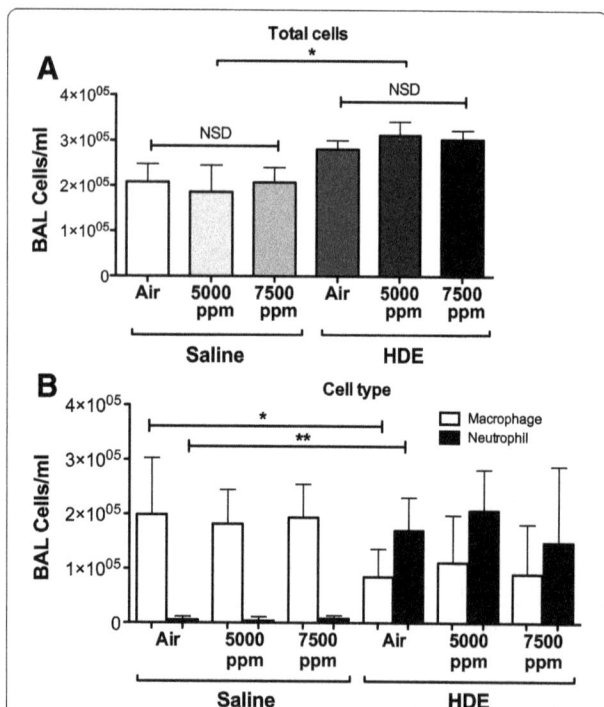

Cytokine expression in response to barn dust is Increased with hypercapnia

BAL was tested first for common markers of inflammation, IL-6 and KC. Both IL-6 (Fig. 2a) and KC (Fig. 2b) were increased in response to barn dust as has been reported previously [5, 13–15] though only IL-6 was significantly elevated by six hours. Exposure to 5000 and 7500 ppm CO_2 caused significant increases in both IL-6 and KC in HDE-exposed animals compared to saline. This effect was only seen with exposure to HDE, as saline-treated mice showed no similar cytokine increases in response to elevated CO_2. No changes were noted in the serum for either (results not shown).

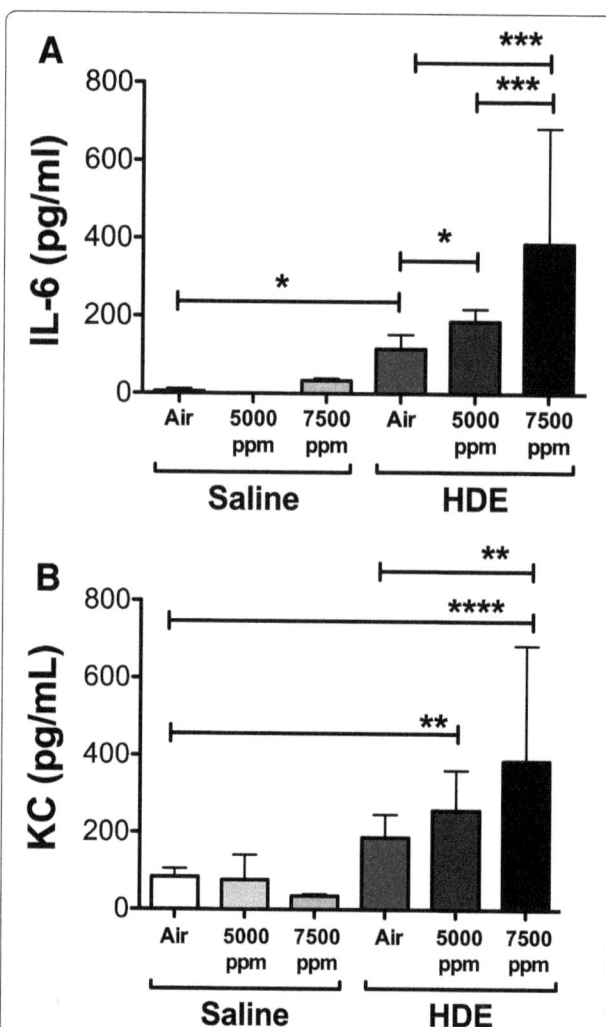

Fig. 1 Effect of HDE on BAL cell counts. Exposure to HDE caused an increase in total BAL cell numbers (**a**) and a shift from predominantly macrophages to neutrophils (**b**). Increasing CO_2 levels (5000 and 7500 ppm) from ambient air (air) had no significant effect on BAL cell number or type in BAL samples. Bar graphs represent standard deviation with error bars shown ($N = 8$ mice/group, $N = 4$ mice/group for 7500 ppm groups). Statistical significance denoted by asterisks (*$p < 0.05$, **$p < 0.01$) as compared to respective saline treatment group

Fig. 2 CO_2 enhances HDE stimulated cytokine expression in BAL. BAL fluid was tested by ELISA for (**a**) IL-6 and (**b**) KC. HDE instillation induces both cytokines. Increasing CO_2 levels (5000 and 7500 ppm) in HDE-treated mice significantly increased production of both cytokines vs ambient air (air). Bar graphs represent standard deviation with error bars shown ($N = 5$-8 mice/group). Statistical significance denoted by asterisks (*$p < 0.05$, **$p < 0.01$, ***$p < 0.001$, ****$p < 0.0001$)

To look for other possible chemokine targets that may be altered in response to the combination of HDE with elevated CO_2, we tested BAL samples using a chemokine dot blot array. Numerous chemokines were altered by HDE (data not shown), however one chemokine, CCL9 showed what appeared to be a noticeable change in response to CO_2. To confirm this result, we tested BAL for CCL9 using ELISA to quantitate the results (Fig. 3a). CCL9 expression was significantly increased by exposure to HDE, and significantly increased over those levels when mice were exposed to HDE plus CO_2. The levels of CCL9 were increased further still at 7500 ppm CO_2 plus HDE, though none of these increases was reflected in serum samples (Fig. 3b), which were uniformly high, as has been shown in other studies [30]. Examination of mRNA showed that increase in CCL9 occurred at the mRNA level as well in lung tissue (Fig. 3c).

CO_2 does not induce significant lung leak

As increased CCL9 levels in the lung may reflect increased leak from the blood, additional mice were treated as in previous experiments, and whole lungs were collected for measure of wet-to-dry ratio. There was no significant increase in wet-to-dry ratio of the lungs of HDE treated or HDE + CO_2 (7500 ppm) treated animals, suggesting extra fluid had not accumulated in the lungs due to leak (Fig. 4).

ICAM-1 expression

ICAM-1 expression is reported to be either increased [26] or decreased [27] in response to hypercapnia. To address this, we performed immunohistochemical staining of mouse lungs. We observed a visible increase in ICAM-1 expression in the bronchial epithelium exposed to saline + 5000 ppm CO_2 alone, which was even more pronounced at 7500 ppm (Fig. 5a–c). ICAM-1 expression was also increased by HDE alone. The addition of CO_2 exposure caused further increases (Fig. 5d–f). To quantitate these visual observations, we examined ICAM-1 mRNA expression. CCL9 mRNA expression in whole lung homogenates showed a similar pattern to what was seen with immunohistochemical staining (Fig. 5g). There was no change in ICAM-1 mRNA in saline-treated animals with increased CO_2, but in HDE + CO_2 treated animals, there were increases in mRNA which became significantly elevated at the 7500 ppm level over that of HDE treatment alone. This was true in both whole lung (Fig 5g) as well as tracheal epithelium (Fig. 5h) for mRNA samples.

MMP-9 mRNA expression

A feature of obstructive lung disease is an increase in MMP-9. We suspected that hypercapnia plus an inflammatory stimulus may have a similar effect. Testing for

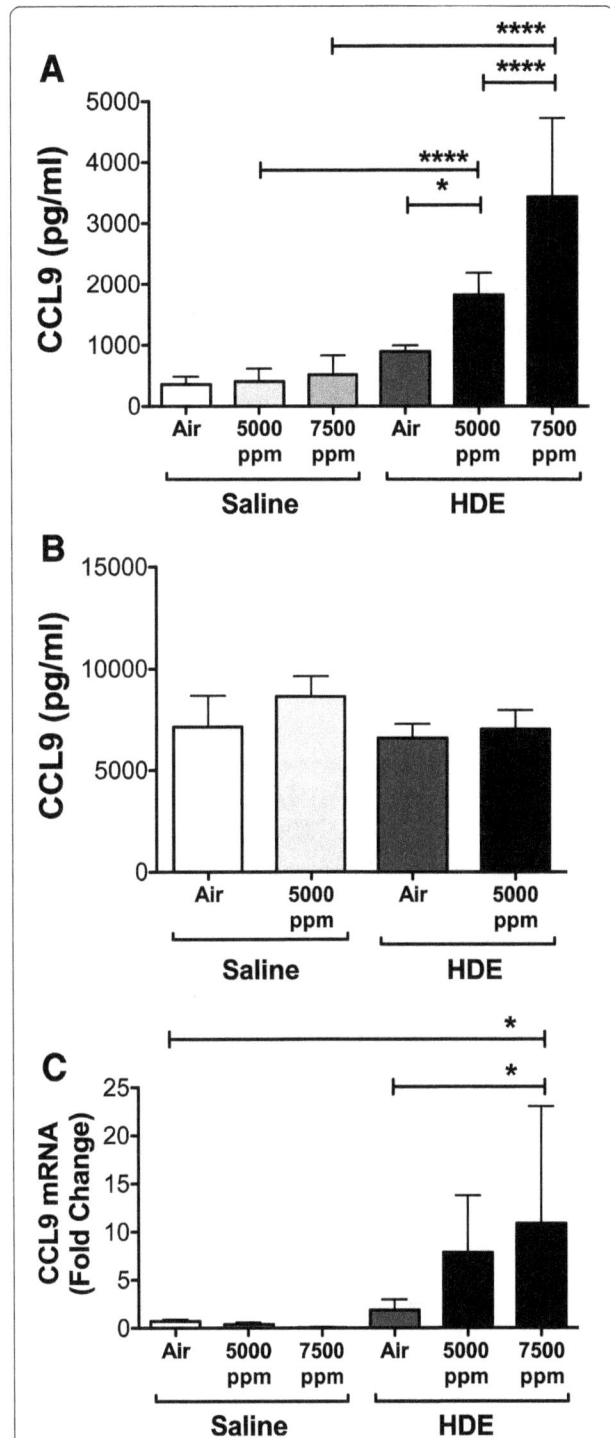

Fig. 3 CCL9 is increased in response to HDE and CO_2. Expression of CCL9 chemokine was examined in BAL (**a**) and serum (**b**) by ELISA. Only the lung showed significant increases in CCL9 in response to HDE. Increase of CO_2 (5000 and 7500 ppm) induced what appeared to be a concentration-dependent increase in CCL9 production vs. ambient air (air) in the lung that was absent in serum as well. Expression in lung was confirmed by mRNA expression (**c**) which showed a similar pattern of CCL9 induction to barn dust and CO_2. Bar graphs represent standard deviation with error bars shown (N = 6-8 mice/group). Statistical significance denoted by asterisks (*$p < 0.05$, **$p < 0.001$, ***$p < 0.0001$)

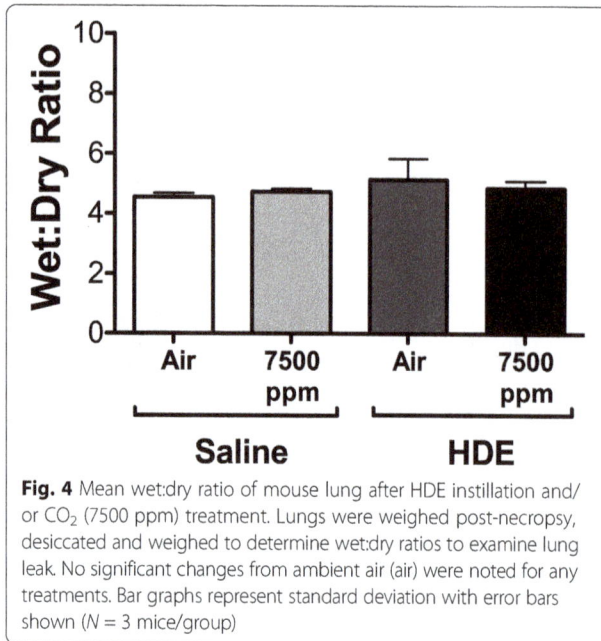

Fig. 4 Mean wet:dry ratio of mouse lung after HDE instillation and/or CO_2 (7500 ppm) treatment. Lungs were weighed post-necropsy, desiccated and weighed to determine wet:dry ratios to examine lung leak. No significant changes from ambient air (air) were noted for any treatments. Bar graphs represent standard deviation with error bars shown ($N = 3$ mice/group)

mRNA expression in whole lung mRNA showed that MMP-9 was not increased by hypercapnia alone, and HDE treatment alone did not induce a significant increase in mRNA (Fig. 6). Combined HDE + hypercapnia treatment, however, showed a significant elevation of MMP-9 mRNA that appeared to be CO_2 dose-dependent (Fig. 6).

Discussion

Workers in CAFOs are exposed to a mixture of organic dusts and gasses in barns. These gasses are produced from the animals living in the building as well as gasses released from wastes and bacterial action. While changes to ventilation may impact dust and gasses in the air, other dust remediation steps such as cleaning or sprinkling [12] may reduce dust, but not gasses. These problems may be greater in colder climates where ventilation must be balanced against heat loss and energy costs.

Of the gasses often studied in CAFOs, three are commonly increased as a result of biological processes in these facilities; NH_3, H_2S, and CO_2 [31–33].

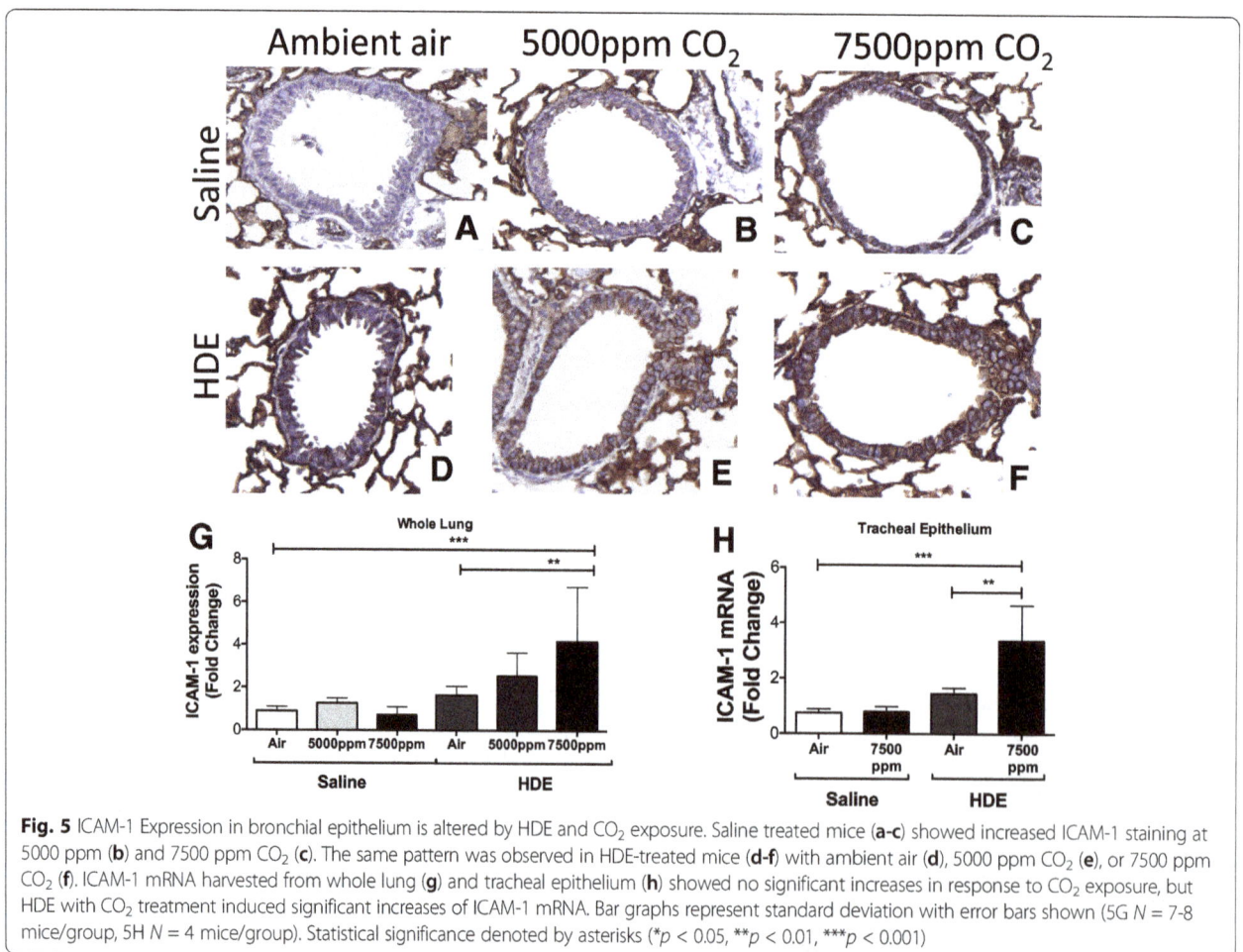

Fig. 5 ICAM-1 Expression in bronchial epithelium is altered by HDE and CO_2 exposure. Saline treated mice (**a-c**) showed increased ICAM-1 staining at 5000 ppm (**b**) and 7500 ppm CO_2 (**c**). The same pattern was observed in HDE-treated mice (**d-f**) with ambient air (**d**), 5000 ppm CO_2 (**e**), or 7500 ppm CO_2 (**f**). ICAM-1 mRNA harvested from whole lung (**g**) and tracheal epithelium (**h**) showed no significant increases in response to CO_2 exposure, but HDE with CO_2 treatment induced significant increases of ICAM-1 mRNA. Bar graphs represent standard deviation with error bars shown (5G $N = 7$-8 mice/group, 5H $N = 4$ mice/group). Statistical significance denoted by asterisks (*$p < 0.05$, **$p < 0.01$, ***$p < 0.001$)

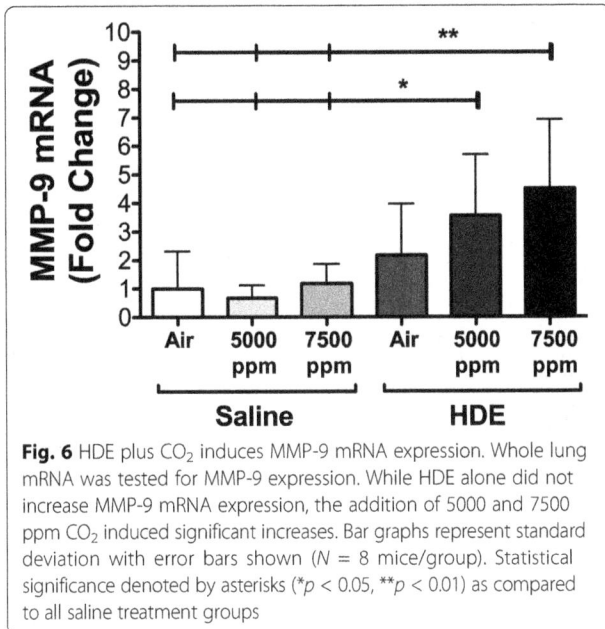

Fig. 6 HDE plus CO_2 induces MMP-9 mRNA expression. Whole lung mRNA was tested for MMP-9 expression. While HDE alone did not increase MMP-9 mRNA expression, the addition of 5000 and 7500 ppm CO_2 induced significant increases. Bar graphs represent standard deviation with error bars shown (N = 8 mice/group). Statistical significance denoted by asterisks (*$p < 0.05$, **$p < 0.01$) as compared to all saline treatment groups

CO_2, while known to cause headaches at higher levels has no current association with known occupational disease. CO_2 is a commonly elevated gas in some work environments such as wastewater treatment [34], and potentially small airtight spaces with several people in them [35]. Many well-ventilated facilities will not reach the 8 h time weighted average exposure (TWA) OSHA limit (5000 ppm), but some facilities tested have been shown to reach these levels [33]. Work by other groups into the effects of permissive hypercapnia show CO_2 alters immune responses to treatments such as endotoxin [36], however the amounts used in many of these experiments are levels not applicable to work exposures. This study addresses this deficiency by examining relatively low dose CO_2 in whole animals using a workplace-relevant inflammatory stimuli (organic barn dust).

Initial examination of cells in the BAL showed HDE treatment increased cell number as well as the number of neutrophils, as has been shown previously [5, 13–15]. Exposure to hypercapnic conditions had no effect on either number or type of cells present other than a mild non-significant increase in total cell numbers in the lung.

When we looked at the release of inflammatory cytokines/chemokines IL-6 and KC, with or without HDE under hypercapnic conditions, hypercapnia had a clear effect. Both cytokines are associated with lung inflammation [14, 15] and in our studies, both were significantly increased in response to HDE + CO_2 exposure. As we did not see a similar increase in saline + CO_2 exposures, this suggests that hypercapnia may alter response to an inflammatory stimuli such as barn dust while not necessarily inducing some of these responses by itself. What

the mechanism is behind such an alteration remains unknown and is the focus of our ongoing studies. The response to HDE may also be changed in other subtle ways. KC is a strong neutrophil chemotactic chemokine [37], and while it is clearly increased in response to HDE + CO_2, we did not see any difference in neutrophil migration.

CCL9 is produced primarily by macrophage cells [38] and typically exist at high constitutive levels in the blood [30]. While little work has examined CCL9 in the lung, a silicosis model shows that challenge with silica induced a specific increase of lung CCL9 [39]. There too they noted very low BAL levels of CCL9 outside of stimulation with particulates. Another paper notes that injection of endotoxin can induce an increase of CCL9 in the heart and lung [30], a key component of barn dusts. In the current study we show that not only is CCL9 induced by HDE, but that it is significantly increased in a CO_2 dose-dependent manner when given with HDE. Given the high constitutive expression of CCL9 in circulation, there was concern that an increase in epithelial leak may be responsible for the elevation in CCL9 in BAL samples. Wet-to-dry ratios of the lungs, however, were unaffected, showing increased lung leak was not a factor. More telling, however, mRNA from lung tissue showed an increase that generally reflected protein levels seen in the lung, suggesting that CCL9 present in BAL is locally produced in response to HDE and HDE + CO_2 while serum levels of protein were unaffected.

CCL9 is chemotactic for Langerhans cells and CD4+ T cells in other tissues [38, 40]. The chemokine binds the CCR1 receptor [30], but is less chemotactic than other ligands for this receptor. The mechanisms by which CCL9 functions are still mostly unresolved, though local production in response to challenge suggests some potential function in the response to inhaled challenges to the immune system. It was discovered that proteolytic cleavage of CCL9 greatly enhances its chemotactic potential [41], suggesting that CCL9 may act as an early response chemokine, responding to local proteolysis that enhances the chemotactic signal. This is of particular interest to our work in that our group has recently demonstrated that HDE is capable of inducing proteolytic cleavage/activation of PAR receptors [42] by HDE. It is therefore possible that CCL9 may be similarly activated in the alveolar space in response to barn dust. We are currently examining this possibility.

Another important marker of increased inflammation is ICAM-1 expression. This cell receptor is vital for migration of neutrophils to the lung [43], and given the lack of significant neutrophil increase, we wondered if CO_2 had any effect on this receptor. Somewhat surprisingly, we did see clear increases in tissue staining for the receptor in the bronchial epithelium with saline + CO_2

alone. Because HDE predictably induced ICAM-1 so significantly in these bronchial cells [44], it was not clear if addition of CO_2 enhanced this effect or not. An examination of lung mRNA showed that mRNA was indeed increased with HDE + CO_2, but not so with saline + CO_2. As whole lung RNA samples may not reflect tracheal mRNA we isolated tracheal epithelial cell mRNA from animals as well, showing a similar pattern of expression to whole lung samples. This may suggest that a process in ICAM-1 protein production may be responsible for the increases we see with CO_2 treatment alone. This may also help to explain the modest increase in ICAM-1 mRNA with HDE treatment alone, despite its clear increase in response to HDE [44].

Finally, we decided to look at MMP-9 due to mention of an unpublished observation that CCL9 increased MMP-9 in the lung [39] and its roles in neutrophil migration and tissue remodeling in the lung [45, 46]. Similar to the other chemokines we examined, there was a clear increase in MMP-9 mRNA in lung tissue as CO_2 was increased. Similar to other factors examined such as CCL9, this increase was only apparent when HDE was present.

Conclusions

These results raise a number of questions with relation to workplace ventilation. Does ventilation need to be considered with relation to common illnesses and contaminants of workplaces and how they may interact? While elevated CO_2 exposure alone in most cases appeared insufficient to induce changes, the lung appears to alter several responses when elevated CO_2 is present in addition to an innate immune stimulus. In this respect, CO_2 might function as a tuning mechanism of innate immunity, or perhaps an indicator of dysfunction, requiring a different or elevated response. Another question remaining regards possible acidosis in the exposed animals, and if this is a factor in altered immune responses. While blood gas sampling was not done, the anesthesia protocol at the end of the experiment had animals out of the chamber long enough to likely skew such readings. This remains a technical issue to address in future studies. What our work clearly does show is that the effects of gas exposures at levels seen in work environments, particularly in CAFOs, can depend on responses to other elements present, in particular organic dust.

While this work is in mice and uses an established laboratory-optimized dust injury model, we do note that dust extracts may not mimic a true dust exposure as encountered in the barn. Work will also have to be done with regards to which signaling pathways are affected by these exposures. We do still feel this work shows the importance of further work in mixed environmental exposures and for testing of workers to dusts and gas exposures in the work environment.

Acknowledgments
Not applicable.

Funding
The work was supported by a pilot grant from the Great Plains Center for Agricultural Health (DS) and the National Institute for Occupational Safety Health and the Central States Center for Agricultural Safety and Health (CS-CASH; U54OH010162) to TAW and R01OH008539 to DJR. Dr. Wyatt is the recipient of a Research Career Scientist award (1IK6 BX003781) from the Department of Veterans Affairs.

Authors' contributions
DS conceived of the study, analyzed data, and carried out most of the experiments and writing of the manuscript. JMD provided technical help and aided with experiments. KLB provided further technical help with regards to mRNA techniques and analysis. DJR and TAW assisted with experimental design, manuscript writing, and guidance of the project. All authors have read and approved of the final manuscript.

Competing interests
The authors declare that they have no competing interests.

Author details
[1]Research Service, Veterans Administration Nebraska Western Iowa Health Care System, Omaha, NE 68105, USA. [2]Pulmonary, Critical Care, Sleep & Allergy Division, Department of Internal Medicine, University of Nebraska Medical Center, 985910 The Nebraska Medical Center, Omaha, NE 68198-5910, USA. [3]Department of Environmental, Agricultural and Occupational Health, University of Nebraska Medical Center, 985910 The Nebraska Medical Center, Omaha, NE 68198-5910, USA.

References
1. Schiffman SS, Studwell CE, Landerman LR, Berman K, Sundy JS. Symptomatic effects of exposure to diluted air sampled from a swine confinement atmosphere on healthy human subjects. Environ Health Perspect. 2005;113(5):567–76.
2. Vogelzang PFJ, Van Der Gulden JWJ, Folgering H, Heederik D, Tielen MJM, Van Schayck CP. Longitudinal changes in bronchial responsiveness associated with swine confinement dust exposure. Chest. 2000;117(5):1488–95.
3. Von Essen S, Romberger D. The Respiratory Inflammatory Response to the Swine Confinement Building Environment: The Adaptation to respiratory Exposures in the Chronically Exposed Worker. J Agric Saf Health. 2003;9(3): 185–96.
4. May S, Romberger DJ, Poole JA. Respiratory health effects of large animal farming environments. J Toxicol Environ Health Part B Crit Rev. 2012;15(8): 524–41.
5. Poole JA, Romberger DJ. Immunological and inflammatory responses to organic dust in agriculture. Curr Opin Allergy Clin Immunol. 2012;12(2):126–32.
6. Donham KJ, Cumro D, Reynolds SJ, Merchant JA. Dose-response relationships between occupational aerosol exposures and cross-shift declines of lung function in poultry workers: recommendations for exposure limits. J Occup Environ Med. 2000;42(3):260–9.
7. Kirychuk SP, Dosman JA, Reynolds SJ, Willson P, Senthilselvan A, Feddes JJ, Classen HL, Guenter W. Total dust and endotoxin in poultry operations: comparison between cage and floor housing and respiratory effects in workers. J Occup Environ Med. 2006;48(7):741–8.
8. Poole JA, Wyatt TA, Von Essen SG, Hervert J, Parks C, Mathisen T, Romberger DJ. Repeat organic dust exposure-induced monocyte inflammation is associated with protein kinase C activity. J Allergy Clin Immunol. 2007;120(2):366–73.
9. Poole JA, Wyatt TA, Oldenburg PJ, Elliott MK, West WW, Sisson JH, Von Essen SG, Romberger DJ. Intranasal organic dust exposure-induced airway adaptation response marked by persistent lung inflammation and pathology in mice. Am J Physiol Lung Cell Mol Physiol. 2009;296(6):L1085–95.

10. Charavaryamath C, Juneau V, Suri SS, Janardhan KS, Townsend H, Singh B. Role of toll-like receptor 4 in lung inflammation following exposure to swine barn air. Exp Lung Res. 2008;34(1):19–35.

11. Bailey KL, Poole JA, Mathisen TL, Wyatt TA, Von Essen SG, Romberger DJ. Toll-like receptor 2 is upregulated by hog confinement dust in an IL-6-dependent manner in the airway epithelium. Am J Physiol Lung Cell Mol Physiol. 2008;294(6):L1049–54.

12. Senthilselvan A, Dosman JA, Kirychuk SP, Barber EM, Rhodes CS, Zhang Y, Hurst TS. Accelerated lung function decline in swine confinement workers. Chest. 1997;111(6):1733–41.

13. Wyatt TA, Slager RE, Heires AJ, DeVasure JM, VonEssen SG, Poole JA, Romberger DJ. Sequential activation of protein kinase C isoforms by organic dust is mediated by tumor necrosis factor. Am J Respir Cell Mol Biol. 2010; 42(6):706–15.

14. Wyatt TA, Slager RE, DeVasure J, Auvermann BW, Mulhern ML, Von Essen S, Mathisen T, Floreani AA, Romberger DJ. Feedlot dust stimulation of interleukin-6 and -8 requires protein kinase Ce in human bronchial epithelial cells. Am J Physiol Lung Cell Mol Physiol. 2007;293(5):L1163–70.

15. Romberger DJ, Bodlak V, Von Essen SG, Mathisen T, Wyatt TA. Hog barn dust extract stimulates IL-8 and IL-6 release in human bronchial epithelial cells via PKC activation. J Appl Physiol. 2002;93(1):289–96.

16. Larsson B, Palmberg L, Malmberg PO, Larsson K. Effect of exposure to swine dust on levels of IL-8 in airway lavage fluid. Thorax. 1997;52(7):638–42.

17. Gustin P, Urbain B, Prouvost J, Ansay M. Effects of atmospheric ammonia on pulmonary hemodynamics and vascular permeability in pigs: Interaction with endotoxins. Toxicol Appl Pharmacol. 1994;125(1):17–26.

18. Donham KJ, Cumro D, Reynolds S. Synergistic effects of dust and ammonia on the occupational health effects of poultry production workers. J Agromedicine. 2002;8(2):57–76.

19. Clark PC, McQuitty JB. Air quality in farrowing barns. Canadian Agricultural Engineering. 1988;30(1):173–8.

20. Langford NJ. Carbon dioxide poisoning. Toxicol Rev. 2005;24(4):229–35.

21. Abolhassani M, Guais A, Chaumet-Riffaud P, Sasco AJ, Schwartz L. Carbon dioxide inhalation causes pulmonary inflammation. Am J Physiol Lung Cell Mol Physiol. 2009;296(4):L657–65.

22. Wang N, Gates KL, Trejo H, Favoreto Jr S, Schleimer RP, Sznajder JI, Beitel GJ, Sporn PH. Elevated CO2 selectively inhibits interleukin-6 and tumor necrosis factor expression and decreases phagocytosis in the macrophage. FASEB J. 2010;24(7):2178–90.

23. Laffey JG, Kavanagh BP. Carbon dioxide and the critically ill–too little of a good thing? Lancet. 1999;354(9186):1283–6.

24. Schneberger D, Cloonan D, DeVasure JM, Bailey KL, Romberger DJ, Wyatt TA. Effect of elevated carbon dioxide on bronchial epithelial innate immune receptor response to organic dust from swine confinement barns. Int Immunopharmacol. 2015;27(1):76–84.

25. Satish U, Mendell MJ, Shekhar K, Hotchi T, Sullivan D, Streufert S, Fisk WJ. Is CO2 an indoor pollutant? Direct effects of low-to-moderate CO2 concentrations on human decision-making performance. Environ Health Perspect. 2012;120(12):1671.

26. Liu Y, Chacko BK, Ricksecker A, Shingarev R, Andrews E, Patel RP, Lang Jr JD. Modulatory effects of hypercapnia on in vitro and in vivo pulmonary endothelial-neutrophil adhesive responses during inflammation. Cytokine. 2008;44(1):108–17.

27. Takeshita K, Suzuki Y, Nishio K, Takeuchi O, Toda K, Kudo H, Miyao N, Ishii M, Sato N, Naoki K, Aoki T, Suzuki K, Hiraoka R, Yamaguchi K. Hypercapnic acidosis attenuates endotoxin-induced nuclear factor-[kappa]B activation. Am J Respir Cell Mol Biol. 2003;29(1):124–32.

28. Poole JA, Dooley GP, Saito R, Burrell AM, Bailey KL, Romberger DJ, Mehaffy J, Reynolds SJ. Muramic acid, endotoxin, 3-hydroxy fatty acids, and ergosterol content explain monocyte and epithelial cell inflammatory responses to agricultural dusts. J Toxicol Environ Health A. 2010;73(10):684–700.

29. Boissy RJ, Romberger DJ, Roughead WA, Weissenburger-Moser L, Poole JA, LeVan TD. Shotgun pyrosequencing metagenomic analyses of dusts from swine confinement and grain facilities. PLoS One. 2014;9(4), e95578.

30. Poltorak AN, Bazzoni F, Smirnova II, Alejos E, Thompson P, Luheshi G, Rothwell N, Beutler B. MIP-1 gamma: molecular cloning, expression, and biological activities of a novel CC chemokine that is constitutively secreted in vivo. J Inflamm. 1995;45(3):207–19.

31. Peters TM, Anthony TR, Taylor C, Altmaier R, Anderson K, O'Shaughnessy PT. Distribution of particle and gas concentrations in swine gestation confined animal feeding operations. Ann Occup Hyg. 2012;56(9):1080–90.

32. Donham KJ, Popendorf WJ. Ambient Levels of Selected Gases Inside Swine Confinement Buildings. Am Ind Hyg Assoc J. 1985;46(11):658–61.

33. Dong H, Kang G, Zhu Z, Tao X, Chen Y, Xin H, Harmon JD. Ammonia, methane, and carbon dioxide concentrations and emissions of a hoop grower-finisher swine barn. Trans ASABE. 2009;52(5):1741–7.

34. Teixeira JV, Miranda S, Monteiro RAR, Lopes FVS, Madureira J, Silva GV, Pestana N, Pinto E, Vilar VJP, Boaventura RAR. Assessment of indoor airborne contamination in a wastewater treatment plant. Environ Monit Assess. 2013; 185(1):59–72.

35. Chan MY. Commuters' exposure to carbon monoxide and carbon dioxide in air-conditioned buses in Hong Kong. Indoor Built Environ. 2005;14(5):397–403.

36. Lang JD, Figueroa M, Sanders KD, Aslan M, Liu Y, Chumley P, Freeman BA. Hypercapnia via reduced rate and tidal volume contributes to lipopolysaccharide-induced lung injury. Am J Respir Crit Care Med. 2005;171(2):147–57.

37. Borish LC, Steinke JW. 2. Cytokines and chemokines. J Allergy Clin Immunol. 2003;111(2 Suppl):S460–75.

38. Hara T, Bacon KB, Cho LC, Yoshimura A, Morikawa Y, Copeland NG, Gilbert DJ, Jenkins NA, Schall TJ, Miyajima A. Molecular cloning and functional characterization of a novel member of the C-C chemokine family. J Immunol. 1995;155(11):5352–8.

39. Brass DM, McGee SP, Dunkel MK, Reilly SM, Tobolewski JM, Sabo-Attwood T, Fattman CL. Gender influences the response to experimental silica-induced lung fibrosis in mice. Am J Physiol Lung Cell Mol Physiol. 2010;299(5):L664–71.

40. Mohamadzadeh M, Poltorak AN, Bergstresser PR, Beutler B, Takashima A. Dendritic cells produce macrophage inflammatory protein-1γ, a new member of the CC chemokine family. J Immunol. 1996;156(9):3102–6.

41. Berahovich RD, Miao Z, Wang Y, Premack B, Howard MC, Schall TJ. Proteolytic activation of alternative CCR1 ligands in inflammation. J Immunol. 2005; 174(11):7341–51.

42. Romberger DJ, Heires AJ, Nordgren TM, Souder CP, West W, Liu X, Poole JA, Toews ML, Wyatt TA. Proteases in agricultural dust induce lung inflammation through PAR-1 and PAR-2 activation. Am J Physiol Lung Cell Mol Physiol. 2015;309(4):L388–99.

43. Tosi MF, Stark JM, Smith CW, Hamedani A, Gruenert DC, Infeld MD. Induction of ICAM-1 expression on human airway epithelial cells by inflammatory cytokines: effects on neutrophil-epithelial cell adhesion. Am J Respir Cell Mol Biol. 1992;7(2):214–21.

44. Mathisen T, Von Essen SG, Wyatt TA, Romberger DJ. Hog barn dust extract augments lymphocyte adhesion to human airway epithelial cells. J Appl Physiol. 2004;96(5):1738–44.

45. Delclaux C, Delacourt C, D'Ortho M, Boyer V, Lafuma C, Harf A. Role of Gelatinase B and Elastase in Human Polymorphonuclear Neutrophil Migration across Basement Membrane. Am J Resp Cell Mol Biol. 1996;14(3):288–95.

46. Shapiro SD. Elastolytic metalloproteinases produced by human mononuclear phagocytes: Potential roles in destructive lung disease. Am J Respir Crit Care Med. 1994;150(6 II):S160–4.

16

Cardiovascular risk factors among industrial workers

Prajjwal Pyakurel[1*], Prahlad Karki[2], Madhab Lamsal[3], Anup Ghimire[1] and Paras Kumar Pokharel[1]

Abstract

Background: Cardiovascular diseases (CVD) are the number one cause of death globally, more people die annually from CVDs than from any other cause. An estimated 17.5 million people died from CVD in 2012, representing 46.2 % of all NCD death globally. An accurate characteristic of the cardiovascular risk factors in a specified population group is essential for the implementation of educational campaign. However, there are no reliable CVD risk factors burden, nor of its awareness and treatment status in Nepal industrial settings. We aimed to assess cardiovascular risk factors among men age 20-59 years in one of the largest industrial corridor of Eastern Nepal.

Methods: A total of 494 industrial workers between ages of 20–59 years, from two industries participated in the study. Pretested semi-structured questionnaire was used to collect the information. Primary outcome was cardiovascular risk factors based on STEPS survey and study on non-communicable disease in Nepal. A semi-structured questionnaire was used to interview 494 industrial workers. Lipid profile and serum blood glucose of 406 workers and electrocardiogram of 400 workers was done.

Results: The prevalence of cardiovascular disease (CVD) was 13.8 %. Those who were >45 years were 2.72 times more likely to develop CVD. Those who smoked more pack year, had family history of hypertension (HTN) and consumed no fruits were 4.32, 1.90.2.47 times more likely to develop CVD. Low density Lipoprotein (LDL) level <130 was found to be protective compared to LDL level above ≥ 130. On adjusted analysis those who did not consume fruits and had high LDL level were 3.32 and 3.03 more likely to develop CVD.

Conclusion: There is high prevalence of CVD risk factors. Although majority of them are literate there is lack of health education and awareness among young male population in an eastern Nepal industrial setting.

Keywords: Cardiovascular disease, Occupational health, Industrial workers

Background

CVD are the number one cause of death globally, more people die annually from CVD than from any other cause. An estimated 17.5 million people died from CVD in 2012, representing 46.2 % of all Non-communicable disease (NCD) death [1]. Of these deaths, an estimated 7.4 million were due to heart attack and 6.7 million were due to stroke [1]. Low middle income country (LMIC) are disproportionally affected by CVD, over 80 % of CVD deaths takes place in LMIC. In 2012 heart disease and stroke were among the top three causes of years of life lost due to premature mortality [1]. The number of people, dying from CVDs, mainly heart disease and stroke, will increase to reach 23.3 million by 2030 [2, 3].

Over the last four decades, the rate of death from CVD has declined in high- income countries, owing to reduction in CVD risk factors and better management. Recent studies indicate that, although the risk-factor burden is lower in low-income countries, the rates of major CVD and death are substantially higher than high-income countries [1]. CVD mortality rates in the South Asian countries are much higher than the East Asian countries [4]. Estimates from the Global Burden of Disease (GBD) study suggest that by the year 2020, India alone will have

* Correspondence: prazzwal@gmail.com
[1]School of Public Health and Community Medicine, B.P.Koirala Institute of Health Sciences, Postal Address: 56705, Dharan, Nepal
Full list of author information is available at the end of the article

more individuals with CVD than in any other region [5]. Unfortunately, no large-scale, methodologically sound, epidemiological studies are available in these populations to estimate the true incidence of cardiovascular events.

In Nepal, 42 % of deaths are caused by NCD and nearly 35 % of deaths are caused by CVD, cancer, chronic obstructive pulmonary disease and diabetes mellitus [6]. Prevalence of coronary heart diseases in eastern region was 5.7 % in 2005. Similarly, prevalence of hypertension was 22.7 % in Dharan municipality [7]. Studies have shown that the prevalence of hypertension in adult population was around 20 % in urban population [8]. According to the data of 'Sunsari Health Survey' of the year 1993, the prevalence of diabetes and hypertension in Sunsari Districtfrom eastern Nepal, was about 6 % and 5.1 % respectively in adults [9]. The NCD risk factors: STEPS survey Nepal 2013 showed prevalence of smoking-18.5 %, alcohol-17.4 %, HTN-23.4 %, diabetes-3 %, hypercholesterolemia-22.7 % and hypertriglyceridaemia-25.2 % [10].

The concept of occupational safety and health (OSH) in Nepal is in initial stage. The government of Nepal has enforced concepts of OSH through its Labor Act 1992; it has highlighted few issues and provisions on working hours, physical infrastructural setup, yearly medical examination and provisions of safety measures in work etc. It has already endorsed 9 conventions passed by International Labor Organization (ILO) but has not yet ratified convention No. 155 which solely bears OSH obligations [11].

An accurate characteristic of the CVDs risk factors in a specified population is essential for the implementation of educational campaigns [12]. Identifying risk factors and implementing certain intervention will definitely help to reduce CVD risk. However, there are no reliable study on burden of risk factors, awareness and treatment of CVD in industrial setting of Nepal. We aimed to assess CVDs risk factors among men age 20–59 years in one of the largest industrial corridor of Eastern Nepal.

Methods

A cross sectional study was conducted among men age 20–59 years in one medium and one large size industries in the industrial Corridor of Eastern Nepal from July 2012 to July 2013. Medium size industries was defined as industries with fixed assets between Nepalese rupees (NRs) 30 million and 100 million whereas large size industries was defined as investment of more than NRs 100 million in fixed assets. Female workers and all the small industries workers were excluded from the study.

The intention was not to select particular type of industry (e.g. metal, beverages etc.) but to select an isolated population whose CVD burden are still hidden and where preventive programmes can be initiated. Industrial setting, with their intramural resources and healthcare infrastructure, are ideal for initiating preventive activities

to increase the awareness and control of CVD. Two industries were selected by simple random sampling through lottery method from the industrial cue sheet of Large and Medium size industries, provided by Morang Merchant Association Biratnagar Nepal, an organization working for the welfare of industries in Eastern Nepal. During lottery method each industry name was transferred from a que-sheet and was put on a piece of paper. The piece of paper were placed in a container and thoroughly mixed. The required number of industries was selected without looking the name of the industries. Industries selected were Hulas Wire Industries Private Pvt. Limited which was the large size industry and Pragati Textile Industries Pvt. Limited which was the medium size industries. Workers were selected through systematic random sampling. List of workers working for various duration of years and various shifts excluding the night shifts were made. Altogether there were 1000 workers from these two industries after exclusion of night workers. Dividing the total population by the required sample size estimated sampling interval of 2.02 was made. Taking round figure of 2 workers, every third workers were selected as the sample. Workers who were unable to provide consent were excluded. If the total sample size was not met due to workers not providing consent, list of workers who were not considered in the initial stage was made and sample was drawn by similar process through systematic random sampling.

According to the study done by Kaur et al. [13] in India the least prevalence risk factor of CVD was diabetes which was 16.3 %.

Prevalence (p) = 16.3 %

Compliment of prevalence (q) = 100−16.3 = 83.7 %

Permissible Error (PE) at 20 %, L =20 % of 16.3 = 3.26

Sample size (n) = (Z1-α) 2× pq/L2

= (1.96) 2× 16.3 × 83.7/(3.26) 2

=493.30 (494)

The study site was the Sunsari-Morang Industrial Corridor of Eastern Nepal which is the 28 km long corridor extending from Khanar of Sunsari District to Rani of Morang district of eastern Nepal, where majority of medium and large sized industries are located.

The data was collected using a pre-tested semi-structured questionnaire. Questions were adopted from WHO STEPS [14] questionnaire and a hospital based study on noncommunicable disease in Nepal [15]. Risk factors were based on self-report, physical and bio-chemical measurement. The questionnaire was used to elicit information from each study participant for socio-demographic characteristics, lifestyle-related factors and physical and bio-chemical measurements.

Cardiovascular positive cases was defined as those cases which had been diagnosed on the basis of documentation, evidence of treatment of CVD, positive rose angina questionnaire and with presence of Electrocardiogram (ECG) abnormalities 1-1-1, 1-1-2, 1-1-3, 1-1-4, 1-1-5, 1-1-6 and 1-1-7 representing major Q wave 4-1-1 and 4-1-2 representing ST-T changes and 5–1 and 5–2 representing T waves changes in the Minnesota coding [16].

Two blood pressure measurements were taken using standard techniques. The measurements were obtained half an hour apart. The lower of the two measurements was used for analysis. Height was measured in meters. Weight was measured in kilogram [17]. Waists circumference (WC) was measured at the centre point of the subcostal margin in the mid-axillary line and the highest point of the iliac crest in the mid-axillary line. Hip circumferences (HC) were measured at the level of the greater trochanter. ECGs were read by cardiologist and coded using the Minnesota coding system [16].

Blood samples were drawn by trained personnel, centrifuged and stored for analysis. Laboratory measurements included estimation of fasting blood glucose, total cholesterol, triglycerides, high density lipoprotein (HDL) and LDL. Glucose was analyzed by oxidase method (GOD-POD), cholesterol by (CHOD-PAP) method, TG by (GPO-PAP) method, HDL by Cholesterol Liquicolor test kit and LDL by Friedewald formula [18–22].

Analysis
All data was entered in Microsoft XP Excel spread sheet and converted into SPSS (Statistical Package for Social Sciences) Version 17 program for statistical analysis. The significance of proportion was used by examining Chi-square test and Fisher Exact test. The probability of significance was set at 5 % level of significance and 95%confidence interval. Odd's ratio was calculated.

Ethical clearance
This study was conducted after obtaining ethical clearance from Institutional Ethical Review Board of B. P. Koirala Institute of Health Sciences, Dharan, Nepal. Approval for conducting the study was obtained both from the management and the employee representative. Written informed consent from the study subject was taken after explaining all the procedure in Nepali.

Results
A face to face semi-structured interview was done among 494 industrial workers over a course of one year. Response rate for face to face interview was 100 %. Lipid profile and serum blood glucose of 406 workers and ECG of 400 workers were done.17.81 % of workers for blood test examination and 19.02 % of workers for ECG examination didn't participated.

Demographic characteristics
The mean age of the participant was 33.56 ± 8.75 years with 40.7 % of the workers in age group of 20–29 years.

Majority of them (97.6 %) were literate with more than half (60.6 %) completed some secondary education. About 2/3rd (74.5 %) were below the poverty line.

Behavioural CVD risk factor profile showed 63.2 % did vigorous intensity exercise. Most of them (90.5 %) were non-vegetarian. More than 1/3rd (38.3 %) did not consume fruits/week. Majority of them (97.4 %) consumed salt more than that recommended by World Health Organization (WHO) of 35 g/week. About 40.2 % were current smoker. Local Rakhsi (Home-made alcohol) was consumed by about 63.9 % of the workers. Almost 30 % of the workers were hazardous drinkers (Table 1).

Physical and biochemical parameter showed mean pulse rate of 75.04 ± 8.85 beats/min. About 41 % were prehypertensive. Body mass index (BMI) was at increased risk and at higher high risk for 46 % of the participants as per the BMI for Asian classification. Almost half of them (46.9 %) had central obesity. Hyperglycaemia was seen in 4.2 % and dyslipidemia in 84.5 % of the workers (Table 2).

Table 1 Behavioural risk factor profile of workers (n = 494)

Characteristics	Percentage
Physical activity	
Vigorous intensity exercise	63.2
Moderate intensity exercise	36.8
Dietary Habit	
Vegetarian	9.5
Non-vegetarian	90.5
Fruit Consumption/week	
None Serving	38.3
1 Serving	25.1
>1 Serving	36.6
Salt individual/week	
≤35 g	2.6
>35 g	97.4
Smoke Product User (n = 251)	
Current	40.4
Former	10.5
Never	49.1
Pack Year (n = 251)	
≤5	94.4
>5	5.6
Alcohol type among user (n = 366)	
Local Rakshi	63.9
Beer	16.7
Whisky, Rum, Gin	19.4
Alcohol amount/week (n = 366)	
<21 units	69.4
≥21 units	30.6

Table 2 Physical and Biochemical profile of workers

Characteristics	Percentage
JNC-7 classification of HTN (n = 494)	
Normal	25
Pre-hypertension	41.4
Hypertension stage 1	24.5
Hypertension stage 2	9.1
BMI For Asian Population (n = 494)	
Underweight (<18.5 kg/m^2)	6.3
Increased but acceptable risk (18.5- 23 kg/m^2)	46.8
Increased risk (23–27.5 kg/m^2)	35.8
Higher High Risk (≥27.5 kg/m^2)	11.1
Waist- Hip Ratio (n = 494)	
Normal (<0.90)	53
Central obesity (>0.90)	47
Serum Biochemistry Profile (n = 406)	
Diabetes (≥126 mg/dl)	4.2
Impaired fasting blood glucose (≥110 mg/dl and <126 mg/dl)	30.5
Hypercholesterolemia	44.1
Hypertriglyceridemia	49.3
Decreased HDL	65.8
Dyslipidaemia	84.5
Cardiovascular disease	13.8

Those who were >45 years were 2.72 times more likely to had CVD compared to those ≤ 45 years. (OR = 2.72, CI 1.35 to 5.40) Similarly, those who did not consume fruits were 2.47 times more likely to develop CVD. (OR = 2.47, 1.47-4.16) More pack year of smoking was related to more chances of developing CVD. Those who consumed more than 5 pack years were 4.32 times more likely to develop CVD compared to those who smoked ≤ 5 pack years. (OR = 4.32, 1.34-13.84). Those who had family history of HTN were 1.90 times more likely to develop CVD compared to those who did not had family history of HTN. (OR = 1.90, CI 1.14-3.19). Similarly those who had a LDL level of <130 were 0.55 times more likely to be protective from CVD compared to those who had LDL level of ≥130. (OR = 0.31-0.99) (Table 3).

Binary logistic regression analysis revealed that those who did not consumed fruit once a week had 3 times more chances of developing CVD compared to those who did consumed fruits (adjusted OR (AOR) 3.58, CI 1.24-8.87), as shown in Table 4. Similary those who had high LDL of < 130 were 0.18 times more likely to be protective from CVD compared to those who had LDL level of ≥130 (adjuster OR (AOR) = 0.35-0.97). Potential confounders were identified through literature search and those variables whose P value was < 0.05 were entered in

the logistic regression model. The following variables were adjusted in the regression model (age, HTN, pack year of smoking, tobacco chewing user, diabetes, physical activity, total cholesterol, triglycerides, HDL, LDL, dietary history, fruit consumption/week, waist-hip ratio, earplug used and working hours/week) (Table 4).

Discussion

This study done in industrial setting among relatively young urban population, found prevalence of cardiovascular risk factors to be high. The study had included industrial workers of age 20–59 years which were similar to study done among industrial workers in one of the large industry in northern India [16]. The mean age of the participants were 33.56 years which were lower than a similar study done among Brazilian industry workers [12]. Bulletin on CVD risk test showed men age 45 years or older were at greater risk of CVD [23].

More than half of the workers had completed some secondary education in our study which were comparatively less than study done by Prabhakharan et al. in Northern India where 66.4 % were graduate/postgraduate/professional [16].

Workers were involved in moderate and vigorous physical activity at any time during work, leisure time and household activities. Although workers showed high physical activity at work presence of risk factors still seemed to be high. In a study done by Mehan et al. in industrial setting none of the subjects, including workers, were found to be engaged in heavy activities at workplace. Majority of subjects were engaged in light activities and moderate activities. This could be due to the differences in characteristics of industrial setting [24].

Non-vegetarian comprised about 90 % of our study population. A study among chemical industrial workers in India showed most of the respondents was vegetarian in contrast to our study. Although there were changes in dietary pattern in both industries, CVD risk factors still seemed to be high. This showed the role of multiple risk factors in the causation of disease. Most of the respondent in our study consumed less fruits. In a similar study done by Mehan et al. the mean daily fruits and vegetables consumption were less than the recommended WHO guideline which were similar to our study [24]. In our study those who consumed no fruits were more likely to develop CVD in comparison to those who consumed fruits. (OR = 2.47, CI 1.47 to 4.16). Similarly careful analysis of INTERHEART data revealed, South-Asians had lower prevalence of vegetables and food intake compared to rest of the world [25].

Respondents consumed more than 35 g of salt/week. Most of them consumed salt and pickle for taste as their regular diet. WHO guideline recommends taking too much salt whether in the form of added salt in meal or

Table 3 Risk factors associated with Cardiovascular Disease (Bivariate analysis)

Variable	Cardiovascular disease			Odd's Ratio	Confidence Interval
	Positive	Negative	Total		
Age					
>45	13 (27.7)	34 (72.3)	47 (100)	2.72	1.35-5.40
≤45	55 (12.3)	392 (87.7)	447 (100)		
Fruits/week					
No fruit consumption	39 (20.6)	150 (79.4)	189 (100)	2.47	1.47-4.16
Fruit consumption	29 (9.5)	276 (90.5)	305 (100)		
Pack year of smoking					
>5 pack year	5 (35.7)	9 (64.3)	14 (100)	4.32	1.34-13.84
≤5 pack year	27 (11.4)	210 (88.6)	237 (100)		
Family History of Hypertension					
Yes	36 (18.6)	158 (81.4)	194 (100)	1.90	1.14-3.19
NO	32 (10.7)	268 (89.3)	300 (100)		
LDL Cholesterol					
<130	22 (10.7)	183 (89.3)	205 (100)	0.55	0.31 -0.99
≥130	34 (17.7)	158 (82.3)	192 (100)		

taking regular salt containing foodstuffs increases blood pressure and subsequent chances of developing CVD [26].

Current smokers comprised of more than 1/3rd of the respondents. In study done by Shields et al. comparing those who had never smoked daily, current daily smokers had 60 % higher risk of incident heart disease during the follow-up period. The relative risk ratio was 1.6 times more in current daily smokers in compared to those who had never smoked [27]. In our study those who consumed >5 pack years of cigarettes were more likely to develop CVD compared to those who consumed ≤5 pack years of cigarettes (OR = 4.32, CI 1.34 to 13.84). In Framingham risk prediction equations for incidence of CVDs using detailed measures for smoking, compared to never smokers the risk of CVD incidence increased with pack-years [28].

About 30 % of the workers drank more than the recommended 21 units/week and were hazardous drinkers, 33.6 % were hypertensive, 11.1 % were considered high to very high risk as per the BMI for Asian Population, 46.96 % had central obesity, 4.2 % had hyperglycaemia and about 85 % had dyslipidemia.

Table 4 [a]Association of cardiovascular disease with risk factors (Multivariate analysis)

Significant variable	Significant values	Adjusted OR	95 % CI
No fruit consumption	0.02	3.58	1.24-8.87
LDL Cholesterol	0.04	0.18	0.35-0.97

[a]Age, HTN, pack year of smoking, tobacco chewing user, diabetes, physical activity, total cholesterol, triglycerides, HDL, LDL, dietary history, fruit consumption/week, waist-hip ratio, earplug used and working hours/week

Study done by Roy et al. on impact of alcohol on CHD in 10 medium-to large size industries from diverse sites found possible harm of alcohol for CHD risk in Indian men. However this relationship needs to be further examined in large, prospective study [29]. Study done by Sharma et al. on general population of Nepal showed prevalence of HTN to be 34 % which is comparable to our study [30]. Similarly other studies done in India showed 12.2 % were in the high to very high risk as per the BMI which is comparable to our study.(15) A review done by Vaidya et al. on obesity prevalence in Nepal showed high levels of central obesity (between 40 % and 60 %) across different demographic groups, which could be comparable to our study [7].

Dyslipidemia were seen among 85 % of the respondents. Most of the industrial population resides in and around Duhabi and Khanar of Sunsari district in Koshi zone of south-eastern Nepal which is rapidly urbanizing. With growing population, changes in lifestyle and food-habit especially in suburban and rural areas of the country, there is a potential threat of increasing risk factor for CVDs especially Coronary Heart Disease (CHD). The healthy traditional plant-based diets are being replaced by cheaper calorie dense high-fat foods. There is high intake of saturated and trans-saturated fatty acid. All factors have led to the occurrence of dyslipidemia especially hypercholesterolemia [30, 31].

Strength of the study

This is one of first attempts to understand CVD risk factors among industrial population in Nepal. We tried to explore occupational sector which is neglected area of research in Nepal. In study methodology we have used pre-tested questionnaire, scientific calculation of sample size, random and systematic sampling and calculation of unadjusted and adjusted Odd's ratio which adds to the strength of our study.

Limitation

The study was carried out in industrial setting and only in males hence it could not be representative of general population. The results could not be generalized to individuals older than 60 years, in whom the risk factors as well as disease burden is higher than this population. Night shift workers were excluded in the study. This is the first kind of study done in industrial sector of Nepal hence comparison could not be made with other industries of the country.

Conclusion

There is high prevalence of CVD risk factors among industrial workers. Although the study population was not representative of general industrial population we believe that it does represent the similar kind of CVD risk factors burden among many of medium and large size industries in Eastern Nepal. Though this seems to be a small occupational health survey but it adds on the risk factors prevalent in the industrial set-up and thus focuses the attention of cardiovascular epidemiologist and researcher to conduct more studies.

Abbreviation

BMI: body mass index; CHD: coronary heart disease; CHOD –PAP: enzymatic colorimetric determination of serum cholesterol; CVD: cardiovascular disease; ECG: electrocardiogram; GBD: global burden of disease; GOD-POD: glucose – oxidase method; GPO-PA method: quantitative estimation of triglycerides in serum or plasma; HC: height circumference; HDL: high density lipoprotein; HTN: hypertension; ILO: international labour organization; LDL: low density Lipoprotein; LMIC: low-middle income country; NCD: non-communicable disease; NRs: nepalese rupees; OSH: occupational safety and health; Pvt.: private; SPSS: statistical package for social science; WC: waist circumference.

Competing interests

The authors declare that they have no competing interests.

Authors' contributions

PP, PKP and ML made substantial contributions to the conception or design of the work or the acquisition, analysis, and interpretation of data for the work. PP, PK and ML and AG revised the work critically for important intellectual content. PP, PKP, PK and AG gave final approval of the version to be published. PP, PK, PKP, AG & ML all agree to be accountable for all aspects of the work in ensuring that questions related to the accuracy or integrity of any part of the work are appropriately investigated and resolved. All authors read and approved the final manuscript.

Acknowledgement

A very special acknowledgement goes to Dr. Sanjiv Kumar Sharma (Prof, Internal medicine) who have always encouraged and supported me during difficult times and without his help this work would have been very difficult to accomplish. Sincere thanks goes to Kidney, Hypertension, Diabetes, Cardiovascular Disease (KHDC) team members Dr. SadikshyaAdhikhariSapkota, Kaji Man Giri and MamitRai. I also consider it very important to offer thankfulness to Dr. VivekKattel (Assistant Professor, Internal medicine), Prakash Chandra Karkee, Anil Khadka, Ram Binay Shah, Bsc MLT (2011batch), Anup, Aastha (interns), Kissan, Safal, Rajendra, Prakash, Jasraj (MBBS final year students) for their cooperation. I also like to thank Dr. Puspanjali Adhikari for grammer and language correction. My earnest appreciation goes to SanjeevJha, Shree Narayan Majhi (Hulas Wire Industries Pvt. Ltd.), PradeepNiraula, BhadduSardar (Pragati textile Ltd.) and to all those factory workers who agreed to be a part of this study. My appreciation also goes to B.P. Koirala Institute of Health Sciences for providing me opportunity of carrying out research in this topic. Lastly I would like to thank all the people who directly or indirectly supported my work.

Author details

[1]School of Public Health and Community Medicine, B.P.Koirala Institute of Health Sciences, Postal Address: 56705, Dharan, Nepal. [2]Department of Internal Medicine, B.P.KoiralaInstitue of Health Sciences, Dharan, Nepal. [3]Department of Bio-chemistry, B.P.KoiralaInstitue of Health Sciences, Dharan, Nepal.

References

1. World Health Organization. Global status report on non-communicable disease 2014. ISBN 9789241564854 Switzerland: WHO Press, World Health Organization; 2014 http://www.who.int/nmh/publications/ncd-status-report-2014/en/(accessed 19 Dec 2015)

2. World Health organization. Global status report on non-communicable diseases 2010. ISBN 978 92 4 068645 8 Switzerland: WHO Press, World Health Organization; 2010 http://www.who.int/nmh/publications/ncd_report_full_en.pdf (accessed 17 Dec 2015)

3. Mathers CD, Loncar D. Projections of global mortality and burden of disease from 2002 to 2030. PLoSMed. 2006;3(11):e442. http://journals.plos.org/plosmedicine/article?id=10.1371/journal.pmed.0030442 (accessed date 19 Dec 2015).

4. Ueshima H, Sekikawa A, Miura K, Turin TC, Takashima N, Kita Y, et al. Cardiovascular disease and risk factors in Asia: a selected review. Circulation. 2008;118(25):2702–9. http://circ.ahajournals.org/content/118/25/2702.full.pdf (accessed date 19 Dec 2015).

5. Christopher J, Murray L, Lopez A. The global burden of disease. United Kingdom: Harvard University Press; 1996. http://apps.who.int/iris/bitstream/10665/41864/1/0965546608_eng.pdf (access date 19 Dec 2015). ISBN 0-9655466-0-8.

6. Government of Nepal Ministry of Health and Population, Nepal Health Research Council, World Health Organization, Country office for Nepal. Non-Communicable diseses risk factors: STEPS Survey Nepal 2013: Ramsapath Kathmandu, Nepal; National Health Research Council;2013 http://www.searo.who.int/nepal/mediacentre/non_communicable_diseases_risk_factors_steps_survey_nepal_2013.pdf (accessed date 19 Dec 2015)

7. Vaidya A, Pokharel PK, Nagesh S, Karki P, Kumar S, Majhi S. Prevalence of coronary heart disease in the urban adult males of eastern Nepal: a population-based analytical cross-sectional study. Indian Heart J. 2009;61(4): 341–7. http://indianheartjournal.com/ihj09/july_aug_09/341-347.html (19th Decmber 2015).

8. Maskey A, Sayami A, Pandey R. Coronary artery disease: an emerging epidemic in NEPAL. Journal of Nepal Medical Association. 2003;42:122–4. http://jnma.com.np/files/archive/2003/vol.42, %20no.146(2003)/Coronary % 20 Artery % 20 Disease. pdf (access date 19 Dec 2015).

9. Bhandari GP, Angdembe MR, Dhimal M, Neupane S, Bhusal C. State of non-communicable disease in Nepal. BMC Public Health. 2014;14(23). http://bmcpublichealth.biomedcentral.com/articles/10.1186/1471-2458-14-23(18th December 2015).

10. Government of Nepal Ministry of Health and Population, Nepal Health Research Council, World Health Organization, Country office for Nepal. Non-Communicable diseses risk factors: STEPS Survey Nepal 2013: Ramsapath Kathmandu, Nepal; National Health Research Council;2013. http://www.searo.who.int/nepal/mediacentre/non_communicable_diseases_risk_factors_steps_survey_nepal_2013..pdf (accessed 19 Dec 2015)

11. Joshi SK. Occupational Safety and Health in Nepal. International Journal of Occupational Safety and Health. 2011;1:1–2. http://nepjol.info/index.php/IJOSH/article/view/5224/4347 (accessed date 20 Dec 2015).

12. Cassani RSL, Nobre F, Filho AP, Schmidt A. Prevalence of cardiovascular risk factors in a population of Brazilian industry workers. Arq Bras Cardiol. 2009; 92(1):16–22. http://www.scielo.br/pdf/abc/v92n1/en_04.pdf (accessed 20 Dec 2015).

13. Kaur P, Rao TV, Sankarasubbaiyan S, Narayanan AM, Ezhil R, Rao SR, et al. Prevalence and distribution of cardiovascular risk factors in an urban industrial population in south India: a cross-sectional study. J Assoc Physicians India. 2007;55:771–6. http://www.japi.org/november2007/O-771. pdf (access date 20 Dec 2015).

14. World Health Organization. The WHO STEP wise approach to chronic disease risk factor surveillance (STEPS).Geneva, Switzerland: WHO Press. http://www.who.int/chp/steps/STEPS_Instrument_v2.1.pdf (access date 20 Dec 2015)

15. Nepal Health Research Council. Prevalence of non-communicable disease in Nepal,Hospital based study2010. Nepal: S.S Printing Press; 2012. http://www. ncf.org.np/upload/files/611_en_Non_Communicable_diseases.pdf (access date 20 Dec 2015).

16. Prabhakaran D, Shah P, Chaturvedi V, Ramakrishnan L, Manhapra A, Reddy KS. Cardiovascular risk factor prevalence among men in a large industry of northern India. Natl Med J India. 2005;18(2):59–65. http://www.nmji.in/ archives/Volume_18-2_March_April2005/Original_articles/59-75_1.pdf (accessed date 20 Dec 2015).

17. Glynn M, Drake W. Hutchison's Clinical Methods:An integrated approach to clinical practice. United Kingdom: Saunders Elsevier; 2007.

18. KEE GAD Biogen Pvt. Ltd. Ver. KGGLU104.1/1GLUCOSE (GOD- POD Method, End Point). New Delhi-110028, India. 2010.

19. N.S. BIOTEC MEDICAL EQUIPMENTS. CHOL-MC-0530. CHOLESTEROL (CHOD-PAP) Enzymatic Colorimetric Determination of Serum Cholesterol. Alexandaria-Egypt

20. MEDICHEM MIDDLE EAST Clinical Chemistry Reagents. Cat. No.15181. Triglycerides GPO/PAP Enzymatic colorimetric method. Syria;2010.

21. HUMAN.SU-HDLDD INF 1008401 GB 09-2002-11. HDL CHOLESTEROL liquicolor HDL.Direct Homogenous Test for the Determination of HDL-cholesterol Enzymatic Colorimetric test; 2002.

22. General Practice Notebook. Friedwald equation. https://www.easycalculation. com/medical/ldl-cholesterol.php (accessed date 20 Dec 2015)

23. Aetna. Cardiovascular Disease Risk Tests. www.aetna.com/cpb/medical/data/ 300_399/0381.html (accessed 20 Dec 2015)

24. Mehan MB, Srivastava N, Pandya H. Profile of non communicable disease risk factors in an industrial setting. J Postgrad Med. 2006;52(3):167–73. http://www.bioline.org.br/pdf?jp06056 (accessed date 20 Dec 2015).

25. Goyal A, Yusuf S. The burden of cardiovascular disease in the Indian subcontinent. Indian J Med Res. 2006;124(3):235–44. http://www.ncbi.nlm. nih.gov/pubmed/17085827 (access date 20th Dec 2015).

26. World Health Organization. Guideline: Sodium intake for adults and children. ISBN 978 92 4 150483 6: Geneva, Switzerland; 2012. http://apps. who.int/iris/bitstream/10665/77985/1/9789241504836_eng.pdf?ua=1&ua=1 (accessed date 20 Dec 2015)

27. Shields M, Wilkins K. Smoking, smoking cessation and heart disease risk: A 16-year follow-up study. Health Reports. 2013;24(2):12–22. http://www. statcan.gc.ca/pub/82-003-x/2013002/article/11770-eng.htm (access date 20 Dec 2015).

28. Mannan H, Stevenson C, Peeters A, Walls H, McNeil J. Framingham risk prediction equations for incidence of cardiovascular disease using detailed measures for smoking. Heart Int. 2010;5(2):e11. http://www.ncbi.nlm.nih.gov/ pmc/articles/PMC3184690/ (accessed date 20 Dec 2015).

29. Roy A, Prabhakaran D, Jeemon P, Thankappan KR, Mohan V, Ramkrishna L et al. Impact of alcohol on coronary heart disease in Indian men. Atherosclerosis 210 (2):531–5. http://www.ncbi.nlm.nih.gov/pubmed/ 20226461 (access date 20 Dec 2015)

30. Sharma SK, Ghimire A, Radhakrishnan J, Thapa L, Shrestha NR, Paudel N, et al. Prevalence of hypertension, obesity, diabetes, and metabolic syndrome in Nepal. Int J Hypertens. 2011;2011:821971. http://www.hindawi. com/journals/ijhy/2011/821971/ (accessed date 20 Dec 2015).

31. Limbu YR, Rai SK, Ono K, Kurokawa M, Yanagida JI, Rai G, et al. Lipid profile of adult Nepalese population. NepalMedCollJ. 2008;10(1):4–7. http://nmcth. edu/images/gallery/Editorial/VoZ2lyrlimbu.pdf (accesses date 20 Dec 2015)).

17

Diagnosis, monitoring and prevention of exposure-related non-communicable diseases in the living and working environment: DiMoPEx-project is designed to determine the impacts of environmental exposure on human health

Lygia Therese Budnik[1*], Balazs Adam[2], Maria Albin[3,4], Barbara Banelli[5], Xaver Baur[6], Fiorella Belpoggi[7], Claudia Bolognesi[8], Karin Broberg[4], Per Gustavsson[4], Thomas Göen[9], Axel Fischer[10], Dorota Jarosinska[11], Fabiana Manservisi[7], Richard O'Kennedy[12], Johan Øvrevik[13], Elizabet Paunovic[11], Beate Ritz[14], Paul T. J. Scheepers[15], Vivi Schlünssen[16,17], Heidi Schwarzenbach[18], Per E. Schwarze[13], Orla Sheils[19], Torben Sigsgaard[17], Karel Van Damme[20] and Ludwine Casteleyn[20]

Abstract

The WHO has ranked environmental hazardous exposures in the living and working environment among the top risk factors for chronic disease mortality. Worldwide, about 40 million people die each year from noncommunicable diseases (NCDs) including cancer, diabetes, and chronic cardiovascular, neurological and lung diseases. The exposure to ambient pollution in the living and working environment is exacerbated by individual susceptibilities and lifestyle-driven factors to produce complex and complicated NCD etiologies.

Research addressing the links between environmental exposure and disease prevalence is key for prevention of the pandemic increase in NCD morbidity and mortality. However, the long latency, the chronic course of some diseases and the necessity to address cumulative exposures over very long periods does mean that it is often difficult to identify causal environmental exposures.

EU-funded COST Action DiMoPEx is developing new concepts for a better understanding of health-environment (including gene-environment) interactions in the etiology of NCDs. The overarching idea is to teach and train scientists and physicians to learn how to include efficient and valid exposure assessments in their research and in their clinical practice in current and future cooperative projects.

DiMoPEx partners have identified some of the emerging research needs, which include the lack of evidence-based exposure data and the need for human-equivalent animal models mirroring human lifespan and low-dose cumulative exposures. Utilizing an interdisciplinary approach incorporating seven working groups, DiMoPEx will focus on aspects of air pollution with particulate matter including dust and fibers and on exposure to low doses of solvents and sensitizing agents. Biomarkers of early exposure and their associated effects as indicators of disease-derived information will be

(Continued on next page)

* Correspondence: L.Budnik@uke.de
[1]Division of Translational Toxicology and Immunology, Institute for Occupational and Maritime Medicine (ZfAM), University Medical Center Hamburg-Eppendorf (UKE), Hamburg, Germany
Full list of author information is available at the end of the article

(Continued from previous page)
tested and standardized within individual projects. Risks arising from some NCDs, like pneumoconioses, cancers and allergies, are predictable and preventable. Consequently, preventative action could lead to decreasing disease morbidity and mortality for many of the NCDs that are of major public concern. DiMoPEx plans to catalyze and stimulate interaction of scientists with policy-makers in attacking these exposure-related diseases.

Keywords: Noncommunicable diseases, Human biomonitoring, Environmental/occupational exposure to xenobiotics

Background

Adverse health outcomes because of exposure received in the living and working environments in combination with lifestyle have been estimated to be responsible for up to 75% of global noncommunicable diseases (NCDs) [1, 2]. Chronic diseases resulting from these exposures provide a major contribution not only to the NCD burden but also to the resulting increase in health costs. Since most of these diseases are preventable, appropriate health policies should concentrate on this major societal challenge.

In 2010, about 40 million people died worldwide from NCDs, including cancer, diabetes, and chronic cardio-vascular, neurological and lung diseases [3]. This represents an increase from 60% of total deaths attributed to these diseases in the year 2000 to 70% (total deaths) within 10 years (see Additional file 1: Info Box 1, for more details). In 2015, the World Health Organization (WHO) ranked environmental exposures among the top risk factors for chronic disease mortality [4]. Pollution (from air, soil, water) is one of the leading causes of death from NCDs (for other environmental factors see Table 1). Worldwide, diseases related to environmental pollution were responsible for 9 million premature deaths in 2015 - three times as many deaths as from AIDS, tuberculosis and malaria combined [5]. Every year, environmental risks – such as indoor and outdoor air pollution, second-hand smoke, unsafe water, lack of sanitation and inadequate hygiene – take the lives of 1.7 million children under 5 years, reported WHO in 2017 [6]. Ambient air pollution alone is estimated to cause 7 million premature deaths per year (recently highlighted in the Global Burden of Disease (GBD project [7]). Data from the GBD study group demonstrate a strong link between both indoor and outdoor air pollution exposure and cardiovascular disease (CVD), as well as between air pollution and cancer [8]. In some parts of the European Union (EU), air pollution causes a reduction in the average life expectancy of more than one year [9, 10].

The concept of the "exposome" as the total of all external exposures, along with individual susceptibility due to genetic, age-related, and other vulnerabilities, is gaining increasing credence from both the scientific and clinical communities [11, 12]. Pollutants, food additives, chemicals found in cosmetic products and therapeutic exposure (chemo–/ radio therapy) are prime examples of such cumulative exposures. Certain pesticides, such as organophosphates, are examples of man-made chemicals to which large populations in agricultural communities are exposed, as well as consumers via their diet, and contribute to neurotoxicity in human populations worldwide [13–15]. The compromising of health (effect

Table 1 Synopsis

The main purpose of the European Cooperation in Science and Technology program is to provide a framework for international cooperation among researchers and other professionals. By bringing together experts in significant areas of human life and development, opens up the possibilities of new ideas, approaches and solutions. The European Cooperation in Science and Technology COST program is founded partially by the member states, who delegate the management committee members. The Action Diagnosis, Monitoring and Prevention of Exposure-related Noncommunicable Diseases (DiMoPEx) fosters capacity-building by bringing together basic scientists, clinical researchers and practitioners in the relevant (sub-)disciplines and organizing interdisciplinary collaboration and training in research that addresses the societal challenges outlined above. Members aim to implement new concepts in joint interdisciplinary research and training initiatives to enhance networking between expert centers and offer a platform for interdisciplinary collaboration between researchers across Europe. DiMoPEx also aims to attract and focus the interests of the next generation of early career investigators on key emerging issues of exposure-related disease burden and various aspects of exposure assessment sciences.

The predominant goal is to help scientists, physicians and health officials to prevent and reduce health impacts associated with various exposure scenarios and train highly skilled researchers of health-environment (including gene-environment) interactions in the etiology of exposure- related NCDs within seven working groups

The overarching idea of the DiMoPEx project (http://dimopex.eu/ working) groups is to teach and train about how to learn to include evidence-based exposure assessment (in research and clinical settings). Using modern methods such as ambient monitoring and human biomonitoring methods (WG1, WG 2), the various biomarkers of effect and susceptibility alongside with the clinical diagnostic methods and biomarker-based evaluation of lifestyle factors (WG3, WG 6) can be combined, resulting in the development of cooperative projects that are too broad for coverage by individual disciplines (i.e. epidemiology or traditional environmental medicine). Within several joint research projects, DiMoPEx partners are already focusing on the impact of pollution on human health. The projects are concentrating on several pollutants (particulate mass fractions PM2.5 and PM10, a range of metals, inorganic gases and organic compounds) in living and working environments and their health impacts [138].

The DiMoPEx Action anticipates initiating health research with important benefits for public health and the healthcare system of the European Community. DiMoPEx will catalyze and stimulate interaction of scientists with policy-makers on exposure-related diseases of concern to society (see below, WG 7 for more details on cooperation with the WHO scientists, implementation of the new knowledge, involving external partners and policy makers). See below for detailed working groups description.

measure modifications, EMM) is possible through lifestyle factors such as smoking, alcohol abuse and bad nutrition/obesity, as well as through interactions between these. For example, smoking increases the risk of lung cancer (through co-exposure to asbestos, radon or arsenic) from < 20% (exposure alone) to over 80% excess risk because of the synergistic effects [16]. Health hazards also arise from the globalization of trade [17] and production processes with direct and indirect environmental and occupational health impacts [18, 19]. Further, new hazards are continuously being discovered, such as those related to the introduction of nanoproducts in industrial and consumer goods [20].

The long latency periods, combined cumulative exposures and chronic course of diseases often makes it difficult to identify environmental/occupational exposure as the cause of NCDs [21, 22]. One source of exposure may cause several outcomes and also different types of exposure may affect the same disease outcome; for example, air pollution has been linked to a number of common diseases, including cardiovascular, cerebrovascular, respiratory, reproductive, neuro-developmental and neuro-degenerative diseases. [23] Conversely, multiple exposures may have a cumulative effect on the same target organ.

At the patho-physiological level, exposure-related NCDs arise as a result of interactions between internal (genetic, epigenetic, hormonal, aging etc.) factors and external (occupational/environmental) influences [24]. In recent years, enormous progress in the exploration of genetic and epigenetic factors and resulting disease risks has been made. This knowledge has already found its way into the contents of academic teaching programs in medical schools and postgraduate courses (e.g. in molecular epidemiology, neurosciences, personalized medicine). In contrast, the other major and modifiable dimension of pathogenesis, the influence of occupational/environmental exposure and lifestyle factors, has received comparatively little attention. Current figures published by WHO (see Additional file 1: Info Box 1) indicate an urgent need for an update in the research and training potential concerning environmental health issues, and in implementing public health research across Europe, with an interdisciplinary evidence-based orientation in the natural sciences, public health and medicine.

Outline

This review assesses the current status and future needs of the multicenter European COST Action DiMoPEx (http://www.cost.eu/COST_Actions/ca/CA15129). The separate sections represent the identified current research objectives and future goals of the DiMoPEx action. It reflects the structure of this multicenter action with 7 working groups (http://dimopex.eu/working), highlighting the role of individual working groups within the DiMoPEx

framework and the specific methods provided by individuals groups for the ongoing and planned collaborative projects. A short description of the ongoing interdisciplinary research projects is also provided demonstrating how the evidence-based exposure data can be applied for the diagnosis and monitoring of exposure-related NCDs (from the perspective of the action partner).

DiMoPEx project goals identified by the project partners
How to improve diagnosis, monitoring and prevention of NCDs?
Current status and future needs to be addressed
DiMoPEx partners recognize an important research need: to link the living and working environment with disease prevalence in order to prevent the pandemic increase in NCD morbidity and mortality. Public health benefits may range from effective preventative measures to early detection of possible adverse health outcomes. Four of the currently identified emerging research tasks pursued by DiMoPEx include the following:

1. **To face the difficulties in NCD diagnosis and monitoring of disease progress**
   Many ongoing long-term studies focusing on early signs of related chronic diseases account insufficiently for environmental/occupational determinants of health. Other studies addressing health outcomes in relation to exposures in the living and working environment do not sufficiently account for existing knowledge regarding appropriate exposure measures in their study designs (i.e. some record ever/never occupational exposure or self-reporting of specific chemicals, leading to exposure misclassification and biased results). The effects of multiple exposures and EMM within the same target organ should also be addressed. It is time now to take a closer look at the living and working environment and focus on evidence-based exposure data that has the potential to correlate exposure with disease, which otherwise provides an obstacle to evidence-based recommendations for primary and secondary NCD prevention.

2. **To focus on biomarkers of early response and appropriate human-equivalent animal models (carcinogenicity bioassays to provide a basis for evidence- based interventions**
   Evidence-based interventions have already successfully limited exposure to many known and probable carcinogens, including tobacco, arsenic, asbestos, benzene, vinyl chloride and air pollution. However, among NCDs, cancer is still the second leading cause of death: in 2014 about 591,699 of people died from cancer in the United States alone

[25]. Cancer is an extremely complex disease, not easy to control, and one about which there is insufficient knowledge in terms of etiology. To provide a solid scientific basis for cancer prevention, it is necessary to increase our knowledge about cancer etiology. Basic as well as preventative and clinical research should be developed. In this research, well-designed experimental animal studies [26] and biomarkers of early response should play a central role (carcinogenicity bioassays).

3. **To focus on air pollution as one of the major factors responsible for NCD mortality**

   There is a strong link between both indoor and outdoor air pollution exposure and CVD, as well as between air pollution and cancer. Knowledge of what it is that makes a particle toxic may provide better exposure metrics in epidemiology studies, lead to more efficient abatement strategies to reduce emissions of the most hazardous air pollutants and allow for production of nanoparticles that can be shown to be benign. Being able to predict the toxicity of particulates based on knowledge of size, composition and material properties would also be a prerequisite for reducing the need for extensive toxicity testing of new nano-materials. The oxidative potential of particles is considered by many to be a promising metric to predict particle toxicity.

4. **To recognize the need for the public-health protection through cooperation with policy-makers**

   To benefit societies and enhance the wellbeing of populations and decrease morbidity and mortality from exposure-related NCDs, there is a need for innovation in public health and environment policy and in the business practices of certain industries, leading to healthier environments, as well as a better understanding of risk communication, including its ethical aspects. There is a need to catalyze and stimulate interaction between scientists and policy-makers in respect of exposure-related diseases of concern to society. The predominant goal should be to help scientists, physicians and health officials to prevent and reduce health impacts associated with various exposure scenarios and to train highly skilled researchers for the future labor market.

Implementation of the research goals within the framework of the 7 WGs

The identification of a xenobiotic chemical and the documentation of the degree and extent of exposure by the WG 1 project is fundamental to the investigation of the disruptive effects of that exposure and its consequences for NCDs, which are the specialist interests of the WG 5, WG 2 and WG 6 projects in determining the

biohazard consequences in carcinogenicity, genotoxicity and health effects. WG 3, WG 4 and WG 7 support other groups with knowledge on epidemiology and/or risk communication and canvassing meetings with policy makers to influence environmental/occupational laws, funding groups, etc.

Detailed descriptions of methods applied, issues to be concentrated on within the project and further examples of current activities are summarized in the following sections.

WG 1 advancing towards evidence-based exposure data

Exposure assessment – From environmental to individual exposure

An accurate exposure assessment needs consideration of a wide spectrum of sources, the different pathways and routes of exposure, and the environmental and physiological effects of the xenobiotics [27] (Fig. 1).

The most prominent sources of xenobiotic chemical exposure are emissions from industrial processes and engine exhausts, emissions from other combustion processes, residues from pesticide and biocide applications, emissions from consumer populations via waste effluents (solid waste or wastewater), and indoor air emissions from building materials, consumer products and furniture. People are mainly exposed to this pollution via outdoor and indoor air, tap water and contaminated food, as well as direct skin contact with contaminated surfaces and dermally-applied products, such as cosmetics and personal care products [28–33]. In some special cases, exposure may also occur during rainfall, from surface water, dermal contact or oral ingestion of contaminated soil, from applications of pesticides, biocides and other chemical products [34]. Moreover, lifestyle behavior such as. smoking and the consumption of functional food, nutriceuticals and the application of pharmaceuticals, exacerbate the broad spectrum of chemical exposure experienced by an individual. The manifold emission sources, polluted materials and exposure scenarios determine that extraneous chemicals gain access to the body using all possible routes, most especially by inhalation, oral ingestion and via the dermis.

The assessment of chemical exposure has two main aims. Firstly, the individual pollution agents have to be clearly identified. Secondly, qualitative detection also requires ascertainment of the hazards inherent in these xenobiotics. For risk assessment, however, both the qualitative character of exposure and the extent of the exposure have to be estimated. Some approaches of exposure assessment already enable the attainment of both of these goals, e.g. by a non-target procedure which may also enable a semi-quantitative determination of the analytes. However, for those approaches in which specific

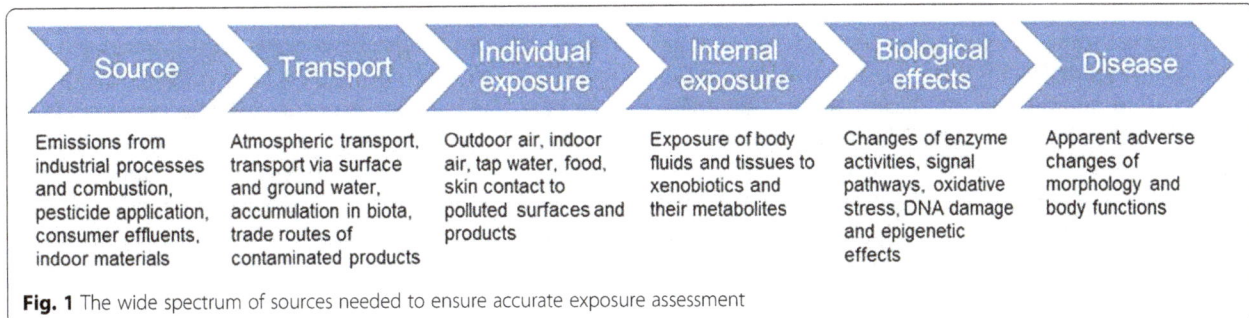

Fig. 1 The wide spectrum of sources needed to ensure accurate exposure assessment

metabolites have to be assessed, the prior identification of the chemical agent is indispensable before targeted measurement can be implemented.

A quantitative estimation of exposure can be performed by a direct or an indirect approach (see Fig. 2). A direct monitoring approach requires determination of the extent of exposure of an individual to a chemical by assessment either externally, internally or as metabolized products. External measurements of ambient exposure can be made from air contamination by that chemical or the contamination of the skin. The internal exposure to a chemical suffered by an individual is by conventional human biological monitoring and the measurement of the unmodified agent, as well as its metabolites and reaction products in blood and urine (see also the later section on human biological monitoring (WG2)). Inevitably, the levels of internal exposure are most strongly connected with the effective dose and the subsequent toxic effects [35]. To use data from individual ambient exposure for risk assessment effectively then it is necessary for an additional calculation about the

absorption efficiency to be made, e.g. by using minute volume, respiratory retention or dermal absorption rate. Indirect approaches of exposure assessment (i.e. dispersion models or other exposure models, questionnaires on exposure scenarios, and questionnaires on food intake or exposure situations) can also be taken as a basis for estimating the levels of environmental contamination. Data from indirect approaches have to be extrapolated to the effective dose in the population by considering pollutant transport processes, accumulation and fate processes in the environment, exposure scenarios, demographic and geographic attributes, lifestyle behavior, human constitution and the pharmacokinetics of the agent. Moreover, an estimation of individual exposure has to include the intra-individual variability of these extrapolation factors within the population [36, 37]. Each extrapolation model should be validated in respect of its performance and uncertainty. Regardless of which approach was used for the assessment of the recent extent of exposure, these might be important for a reasonable risk assessment and for contemplation of the duration of exposure [38].

The tasks of the WG1 "Exposure assessment" project encompass the analysis of skills, expertise and capacities regarding exposure assessment within the consortium, the dissemination of resources and information on assessment procedures and quality assurance, as well as the development and expansion of capabilities and capacities. The most important tasks are the identification of limitations or crucial gaps in knowledge about exposure quantitization and exposure-effect associations, as well as preparing effective solutions for closure of these knowledge gaps. In particular, the WG 1 and WG 2 project groups are providing a sustainable research and training program in the field of exposure science (human biomonitoring, ambient monitoring) for the other DiMoPEx partners.

WG 5 hazards characterization, risk identification: Carcinogenicity bioassays
Diagnosis of cancer as NCD needs biomarker(s) of early effect (detection of preclinical lesions) and new animal study approaches
There is a need for human-equivalent animal models mirroring human lifespan and low dose cumulative

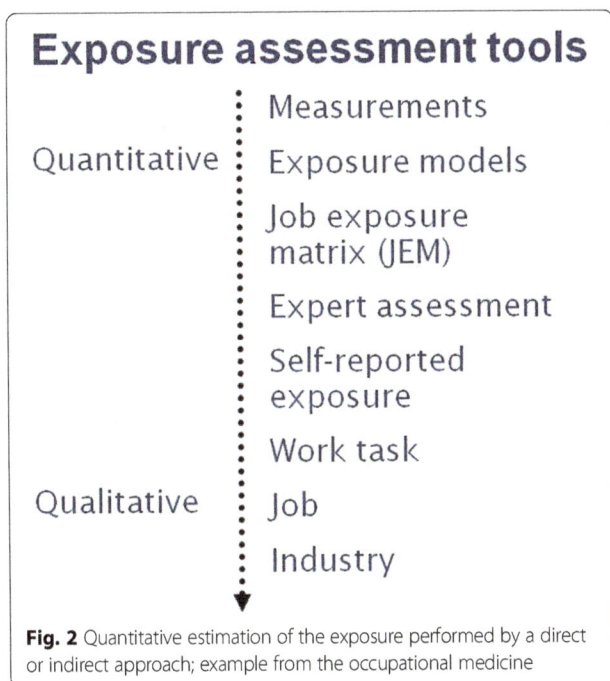

Fig. 2 Quantitative estimation of the exposure performed by a direct or indirect approach; example from the occupational medicine

exposures. The laboratory rat has served as the traditional animal model of choice for research and regulatory developmental and reproductive toxicity testing conducted to support human health hazard identification and risk assessment. The laboratory rat has been more thoroughly characterized than have other species in these research fields, especially when identifying likely human carcinogens. However, with new insights into toxicology, novel integrated experimental approaches for hazard identification are needed with human-equivalent animal models in rodent bioassays for primary prevention (see Additional file 1: Table S1; [39, 40] and Info Box 2) for more information on animal models and Organisation for Economic Co-operation and Development (OECD) guidelines [41].

When conducting cancer bioassays, it is important to investigate the effect of low doses and a systematic dose-calibration study should be performed in an appropriate rodent model in order to identify the relevant administered oral dose of the test substance that results in biomarker concentrations (e.g. urine, serum) comparable to those observed in a human population [42]. Cancer is a complex disease with diverse etiology; see examples of exposure related cancer in Additional file 1: Info Box 3, Table S2 in the supplementary). The neoplastic response depends not only on the kind of agent, its physicochemical and toxicological properties, the mode of exposure, and the type of animal but also, to a great extent, on the latency of the tumor, which varies widely and may be very long. Experimental findings indicate that the latent neoplastic potential for causing a tumor increases with the length of the observation time or age. Thus, experimental carcinogenicity trials should continue until spontaneous animal death and not be cut short. To give a clearer explanation, one of the the DiMoPEx partners compared, in preliminary research, human deaths from malignant tumors at the Hospital of Trieste, in 1989, with rat deaths from malignant tumors in the RI animal facility belonging to control groups, in 1984–1994. Figure 4, which refers to the cumulative prevalence of animals and humans with malignant tumors, histopathologically observed by age at death, shows that 80% of tumors arise after the age of 65 years in humans, which corresponds to 104 weeks in rats [43]. According to the OECD, rats should be sacrificed at 112 weeks of age at death [43], which corresponded to 104 weeks after the start of the treatment. If these animals had been sacrificed at 112 weeks of age (comparable to 65 + age in humans) then the majority of tumors would have been missed. At the Cesare Maltoni Cancer Research Center (CMCRC), studies have been conducted on more than 200 compounds present in the industrial and the general environment, including vinyl chloride, benzene, formaldehyde, trichlorethylene, fuels and their components and

additives, pesticides, and recently aspartame, the most widely diffused artificial sweetener in the world. The results from the CMCRC studies have provided the scientific basis for lowering exposure levels to various agents present in places of work and in daily life. They have also formed the basis for rules and regulations of primary prevention, even if sometimes many years have passed before confirmation of their carcinogenicity in humans (see Additional file 1: Table S3).

Current two-year experimental schemes may mask a carcinogenic response

Cutting short an experiment after two years may mask a possible carcinogenic response, as in the following cases with xylene and mancozeb (see Additional file 1: Table S4) The increase in total malignant tumors, oral cavity carcinomas and hemolymphoreticular neoplasias was only observed for xylene administration after 112 weeks of age (Fig. 3). It should be noted that during exposure tests for xylene, performed by the United States National Toxicology Program, the rats were sacrificed after 104 weeks of treatment without any carcinogenic effect being found [44, 45]. With mancozeb administration, a strong increase in malignant tumors of the thyroid gland in males and female rats was also observed after 112 weeks of age [46]. In demanding that chronic animal studies be terminated after 2 years, regulatory agencies may lose information that is important for extrapolation of the data from animals to humans, most especially for chronic diseases with a long latency time.

An integrated experimental approach

To satisfy the need to consider multiple effects (e.g., cancer and non-cancer) across multiple life stages and to reduce the overall number of animals required for separate studies of these end-points, the adaptation of the carcinogenicity bioassay to integrate additional protocols for comprehensive long-term toxicity assessment was recently proposed. The central aim of the methodology proposed in the integrated experimental approach was to maximize the breadth of outcomes assessed and to increase the sensitivity of testing beyond that in commonly used protocols. This should yield more reliable and inclusive information on many important end-points. In this experimental design, rats from the same generation are used for studying chronic toxicity and carcinogenicity outcomes and distributed into parallel satellite experiments for detecting reproductive/developmental toxicity, thus minimizing variables between different arms of the multi- end-point investigation [47]. This protocol is a incentivizing proposal to regulatory scientists and the scientific community in general. By conducting such integrated bioassays, scientific evidence of risk assessment would be enhanced and expanded, by

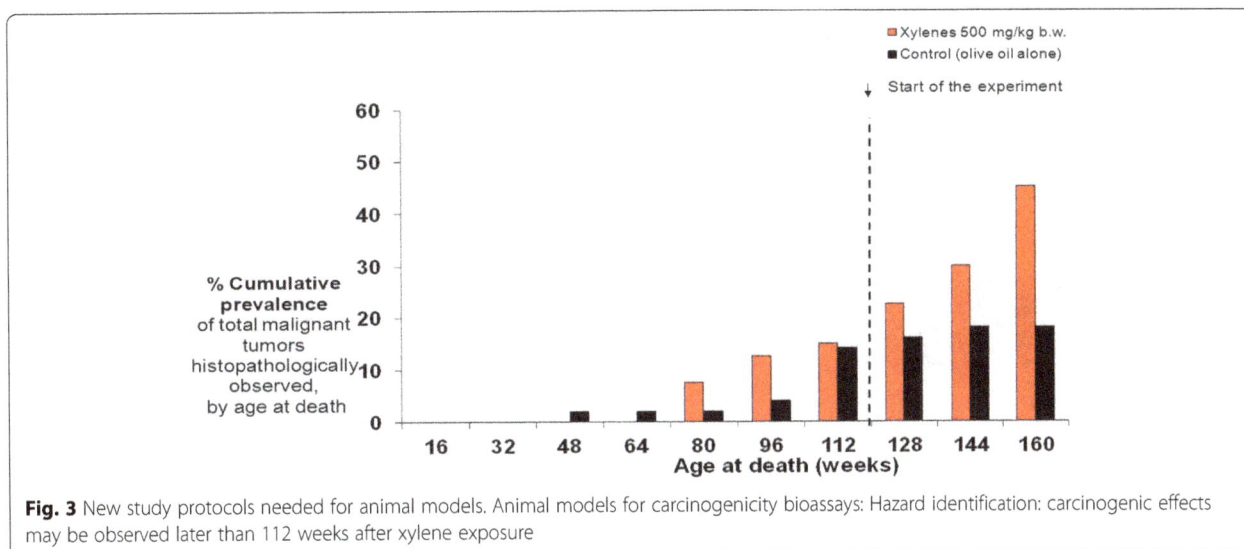

Fig. 3 New study protocols needed for animal models. Animal models for carcinogenicity bioassays: Hazard identification: carcinogenic effects may be observed later than 112 weeks after xylene exposure

gathering sufficient and rapid information about several adverse effects in a unique protocol for protecting public health.

Biomarker of early response to assess the effects of preventive measures and identify individuals at high risk of developing a particular NCD

Efficient patient management relies on early diagnosis of diseases and monitoring of disease progression. In this respect, significant efforts have been made to find informative, blood-based biomarkers or liquid biopsy. As the individual genomic, epigenomic and transcriptomic profiles of diseases become more and more elucidated, the applicability of circulating nucleic acids and exosomes have the potential to complement the existing blood biomarkers in future. In addition, the blood-based detection of disease-specific genetic aberrations, such as mutations, microsatellite alterations and epigenetic modulations in circulating free DNA (cfDNA), or quantitative changes in cfDNA, RNA, microRNAs (miRNAs) and exosomes, represent highly promising approaches for the risk assessment of various diseases. Investigations of these molecular alterations have also revealed an impact on gene expression, resulting in aberrant regulation of disease-specific signal transduction pathways. For the most acute clinical syndromes, it is likely that multiple markers rather than a single marker will give the best diagnosis and prognosis.

The use of the cytokinesis-block micronucleus (CBMN) cytome assay could also be relevant for clinical and epidemiological studies and for preventative interventions, because it could allow the identification of individuals at high risk of developing a given disease and could even qualify as an intermediate biomarker to assess the effects of preventative measures. In prospective studies evaluating large cohorts of disease-free subjects, an increase in

micronucleus frequency (MN) in peripheral blood lymphocytes was associated with an increased cancer risk at the population level, providing suggestive evidence that this biomarker may be predictive of cancer risk [48]. Increased MN frequency was also detected in peripheral lymphocytes of subjects affected by cancer-associated congenital syndromes characterized by deficiencies in the DNA damage response [49]. Many studies also showed an increased MN frequency in peripheral lymphocytes in untreated patients with cancer or pre-neoplastic lesions [50], neurodegenerative diseases [51], CDV and diabetes [52].

Potential biological effect markers – Circulating nucleic acids in human blood

Circulating nucleic acids are promising blood-based biomarkers because of their informative and disease-specific features. Their deregulated levels are associated with tumor genesis, tumor progression, metastases and drug resistance in cancer patients, and reflect physiological and pathological processes of different diseases. Circulating nucleic acids (in plasma or serum) may serve as a "liquid biopsy" that is useful for numerous diagnostic and prognostic applications of different (malignant and benign) diseases, while avoiding tissue biopsies by invasive methods. This minimally invasive procedure allows the repeated taking of blood samples, providing the ability to follow quantitative measurements and genetic or epigenetic changes during the natural course of the disease, facilitating treatment decisions [53, 54].

Nucleic acids are usually released (Fig. 4) during cellular stress or tissue injury into the blood circulation. Their release is associated with inflammatory responses caused by a coordinated expression of numerous genes that initiate, sustain and propagate immune responses and tissue remodelling [55]. This increased cell turnover and impaired blood clearance are possible reasons for

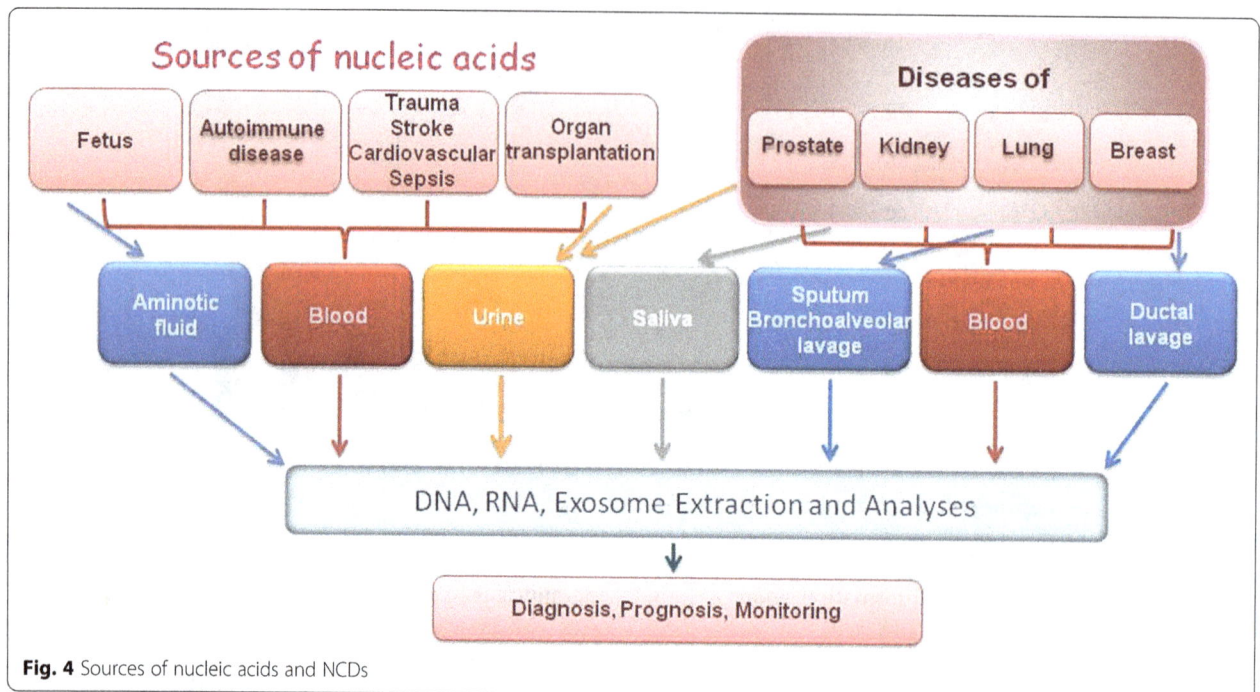

Fig. 4 Sources of nucleic acids and NCDs

the elevated or deregulated levels of circulating nucleic acids in critical disease conditions where organs responsible for elimination of by-products are damaged (as a consequence of systemic inflammation). The release of nucleic acids into the blood circulation occurs during the processes of apoptosis and necrosis. While apoptotic cell death leads to controlled inter-nucleosomal cleavage of genomic DNA, necrotic cell death leads to a discharge of large genomic DNA fragments [56]. Apart from their passive release during cell death, nucleic acids can also be actively excreted into the blood circulation by microvesicles, such as exosomes. Exosomes and their cargo are thought to play an important role in cell-to-cell communication by influencing the recipient cell phenotype [57].

The concentrations of cfDNA are elevated (as an early signal) in the blood circulation after onset of disease and reach the highest level in patients with disease-specific complications and a high mortality risk. Accordingly, the elevation in cfDNA levels is not specific for a specific disease and varies among patients within a patient cohort, but may correlate with the severity of disease. Since cfDNA levels may change during the course of disease and in parallel with the severity of disorder, they could provide a useful marker for the assessment of adverse outcome, allowing clinicians to make a rapid risk stratification for more rational therapeutic decisions [58].

Apart from cfDNA, much attention and effort have been put into the study of cell-free microRNAs (miRNAs) (see Additional file 1: Table S5, [59–61]). The expression of these small, non-coding RNA molecules is often tissue-specific and in many pathological conditions characteristically

deregulated. The clinical relevance of cell-free miRNAs [59] as diagnostic and prognostic markers has been documented for a variety of diseases [60]. Besides, miRNAs that are actively released in exosomes into the blood circulation, can be transferred to recipient cells [61] and can be functional there by respressing their mRNA targets [62]. Thus, exosomes may serve as suppliers of disease-derived genetic information and, consequently, transform their host cell as well. Moreover, exosomal miRNAs stimulate cellular signalling and regulate metabolic functions and homeostasis. The amounts of secreted exosomes as well as their contents of miRNAs have been associated with tumor development and progression, cell migration and proliferation of tumor cells leading to metastasis [63] . (see Additional file 1: Table S5).

Epigenetic markers in early detection of NCDs

Unlike genetic alterations, which can be stably acquired during the life-course, epigenetic modifications (see Additional file 1: Table S6) are dynamic, tissue-specific and can be characteristic of a disease. In this respect, epigenetic alterations may be utilized as biomarkers of exposure and disease and serve as biomolecular sensors for preventive surveillance [64].

Environmental and occupational factors induce epigenetic alterations that can contribute to the onset of NCDs, of which cancer is one of the most prevalent. Occupational exposure to chemicals (e.g. benzene), dusts (e.g. from manufacturing of leather or woods) and/or industrial processes (welding, metallurgy) can be related to cancer and the carcinogenic process is linked to changes in DNA methylation, particularly in its early phases.

Recently, the epigenetic involvement and contribution of 12 chemicals and associated occupations were evaluated from the literature by the International Agency for Research on Cancer (IARC). Human carcinogens related to environmental occupational hazards classified as Group 1 were considered, specifically the three carcinogens aflatoxin, benzene and benzo[a]pyrene), where several studies have reported an epigenetic effect [65]. Increasing scientific evidence has linked diseases other than cancer with epigenetic alterations and exposure to toxic substances. As an example of trans-generational effects, exposure to toxicants during fetal life could be correlated with neurodevelopmental disorders, and epigenetics was considered to be the probable functional phenotype that communicated these diseases [66].

Occupational exposure to specific industrial processes, such as the production and use of nanotubes or fullerenes, can induce epigenetic alterations directly or indirectly through reactive oxygen species (ROS) [67–69]. Occupational asthma [70] and some metabolic diseases can modify the epigenetic status and can contribute to modification of the epigenome. Some neurological diseases, such as Alzheimer's [71] and Parkinson's disease [72], have been linked with occupational exposure to organophosphates and to alteration of the DNA methylation landscape in exposed subjects, underlining a possible cause-effect relationship that needs to be further explored.

Enhancement of genotoxicity and susceptibility markers
Human MN

The MN test is a measure of the increase in micronucleus frequency in cells and is one of the most successful assays in genetic toxicology because of its ability to detect both structural and numerical chromosomal aberrations [73]. It is one of the most widely applied methods for biomonitoring human populations for evaluating exposure to genotoxic agents and genetic instability. The test was established in different surrogate tissues: peripheral blood lymphocytes and erythrocytes, buccal-exfoliated cells and urine-derived cells (Fig. 5). However, the CBMN cytome assay in peripheral blood lymphocytes is the most validated of the methods.

The MN assay, applied in vitro with different established cell lines and in human cultured peripheral lymphocytes, is recommended as part of the basic battery of tests to screen new chemical agents for genotoxicity, allowing the detection of both clastogenic and aneugenic compounds. Indeed, the OECD has published guidelines for the testing of chemicals using the in vitro and in vivo MN assays [74, 75].

Biomonitoring human exposure to genotoxic agents –- CBMN cytome assay in peripheral blood lymphocytes

The CBMN assay is a standard biodosimetry method endorsed by the International Atomic Energy Agency and WHO for measuring exposure to ionizing radiation [76]. The use of the MN test in other exposure scenarios needs to be considered case by case on the basis of the mechanisms of action of the genotoxic agents.

The CBMN assay was largely applied in human populations to evaluate occupational and environmental exposure to genotoxic agents belonging to different chemical classes, with more than 500 associated papers available in the scientific literature. The most frequently investigated groups are hospital personnel, followed by

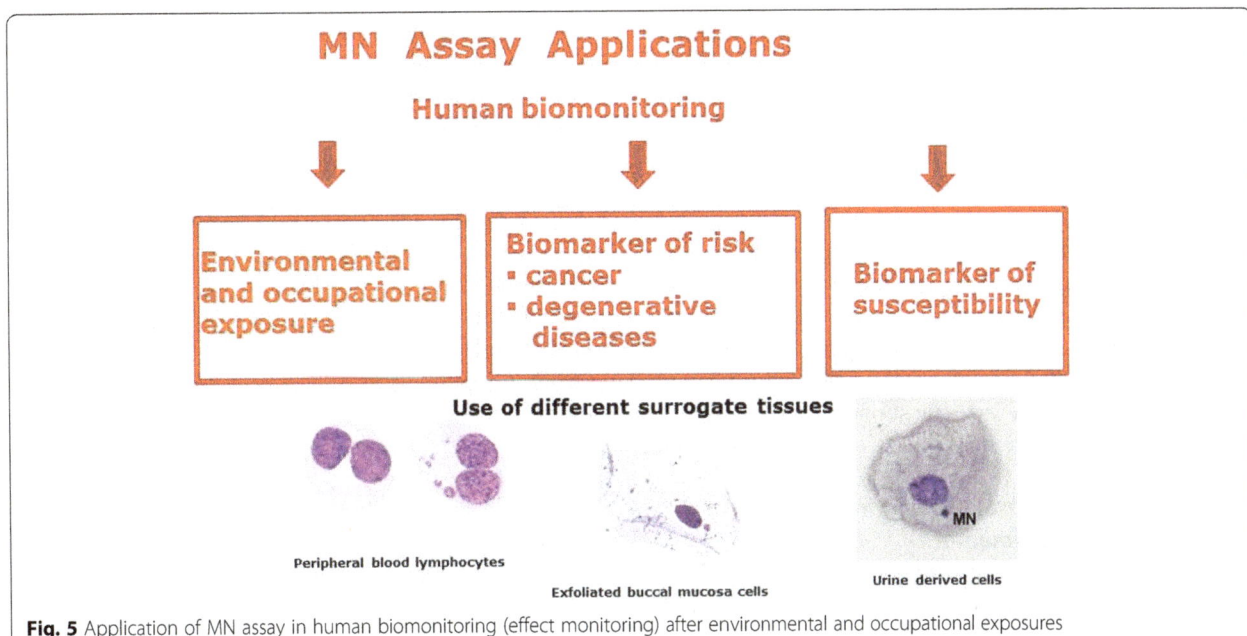

Fig. 5 Application of MN assay in human biomonitoring (effect monitoring) after environmental and occupational exposures

workers in the chemical industry and agricultural workers. The use of the lymphocyte CBMN assay in different exposure scenarios was recently evaluated in the framework of the International Collaborative Project on Micronucleus Frequency in Human Populations (Human Micronucleus project, HUMN) using the systematic review approach [77].

All of the different exposures considered in this review were associated with increased MN frequencies: the average value calculated was 2.5-fold over the background, although the heterogeneity of the available studies and the relevant differences in the quality of the studies do not allow clear conclusions to be drawn. The most pronounced effects, evaluated as increases with respect to the control values, were detected in individuals exposed to metals such as arsenic (6.5-fold), lead (3.8-fold), and chromium (3.5-fold) [78].

Overall, many of the evaluated studies had limitations in study design, recruitment strategy to enrol exposed and control subjects, low statistical power and/or lack of reliable exposure data. The subject selection in many cases did not consider the different tasks in which the workers were involved, the use of protective devices and the known confounding factors for exposed-control matching. Further analyses are needed to elaborate guidelines for the use of the CBMN assay in biomonitoring studies.

MN assay in buccal-exfoliated cells

The MN) cytome assay in uncultured buccal-exfoliated epithelial cells is a minimally invasive approach for evaluating genomic damage and cell death in the human aero-digestive tract (for more information on MN assay in buccal-exfoliated cells, see Additional file 1: Info Box 4) [79–83]. Our recent meta-analysis provides evidence for the utility of the MN assay using buccal-exfoliated cells in the pre-screening as well as in the follow- up of pre-cancerous oral lesions. A significant excess of MN in patients compared with matched controls was observed for patient subgroups with oral and neck cancer (meta-mean ratio (MR) of 2.40, 95% CI: 2.02–2.85) or leukoplakia (meta-mean ratio MR 1.88, 95% CI: 1.51–2.35) [84].

The overall objective of the WG 5 project group is to provide research and training programs covering hazard characterization, risk identification and various early effects biomarkers, including carcinogenicity bioassays. The leader of the WG 5 group are acknowledged expert in the field and provide valuable support for the interdisciplinary projects where needed.

WG 2 human biological monitoring – More than (just) analysis of biomarkers
Exposures to chemicals and particles
A generic view that can be applied to most uses of biomarkers is their contribution to an understanding of the causal link between environmental exposure(s) and the onset and morbidity of disease. From the perspective of epidemiology, the gaps between cause and health outcome may be bridged by the use of biomarker-based research (WG 2). In occupational and environmental health, the use of biomarkers is embedded in a process termed "human biological monitoring" and defined as "the standardized and repeated systematic collection, pretreatment, storage and analysis of body tissues to assess the internal dose of a xenobiotic substance by analysis of the parent substance and/or a product of biotransformation" [85]. A much wider definition of biomonitoring also includes biomarkers that do not carry chemical structure information (a "unique signature") that enables the researcher to link a biomarker value to a specific external factor.

Biomonitoring consists of standardized protocols for the periodic detection of early, preferably reversible, biological signs that are indicative, when compared with adequate reference values, of an actual or potential condition of exposure, effect or susceptibility, possibly resulting in health damage or disease. These signs are referred to as biomarkers [86]. In 1986, Henderson and Zielhuis defined the three types of biomarkers as biomarkers of exposure, of effect, and of susceptibility. Not all biomarkers can be easily classified in this system but it is useful to have a discussion as to how a specific biomarker can be effectively employed in a study design (see Additional file 1: Tables S6 and S7). The functional property of an exposure biomarker is that they carry the signature of a chemical/environmental contaminant marker that can be interpreted in the context of an exposure [87]. Effect biomarkers can provide information on the impact of environmental exposure on molecular, cellular or tissue levels. This 'effect' can be interpreted as an 'adverse' outcome but it often indicates a 'response' that can also be interpreted as a beneficial event, protecting the exposed individual, such as in enzymatic DNA repair. Thus, the terms "biomarker of response" or "biomarker of early effect" can also be used (see Fig. 6). A biomarker cannot always be attributed to a specific causative factor because most of these biomarkers lack chemical structural information, making them non-specific for the causative agent. The contextual information is important for making inferences about the possible involvement of one or more environmental exposures and the use of these biomarkers requires study formats that are particularly well thought-through in their design (Fig. 6).

Susceptibility biomarkers can be used to identify a person for a specific property that may be the result of genetic constitution, acquired properties or both. With these biomarkers, it is possible to classify an individual as "susceptible"or "resistant"to an exposure. The term

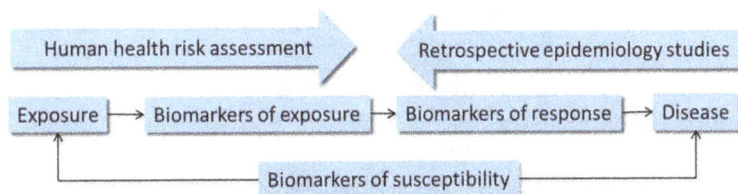

Fig. 6 Human biomonitoring: how a specific biomarker can serve as specific aim in a study design. The "meet-in-the-middle" principle to show how biomarkers can be used prospectively to contribute to human health risk assessment and retrospectively in population-based studies to identify molecules for suitability as intermediate biomarkers of "early effect"'effect' to link exposure biomarkers with disease endpoints

"susceptibility"'is also given a wide interpretation and, at a group level, it is possible to determine an effect measure, such as an Odds Ratio, to assess health risk for a subgroup with one (or more) susceptibility characteristics for comparison with another subgroup with a different susceptibility profile. It is not very useful to interpret a susceptibility outcome for an individual. As for the use of effect biomarkers, the interpretation of susceptibility biomarkers relies on a study designed to support interpretation of susceptibility data in a population.

Nowadays, biomarkers are often applied in population-based studies. Many years of experience have demonstrated that the laboratory-based analysis of biomarkers is usually performed well, because of well-established and rigorous quality assurance. Comparatively, other tasks are performed less successfully and are often suboptimal, e.g. sample collection and data interpretation may have weak spots that contribute to an overall moderate outcome (see Additional file 1: Table S8). As a consequence, biomonitoring studies sometimes do not provide useful results. In a recent study performed in response to the 9/11 Twin Towers terrorist attack in New York, the authors concluded that "'...this study cannot provide any information about exposure or potential health effects" [88]. One of the problems was that insufficient consideration was given to the timing of sample collection relative to the time point of suspected exposure. Also, the groups that were selected for comparison of their biomarker levels were not well suited to the aims of the study.

The availability of a factsheet with the most relevant characteristics of a chemical substance may support well-informed decision-making during the preparation phase. During the EU FP7 project Biomonitoring of Exposure to Carcinogenic Substances (BIOMONECS), a format was developed for this purpose, with the biomonitoring application datasheets (BADS) providing the most relevant information in a concise format. For 15 chemical substances, BADS are available on www.humanbiologicalmonitoring.eu (last updated in 2010). The most recently published BADS are for mercury and methyl mercury [89]. This structured presentation may be useful if time is limited for the deployment of bio-monitoring following a chemical incident.

The WG 2 group also supports the research and training of toxicology knowledge (including nanotechnology and particle toxicology, see below) and with knowledge about the management and risks of chemicals.

Air pollution and particulate matter
Oxidative potential – a possible metric of particle toxicity
Air pollution is a complex mixture of chemically different components. Particulate matter (PM) has been designated as one of the most important components of the burden of disease from air pollution. How particles elicit their responses has not been fully elucidated but many studies have implicated the importance of reactive oxygen species (ROS) formation and oxidative stress in particle toxicity. The oxidative potential of a particles – their ability to generate ROS in cell- free systems – has been suggested as a promising metric for predicting particle toxicity. The oxidative potential could provide a simple screening tool for new nano-materials and a more relevant dose metric in epidemiological studies.

ROS and oxidative stress in particle-induced toxicity
The role of ROS and oxidative stress in particle toxicology has been based, at least partly, on the observation that particles generate ROS in cell-free systems such as aqueous buffers, that increased ROS levels are measured within particle-exposed cells, and that antioxidants inhibit various cellular responses induced by particles [90–94]. Figure 7 presents an overview of cellular ROS production in particle-exposed cells [95] (see also Additional file 1: Table S9, [90–94, 96–100]). An overview of the endogenous components involved in cellular redox -regulation is presented in an attachment (Additional file 1: Table S10).

Beyond oxidative potential – the role of redox signaling in cellular responses to PM
Oxidative stress and redox responses are considered to play a central role in particle-induced toxicity. It is often assumed that the biological reactivity of a particle is because of its oxidative potential: the ability to produce ROS or be able to oxidize target substrates directly in contact with biological fluids or cellular molecules.

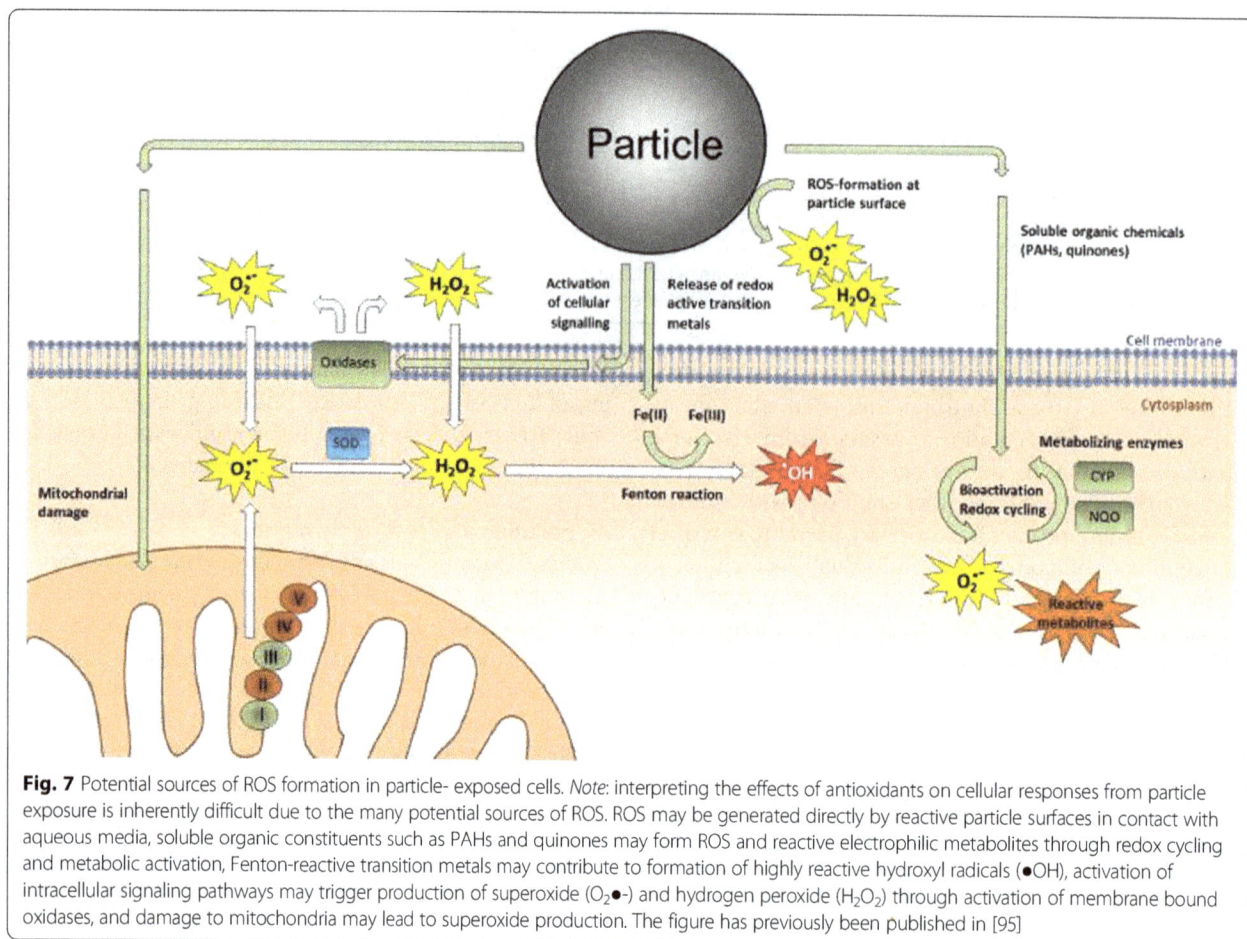

Fig. 7 Potential sources of ROS formation in particle- exposed cells. *Note*: interpreting the effects of antioxidants on cellular responses from particle exposure is inherently difficult due to the many potential sources of ROS. ROS may be generated directly by reactive particle surfaces in contact with aqueous media, soluble organic constituents such as PAHs and quinones may form ROS and reactive electrophilic metabolites through redox cycling and metabolic activation, Fenton-reactive transition metals may contribute to formation of highly reactive hydroxyl radicals (•OH), activation of intracellular signaling pathways may trigger production of superoxide ($O_2\bullet-$) and hydrogen peroxide (H_2O_2) through activation of membrane bound oxidases, and damage to mitochondria may lead to superoxide production. The figure has previously been published in [95]

However, particle exposure may also initiate a number of endogenous redox responses in cells or tissues. Inflammatory responses are considered to be contributory in the development or exacerbation of health effects from exposure to all types of particulates and they involve multiple levels of ROS-production and redox regulation. Clearly, inflammatory processes lead to oxidative stress, as activated immune cells produce and release ROS [96–99]. However, several pro-inflammatory genes are regulated through autocrine or paracrine signaling loops initiated by early cytokines such as interleukin (IL)-1α/β and tumor necrosis factor-α [101, 102]. Both the transcriptional activation and maturation/release of these pro-inflammatory mediators, as well as signaling from their respective receptors, involves multiple redox-regulated processes that could be affected by antioxidant treatment [91, 103–105]. The pathological importance of the oxidative potential of the particles versus these secondary redox responses of exposed cells may not be easy to disentangle, and may require much more sophisticated approaches than mere antioxidant treatment. An in-depth understanding of the role of endogenous redox regulation in these cellular responses is important,

therefore, in order to clarify the relevance of oxidative potential as a metric for predicting particle toxicity.

Rapid methods for the detection of disease/exposure biomarkers, infections, food and environmental contaminants

Previous sections have described the importance of detection of both hazardous materials and exposure-related markers for our understanding of the associated diseases and their development and for optimization of early detection and clinical interventions. This cannot be effectively achieved without high sensitivity, specific and multi-target analytical platforms that are robust and easy-to-use, can generate appropriate measurements very rapidly, and can be applied in non-laboratory settings. This approach will facilitate near-patient testing and is cognizant of the imperative to develop testing regimens that are accessible, minimally invasive and ameliorate the overburdening of health care services. This will require a variety of approaches and will definitely involve the integration of the measurement of different targets including proteins, miRNAs, circulating nucleic acids, cells, exosomes and many other molecular species. Thus, what is required is the capability to handle multiple matrices as sample sources, integration of binders to monitor specific targets (e.g. antibodies, nucleic acid probes) and highly sensitive detection strategies.

The focus of this DiMoPEx partner is the development of rapid diagnostic systems for the detection of a variety of targets using polyclonal, monoclonal and recombinant antibodies. The strategies used include electrochemical and optical detection (surface plasmon resonance, fluorescence, chemiluminescence and absorbance) mainly on microfluidics-based platforms. We generate recombinant antibody-derived structures highly customized for the specific application. We also run an international master's program in biomedical diagnostics and are very involved in scientific approaches for antibody isolation, characterization and subsequent assay development.

In respect of outreach, a DiMoPEx training partner is the Applied Biochemistry Group, Dublin City University, which has a unit (AbYBiotech) that develops customized recombinant antibodies and has all the necessary equipment and developmental pipelines for antibodies and assays (see Additional file 1: Table S11). The successful antibodies need to be fully characterized, with the entire sequence defined and published or available, and this is now facilitated through the use of recombinant antibodies. In relation to DiMoPEx, the group provides opportunities for collaboration in a number of areas, including antibody generation, assay use and validation, exchange of researchers for training, development of education and science outreach. Examples of the research and the potential for collaboration within DiMoPEx can be gleaned from the literature published by the group [106–112].

WG 3: Environmental and occupational epidemiology overarching other WGs

Epidemiology is the branch of science that deals with the study of the causes, distribution, and control of disease in populations. Occupational and environmental epidemiology deals specifically with the impact of occupational and environmental exposures on health and disease in populations. Although experimental and toxicological methods to establish mechanisms for a certain exposure and its impact on organisms are available, most often the only way to confirm the link between an exposure and the outcome is observational epidemiologic studies addressing disease occurrence in human populations. Such population-based studies are the only way to address the exposure-response relationship and to explore susceptibility and societal exposures simultaneously.

Radon exposure, for example, affects smokers and non-smokers equally but, because smokers have a higher basic risk, the total burden is dominated by lung cancer in smokers. As an example, the International Agency for Research on Cancer (IARC) evaluates whether a certain

exposure can cause cancer in humans based on epidemiological evidence or a combination of evidence from epidemiological and animal or mechanistic studies (www.IARC.fr).

The objectives of the Epidemiology WG (WG3) are to:

- provide a sustainable research and training program in the field of environmental and occupational epidemiology for early career investigators;
- In collaboration with other WGs, provide opportunities for participation in environmental and occupational epidemiological research, more specifically in the development of novel exposure–response relationships, in the area of exposure-related diseases;
- provide training in the epidemiology of exposure-related diseases – computer skills training will focus on epidemiological modelling. Including spatio-temporal, exposure-response and interaction modelling.

In DiMoPEx, WG3 provides input and expertise with regards to study design for the other WGs. In collaboration with WG1 and WG2 for example, the WG3 contributes with knowledge about exposure assessment strategies and how to utilize the available data in the most efficient way by exploring alternative exposure metrics (for example, individual measurements versus group-based measurements, cumulative exposure versus period-specific exposure). The members of WG3 share experience with the use of large register-based population studies, in combination with individual exposure measurements obtained from industry-based cohort studies, in order to learn about the advantage of both types of data. WG3 includes researchers with experience in different kinds of exposure-assessment tools in individuals, groups or large populations, including biomarkers, individual- and area- based exposure measures in the environment, and questionnaires. Figure 2 displays the major tools for exposure assessment.

We have introduced register data sources from Denmark – (Danish Occupational Cohort DOC*X (www.DOC-X.dk) and register resources at Aarhus University (http://cirrau.au.dk/). Furthermore, in collaboration with other WGs, the WG Epidemiology WG3 group has submitted a number of spin-off research project proposals, including "Can pyrethroid pesticides cause diabetes?" and "The effect of organic dust and endotoxin exposure on CVD, lung cancer and interstitial lung disease".

WG 4 provides solutions for ethical aspects of data collection and communication for other groups

WG 4 supports the research of other groups and provides training programs for all ethical aspects of data collection, communication and publication ethics. Focusing on early carrier investigators (which are in focus of COST program actions), the DiMoPEx project aims to provide knowledge about data privacy regulations.

Ethics framework

An international ethics reference framework for biomedical research involving human subjects already exists and the researchers can and must be able to refer to this in their work (see Additional file 1: Table S12). While this reference framework is international, the legal anchoring of principles to which this framework refers is provided by national law. National regulations are mostly based on the Oviedo Convention and its Additional Protocol on biomedical research that emphasize: the necessity of obtaining informed consent, the requirement that a research project is submitted to an ethics committee for independent examination of its scientific merit and multidisciplinary review of its ethical acceptability (in each country in which any research activity is to take place).

Some challenges must be considered carefully: the authenticity of informed consent, data protection as a possible obstacle for research, the secondary use of data/samples, the right of an individual to know or not to know, and dealing with communication at a collective level.

Informed consent

In general, the authenticity of informed consent can be questioned for several reasons.:

- The authority or status of the person providing the information may decisively affect the outcome.
- The accuracy of the information provided can be limited.
- Correct understanding of the information is a prerequisite and cannot be assumed if not checked.
- The right to decide is not always synonymous with the ability to decide for oneself.
- Decisional autonomy can be in conflict with social constraints.
- The consequences of a decision may be affected by a perception of power inequality, for instance, when access to a right can be denied as a consequence of the outcome.

The process of obtaining informed consent is the outcome of a complex interaction of personalities. Awareness and understanding is necessary for correctly implementing the process. In a pragmatic way, one may consider consent as authentic when the person is: clearly free in the decision to participate, is equal in relationship with the recruiter, is listened to and receives answers at his or her personal level of understanding, and comprehends what s/he consents to.

Communication/right-to-know

The research subjects might have a legally embedded right to know their individual results from the research, if they wish. IIndividual results are often not provided to the study participants because of:

- lack of relevance of the results at an individual level,
- limited time and/or resources,
- fear of causing (unnecessary) alarm,
- scientific uncertainty,
- lack of possible remediation.

Participatory (community engagement) approaches

From an ethical perspective and from a perspective of increasing confidence and trust in researchers and their research, it is often not sufficient to leave the decision to participate in a study to every single individual. The involvement of community members or representatives of the relevant community in consultation, as a complement to decision-making autonomy, may also be needed. This requires the development of methods to include community consultation, community-based participatory research, and community consent to research. This can be done through processes of cooperative inquiry.

Communication

Spreading information about research outcomes is essential and must occur at the individual as well as at the collective level. Sufficient information is necessary at recruitment, during the study, and while disseminating results (individual and collective, including policy).

There are many challenges for protecting human dignity and the right of the individual research participant, whilst at the same time not hampering the progress of research. Practices show a strong belief in scientific work. Societal acceptance of practices will depend on good communication at all levels. The future of research with human subjects will, to a large extent, depend upon the trust and confidence which is generated in the perception of these (potential) research participants.

Human data sampling and collection: Imminent new OECD and EU data privacy regulations

The last few years have witnessed an important expansion of human DNA sampling and data collecting in order to exploit and study the genetic information collected. The strategic importance of this activity for genetic research and its applications is obvious, yet many DNA banks are concerned about how to obtain valid informed consent and how to deal with retrospective collections (see Additional file 1: Info Box 5, on new OECD, Global Science Forum and on EU-The General Data Protection Regulation, which will become law across the EU in May 2018).

WG 6 steps towards NCD diagnosis and monitoring

Since NCDs not only cause premature deaths and increased morbidity but also have a significant economic impact, the cost-effective and evidence-based interventions and tools to prevent and control various NCDs must include:

- reduction of causative exposures/risk factors;
- early detection and management of respective disorders;
- surveillance of endangered populations to monitor trends in risk factors and diseases (WG6 in cooperation with other WGs).

Such interventions are feasible, but they do necessitate a paradigm shift, away from considering each singular exposure towards the addressing disease clusters collectively in an integrated manner ("exposome"), moving away from a purely clinical approach towards a fully integrated public health approach.

An integrated approach targeting all major common risk factors, with the aim of reducing premature mortality and morbidity of chronic NCDs, is clearly the most cost-effective way to prevent and control the common NCDs. This requires the integration of primary, secondary, and tertiary prevention, health promotion and related programs across numerous sectors and different disciplines. In order to enhance interdisciplinary cooperation, a clinical network concentrating on exposure-related diseases will work with DiMoPEx partners in order to 1) develop common diagnostic scheme guidelines to aid physicians and public health workers to make best use of the evidence; and 2) integrate NCDs intervention initiatives in the health system based on primary health care. The interdisciplinary team of young European researchers will have the opportunity to use the analyses within the framework of the DiMoPEx project to generate risk assessment and prevention models to improve health and safety in Europe for the general public, and, more specifically, for workers and consumers.

Current human studies applying outlined methods on various exposure scenarios

Exposure to welding fumes and cardiovascular toxicity

DiMoPEx partner, Unit Metals and the Health Unit of the Institute of Environmental Medicine, Karolinska Institutet, Sweden, is currently performing research on health problems in the work environment (welding fumes and exposure to soot particles) and early-life exposure to metals and health effects during childhood). The projects are described in brief below:

Exposure to welding fumes increases the risk of CVD and workplace exposure to welding particles occurs frequently in Sweden and worldwide. However, we still do not know what levels of exposure are sufficient to increase the risk of CVD, and whether current welders remain at increased risk ot not. In 2010, the group enrolled welders and controls, all male non-smokers, in southern Sweden, who were characterized for exposure to particles and received medical examinations. The authors found that low-to-moderate exposure to welding fumes can be a risk factor for hypertension [113, 114]. Moreover, the data indicate that welding fumes cause premature ageing of the cardiovascular system [115], possibly by increasing oxidative stress [114, 115] from the high metal content of the welding fumes, as well as epigenetic changes of the F2RL3 gene, a CVD marker [116].

In contrast, the authors did not find signs of other previously suggested mechanisms for cardiovascular damage involving exposure to particles [112]. Our group is now re-examining welders and controls to validate our cross-sectional findings and quantify the effects of welding particle exposure on the cardiovascular system, as well as to explore mechanisms of action, by using a longitudinal approach. The information about medical and occupational histories from the welders and controls is being collected and their heart-rate variability and endothelial function measured. Further, blood and urine samples are being collected for measurement of markers of premature ageing and oxidative stress, as well as markers of inflammation and one-carbon metabolism and of coagulation. The approach will address novel hypotheses, help explain findings from previous studies, assist in risk assessment, and improve advice to welders on the safety of working with welding fumes.

Chimney sweeping and risk of cancer

Chimney sweeps in Sweden have an excess risk of bladder, liver, lung and esophagus cancer. The increase in risk is likely due to exposure to polycyclic aromatic hydrocarbons (PAHs) [117]. It is necessary, therefore, to clarify to what extent contemporary Swedish chimney sweeps exhibit cancer-related DNA changes and if current levels of PAH exposure are genotoxic. 1-hydroxypyrene (1-OHP) has traditionally been used as a proxy for total PAH exposure, although 1-OHPHP is itself not carcinogenic. A more relevant marker of carcinogenic PAHs, but much less studied, is 3-hydroxybenzo(a)pyrene (3-OHBaP) [118]. The aim of the study is to determine early carcinogenic DNA changes in Swedish chimney sweeps and to investigate the association between current exposure and genotoxicity. Chimney sweeps have been recruited for determining exposure, for medical examinations and for the sampling of biomarkers of DNA damage in blood and urine. Biomarkers and medical information are also collected in a control set of male warehouse workers with low exposure to PAHs.

The study will clarify whether current exposure experienced by chimney sweeps is carcinogenic. If there are stronger associations for 3-eOHBaP than for 1-OHP with genotoxicity, this may affect methods used for risk assessment of PAHs in general, which is important for the workplace as well as for the general population.

Pesticides exposure and GxE testing in Parkinson's disease

Parkinson's disease (PD) is a chronic progressive neurodegenerative movement disorder that affects 1% of the population over the age of 60 years and both genetic and environmental factors contribute to its etiology. Specifically, occupational pesticide exposures have been identified as risk factors for PD, but the quality of exposure assessment varies considerably between studies with only a few identifying exposure to specific chemicals.; Some studies recorded ever/never occupational exposure or self-reports of specific pesticides [119] while others created job exposure matrixes (JEMs) [120–125], and only one –- the USA Agricultural Health Study (AHS) cohort of licensed pesticide applicators –- used a prospective design and collected specific pesticide use in great detail [126]. Our own California study (known as the Parkinson's, Environment and Genes PEG study) recently provided some of the strongest evidence yet that specific pesticides in combination with genetic susceptibility contribute to the etiology of PD in humans and that certain pesticides affect pathogenic pathways that have been related to neurodegeneration. In this population-based case control study that was conducted in the heavily agricultural central valley of California, [127], detailed historical data for active occupational and household pesticide use was collected and, most importantly, we were able to employ a geographic information system to assess ambient pesticide exposures from agricultural applications at workplaces and residences. To generate these exposures to pesticides, we were able to rely on the state-mandated California Pesticide Use Reporting (PUR) system (active since 1974), digitized historical land-use maps and address histories of the participants [128]. Combining these data sources, we pinpointed pesticide applications at a precise agricultural site and related these to the home and work addresses of the participants to calculate time-specific pesticide exposures based on application rates per acreage or pounds of pesticide per acre applied annually in the proximity of their homes or workplaces. Using this unique exposure assessment tool and the data and bio-samples collected from almost 1800 study participants, the PEG study provided the first human evidence that a specific combination exposure (paraquat and maneb) increased the risk of PD, confirming animal model findings [129] from toxicological research. We also found that both residential and workplace exposures contribute to PD risk [130], as

did household use of organophosphate pesticides [131] and consumption of contaminated well-water [132]. Importantly, we identified gene-environment interactions for genes in molecular pathways that contribute to PD pathology according to animal/ cell studies. The major pathophysiologic mechanisms we addressed included: 1) dopamine transporter activity, (*DAT*); dopamine metabolism pathways (aldehyde dehydrogenase 1 family, member A1 gene -*ALDH1* [133]) relevant to PD; and mitochondrial dysfunction due to oxidative/nitrosative stress (nitric oxide synthase 1 (neuronal) gene – n*NOS*) [134]. We also identified genetic susceptibility in the proteasomal pathways (*SKP1*-gene [135]), especially when combined with exposure to proteasome-inhibiting pesticides (di-thiocarbamates): genetic susceptibility related to the response of the innate immune system among those exposed to pyrethroid pesticides (MHC class II cell surface receptor encoded by the human leukocyte antigen - *HLA-DR*) [136]; DNA repair gene variants (DNA (apurinic or apyrimidinic site)-lyase gene, 8-Oxoguanine glycosylase 1 (DNA glycosylase) gene, *APEX1, OGG1* [136]) that affect mitochondrial function via oxidative stress; and, finally, genetic susceptibility to the neurotoxic action of organophosphate pesticides for carriers of variants in the pesticide metabolism gene serum paraoxonase/arylesterase1, *PON1* [137]). A summary of our findings has been published recently in the journal *Current Environmental Health Reports* [127], in which the importance of integrating genetic information with advanced exposure assessment methods to describe the combined impact of genes and environment on biologic pathways relevant to disease was praised.

Further joint research projects from DiMoPEx partners that focus on the impact of the pollution on human health are presented in reference [138].

WG 7: Public health protection – how to stimulate interaction between scientist and policy makers

Collaboration with WHO

In the WHO European Region, diabetes, CVD, cancer, chronic respiratory diseases and mental disorders cause no less than 86% of deaths and 77% of the disease burden, with marked inequalities reflecting a social gradient (WHO, 2012, see Additional file 1: Info Box 1). The regional strategy and action plan, frame prevention and control efforts do focus on the proximal risk factors, while acknowledging the relevance of environmental and occupational factors (WHO, 2012, see Additional file 1). DiMoPEx partner(s) aim to collaborate with the WHO, focusing on environmental determinants of health (with a spotlight on chemical, fume and dust exposures in living and working environments). Of mutual interest, is the analysis of and action on modifiable environmental conditions or their modifiable components (http://dimopex.eu/ncds/).

In the context of human health and disease, consideration of the environment focuses on the aspects that can be modified through intervention, leading to reduced human exposure and health impacts, hence offering opportunities for preventative measures. When assessing the GBD, WHO analyses modifiable environmental conditions, including: pollution of air, water or soil by chemical or biological agents; occupational risks; ultraviolet and ionizing radiation; noise; electromagnetic fields; built environments and housing; land-use patterns; roads; major infrastructural and engineering works (roads, dams, railways); agricultural methods; irrigation schemes; man-made vector breeding places; climate and ecosystem change; environment-related behavior (WHO, 2016, see Additional file 1).

A resolution on the health impact of air pollution, adopted at the Sixty-eighth World Health Assembly in May 2015, and a road map for an enhanced global response to air pollution by the health sector provide a framework to guide actions by Member States, WHO and stakeholders globally. In the WHO European Region, the Health 2020 policy, as well as policy commitments from the Sixth Ministerial Conference on Environment and Health (Ostrava, June 2017), combine to guide regional efforts designed to reduce environmental burdens on health and to promote environment-related health benefits (WHO, 2013; WHO, 2017, see Additional file 1). Occupational risks contribute to the burden of NCDs (WHO, 2016, see Additional file 1). The burden of disease because of occupational risk factors, estimated by the GBD project group, included 304,000 deaths from occupational carcinogens (largely asbestos), 205,000 deaths from occupational PM, gases and fumes, with 52,000 deaths from occupational asthmogens (GBD 2013 Risk Factors Collaborators, 2015, see Additional file 1). Important occupational diseases induced by mineral dust and fiber exposure are pneumoconioses. This group of chronic respiratory diseases, including silicosis, asbestosis and coal-workers' pneumoconiosis, is estimated to cause 260,000 deaths per year globally (GBD 2013 Mortality Causes of Death Collaborators, 2015, in WHO (2016, see Additional file 1). Since these NCDs are also our focus, the DiMoPEx partners intend to implement the methodological approaches from WHO and contribute to the process of producing an estimate of the environmental burden of diseases. The common approaches include: comparative risk assessment, calculations based on epidemiological data and expert opinion to fill current gaps in knowledge.

Dissemination and implementation of new knowledge within a scientific network

The DiMoPEx COST Action is dedicated to catalyze a joint effort of European scientists to address the issue of adverse health effects of environmental exposures and to suggest ways of evaluating and managing them. The WG 7 is committed to these goals. In this process, facilitation and coordination of information transfer among the participants, such as between the action core group and external partners, and effective wide-scale dissemination and implementation of the new knowledge produced by the project are essential features.

The first opportunity for networking and for exchange of knowledge and ideas was the combined meeting of DiMoPEx WGs in Hamburg in June 2016, when participants had the opportunity to present their expertise and backgrounds using posters and thematic oral presentations. The second working groups meeting was in Bentivoglio, Italy in October 2017 [138]. In future, specific WG meetings will serve the purpose of formulating concrete plans for joint projects between the partners and affiliates and will prepare the ground for formulating new projects. Another important tool of internal knowledge dissemination is the organization of training schools (e.g. on exposure assessment, occupational and environmental epidemiology, MN methods) and short-term scientific missions of individual institutional and laboratory visits that provide an opportunity for building capability in early career investigators, primarily.

The involvement of external partners in the activities of the Action, such as the European Society for Environmental and Occupational Medicine, the Collegium Ramazzini (http://www.collegiumramazzini.org/about.asp) and the WHO European Centre for Environment and Health, is an important priority. In collaboration with WHO and the International Labour Organization, the DiMoPEx partners perform a systematic review of the relationship between pneumoconiosis and occupational dust and fiber exposures, the results of which allow the estimation of the related burden of disease.

The DiMoPEx website serves as the main platform for informing participants (http//dimopex.eu), external partners, and the wider-scale scientific and decision-making community about the research backgrounds of the participants, plans for cooperation, events, activities, grant applications, formulating and ongoing projects, and results that can be related to the Action.

A further goal of the WG 7 is assembling and critically assessing information, creating new knowledge, and implementing this knowledge, by testing and formulating feasible recommendations for the evaluation and management of health risks of environmental exposures and publishing the results in various electronic and printed media. Apart from the scientific community, the decision- makers of topic-related sectoral policies and industries, as well as the general public, are considered important targets for the dissemination of DiMoPEx results. The research community is primarily informed through peer-reviewed scientific publications, research articles, textbooks and guidelines. At the end of the

COST-Action, a conference will be organized that will address not only scientists but also decision- makers and the general public, with sessions directed to them appropriately, and the relevant messages will be disseminated by an appropriate media coverage.

To ensure the effective and sustainable implementation of the new knowledge produced, tailored information will directly be delivered to decision-makers by printed and electronic leaflets and via the DiMoPEx website.

Summary and conclusions

- Environmental hazardous exposure is among the top risk factors for chronic disease mortality. A better understanding of the health-environment (including the gene-environment) and its interactions in the etiology of NCDs allows more adequate preventative actions that could decrease disease morbidity and mortality for many of the NCDs that are of major public concern.

- Within the COST action DiMoPEx, models will be developed for the assessment of hazardous exposures and their potential health consequences using collected data and available toxicological/ epidemiological evidence.

- DiMoPEx partners believe that combining state-of-the-art exposure assessment methods with clinical efforts should grant a more solid basis for both early recognition and diagnosis strategies, as well as for the advancement of preventive strategies in Europe.

- The predominant goals of the DiMoPEx project arinclude helping scientists, physicians and health officials in preventing and reducing health impairments associated with various exposure scenarios and to train highly researchers in these disciplines with the requisite skills.

- Risk communication expertise developed within the DiMoPEx action and tools to inform exposed subjects and the general public are expected to benefit society.

antigen; HP: Hydoxypyrene; IARC: International Agency for Research on Cancer; ILO: International labour organization; JEM: Job exposure matrix; miRNA: micro RNA; MN: Micronucleus; NCD: Noncommunicable diseases; nNOS1: Nitric oxide synthase 1 (neuronal) gene; NOEL: No Observed Adverse Effect Level; OECD: Organization for Economic Cooperation and Development; OGG1: 8-Oxoguanine glycosylase 1 (DNA glycosylase) gene; PAH: Polycyclic aromatic hydrocarbons; PD: Parkinson's disease; PEG: Parkinson's Environment and Genes Study; PM: Particulate matter; PON1: Gene coding for serum paraoxonase/ arylesterase 1; PUR: California Pesticide Use Reporting; RI: Ramazzini Institute; RNA: Ribonucleic acid; ROS: Reactive oxygen species; SD: Sprague-Dawley (rats); TNF: Tumor necrosis factor; UTR: Untranslational region; WG: Working group; WHO: World Health Organization

Acknowledgements
The support of the COST Association and COST scientific and administrative staff to this DiMoPEx project is gratefully acknowledged.
The authors thank Dr.Kevan Willey, Hamburg for critical appraisal of the manuscript and language corrections.
The authors also thank all DiMoPEx colleagues not involved in the current publication for support and input to the Action.
The WHO regional office for Europe has granted the permission for the reproduction of this article.© World Health Organization 2017.

Funding
The project is funded by the EU -COST Association (under Grant no, CA 15129).

Authors' contributions
Conceived and designed the DiMoPEx project concept: LTB, MA, FB, CB, AF, PTJS, VS, PG, TS, KVD, LC; wrote the introductory parts of the paper: LTB, LC; harmonized the whole manuscript: LTB; Wrote the section: "Exposure assessment – from environmental to individual exposure" part and prepared indicated figure: TG; wrote the section ": Human biological monitoring – more than (just) the analysis of biomarkers" and prepared indicated figure: PTJS; wrote the section "New insights into toxicology: an integrated experimental approach" and prepared indicated figure: FB, FM; wrote the section "Intermediate biomarker to assess the effects of preventive measures and identify individuals at high risk of developing a given NCD": CB, HS; Wrote the section "Potential biological effect markers – circulating nucleic acids in human blood" and prepared indicated figure: HS; wrote the section "Enhancement of genotoxicity and susceptibility marker" and prepared indicated figure: CB, BB; Wrote the section "Oxidative stress and redox responses in particle- induced toxicity" and prepared indicated figure: JØ, PES; wrote the section "Rapid methods for the detection of disease/exposure biomarkers, infections, food and environmental contaminants": RO'K, OS; Wrote the section "Environmental and occupational epidemiology is overarching other working groups and prepared indicated figure: VS, PG; KB: wrote the sections Exposure to welding fumes and cardiovascular toxicity" and "Chimney sweeping and risk of cancer": BR; wrote the section on "Pesticides exposures and GxE testing in Parkinson's disease": BR; wrote the section "Ethical group: data collection and communication": KVD; OS; Collaboration with the WHO: DJ, EP; wrote the section "DiMoPEx: Dissemination and implementation of new knowledge within a scientific network: BA. All authors have accepted the final version of the manuscript.

Abbreviations
1-OHP: 1-hydroxypyrene; AHS: Agricultural Health Study; ALDH1: Aldehyde dehydrogenase 1 family, member A1 gene; APEX1: DNA-(apurinic or apyrimidinic site) lyase gene; BADS: Biomonitoring application datasheets; CBMN: Cytokinesis-block micronucleus; cfDNA: Circulating free DNA; CMCRC: Cesare Maltoni Cancer Research Center; COST: EU programme, European Cooperation in Science and Technology; CVD: Cardiovascular disease; DAT: Dopamine transporter activity; DiMoPEx: Diagnosis, Monitoring and Prevention of Exposure-related Noncommunicable Diseases; DNA: Desoxyribonucleic acid; EMM: Effect measure modifications; EUEFSA: European Union Food safety Authority; GBD: Global Burden of Disease; HLA-DR: MHC class II cell surface receptor encoded by the human leukocyte

Competing interests
The authors report no conflicts of interest in this work.
Disclosure: The manuscript presents the views of the authors and not necessarily the opinions of organizations they represent. DJ and EP are staff members of the World Health Organization (WHO) Regional Office for Europe. The authors alone are responsible for the views expressed in this publication and they do not necessarily represent the decision or stated policy of the World Health Organization.

Author details

[1]Division of Translational Toxicology and Immunology, Institute for Occupational and Maritime Medicine (ZfAM), University Medical Center Hamburg-Eppendorf (UKE), Hamburg, Germany. [2]Faculty of Public Health, Department of Preventive Medicine, University of Debrecen, Debrecen, Hungary. [3]Division of Occupational and Environmental Medicine, University of Lund, Lund, Sweden. [4]Karolinska Institutet, Institute of Environmental Medicine (IMM), Stockholm, Sweden. [5]Tumor Epigenetics Unit, Ospedale Policlinico San Martino, National Cancer Institute, IRCCS and University of Genoa, DISSAL, Genoa, Italy. [6]European Society for Environmental and Occupational Medicine, Berlin, Germany. [7]Cesare Maltoni Cancer Research Center, Ramazzini Institute, Bentivoglio, Bologna, Italy. [8]San Martino-IST Environmental Carcinogenesis Unit, IRCCS, Ospedale Policlinico San Martino, National Cancer Institute, Genoa, Italy. [9]Social and Environmental Medicine, Institute and Outpatient Clinic of Occupational, Friedrich-Alexander-University Erlangen-Nurnberg, Erlangen, Germany. [10]Institute of Occupational Medicine, Charité Universitäts Medizin, Berlin, Germany. [11]WHO European Centre for Environment and Health, Bonn, Germany. [12]Biomedical Diagnostics Institute, Dublin City University, Dublin, Ireland. [13]Norwegian Institute of Public Health, Oslo, Norway. [14]Center for Occupational and Environmental Health, Fielding School of Public Health (FSPH), University of California Los Angeles (UCLA), Los Angeles, USA. [15]Radboud Institute for Health Sciences, Radboudumc (Radboud university medical center), Nijmegen, the Netherlands. [16]National Research Center for the Working Environment, Copenhagen, Denmark. [17]Department of Public Health, Section Environment, Occupation & Health & Danish Ramazzini Centre Aarhus, Aarhus University, Aarhus, Denmark. [18]Department of Tumor Biology, University Medical Center Hamburg-Eppendorf (UKE), Hamburg, Germany. [19]Department of Histopathology, Central Pathology Laboratory, St James's Hospital, Trinity translational Medicine Institute, Dublin, Ireland. [20]Center for Human Genetics, University of Leuven, Leuven, Belgium.

References

1. World Health Organization. Global health risks: mortality and burden of disease attributable to selected major risks. http://www.whoint/healthinfo/global_burden_disease/GlobalHealthRisks_report_fullpdf 2009.
2. Centers of Disease Control and Protection (CDC). Global Health Protection and Security: Global Noncommunicable Diseases (NCDs). http://www.cdcgov/globalhealth/healthprotection/ncd/ 2017.
3. Lim SS, Vos T, Flaxman AD, Danaei G, Shibuya K, Adair-Rohani H, Amann M, Anderson HR, Andrews KG, Aryee M, et al. A comparative risk assessment of burden of disease and injury attributable to 67 risk factors and risk factor clusters in 21 regions, 1990-2010: a systematic analysis for the Global Burden of Disease Study 2010. Lancet. 2012;380:2224–60.
4. World Health Organization: 7 million premature deaths annually linked to air pollution. http://www.whoint/mediacentre/news/releases/2014/air-pollution/en/ 2015.
5. Landrigan PJ, Fuller R, Acosta NJR, Adeyi O, Arnold R, Basu NN, Balde AB, Bertollini R, Bose-O'Reilly S, Boufford JI, et al. The Lancet Commission on pollution and health. Lancet. 2017;
6. WHO: The cost of a polluted environment: 1.7 million child deaths a year. http://www.whoint/mediacentre/news/releases/2017/pollution-child-death/en/ 2017.
7. The WHO Global Health Estimates. http://www.whoint/healthinfo/global_burden_disease/en/ 2014.
8. Institute for Health Metrics and Evaluation (IHME), Seattle, WA, USA. http://www.healthdataorg/data-visualization/gbd-compare 2017.
9. Raaschou-Nielsen O, Andersen ZJ, Beelen R, Samoli E, Stafoggia M, Weinmayr G, Hoffmann B, Fischer P, Nieuwenhuijsen MJ, Brunekreef B, et al. Air pollution and lung cancer incidence in 17 European cohorts: prospective analyses from the European Study of Cohorts for Air Pollution Effects (ESCAPE). Lancet Oncol. 2013;14:813–22.
10. Burnett RT, Pope CA 3rd, Ezzati M, Olives C, Lim SS, Mehta S, Shin HH, Singh G, Hubbell B, Brauer M, et al. An integrated risk function for estimating the global burden of disease attributable to ambient fine particulate matter exposure. Environmental health perspectives. 2014;122:397–403.
11. Rappaport SM. Implications of the exposome for exposure science. J Expo Sci Environ Epidemiol. 2011;21:5–9.
12. Rappaport SM, Smith MT. Epidemiology. Environment and disease risks. Science. 2010;330:460–1.
13. Manthripragada AD, Costello S, Cockburn MG, Bronstein JM, Ritz B. Paraoxonase 1, agricultural organophosphate exposure, and Parkinson disease. Epidemiology. 2010;21:87–94.
14. Ritz BR, Manthripragada AD, Costello S, Lincoln SJ, Farrer MJ, Cockburn M, Bronstein J. Dopamine transporter genetic variants and pesticides in Parkinson's disease. Environmental health perspectives. 2009;117:964–9.
15. Blair A, Ritz B, Wesseling C, Freeman LB. Pesticides and human health. Occup Environ Med. 2015;72:81–2.
16. Hertz-Picciotto I, Smith AH, Holtzman D, Lipsett M, Alexeeff G. Synergism between occupational arsenic exposure and smoking in the induction of lung cancer. Epidemiology. 1992;3:23–31.
17. Budnik LT, Austel N, Gadau S, Kloth S, Schubert J, Jungnickel H, Luch A. Experimental outgassing of toxic chemicals to simulate the characteristics of hazards tainting globally shipped products. PloS one. 2017;12:e0177363.
18. Budnik LT, Wegner R, Rogall U, Baur X. Accidental exposure to polychlorinated biphenyls (PCB) in waste cargo after heavy seas. Global waste transport as a source of PCB exposure. International archives of occupational and environmental health. 2014;87:125–35.
19. Budnik LT, Kloth S, Baur X, Preisser AM, Schwarzenbach H. Circulating mitochondrial DNA as biomarker linking environmental chemical exposure to early preclinical lesions elevation of mtDNA in human serum after exposure to carcinogenic halo-alkane-based pesticides. PloS one. 2013;8: e64413.
20. Sass J, Heine L, Hwang N. Use of a modified GreenScreen tool to conduct a screening-level comparative hazard assessment of conventional silver and two forms of nanosilver. Environmental health : a global access science source. 2016;15:105.
21. Weisel CP. Assessing exposure to air toxics relative to asthma. Environmental health perspectives. 2002;110(Suppl 4):527–37.
22. Abrahamsen R, Fell AK, Svendsen MV, Andersson E, Toren K, Henneberger PK, Kongerud J. Association of respiratory symptoms and asthma with occupational exposures: findings from a population-based cross-sectional survey in Telemark. Norway. BMJ Open. 2017;7:e014018.
23. Thurston GD, Kipen H, Annesi-Maesano I, Balmes J, Brook RD, Cromar K, De Matteis S, Forastiere F, Forsberg B, Frampton MW, et al. A joint ERS/ATS policy statement: what constitutes an adverse health effect of air pollution? An analytical framework. The European respiratory journal. 2017;49
24. Brauer M, Amann M, Burnett RT, Cohen A, Dentener F, Ezzati M, Henderson SB, Krzyzanowski M, Martin RV, Van Dingenen R, et al. Exposure assessment for estimation of the global burden of disease attributable to outdoor air pollution. Environ Sci Technol. 2012;46:652–60.
25. CDC. National Center for Health Statistics: Leading Causes of Death. http://www.cdcgov/nchs/fastats/leading-causes-of-deathhtm 2017.
26. Soffritti M, Belpoggi F, Minardi F, Maltoni C. Ramazzini Foundation cancer program: history and major projects, life-span carcinogenicity bioassay design, chemicals studied, and results. Annals of the New York Academy of Sciences. 2002;982:26–45.
27. World Health Organization. Environmental Health Criteria 214. Human exposure assessement. International Programme on Chemical Safety. http://www.inchemorg/documents/ehc/ehc/ehc214htm 2000.
28. Den Hond E, Paulussen M, Geens T, Bruckers L, Baeyens W, David F, Dumont E, Loots I, Morrens B, de Bellevaux BN, et al. Biomarkers of human exposure to personal care products: results from the Flemish Environment and Health Study (FLEHS 2007-2011). Sci Total Environ. 2013;463-464:102–10.
29. Huang L, Ernstoff A, Fantke P, Csiszar SA, Jolliet O. A review of models for near-field exposure pathways of chemicals in consumer products. Sci Total Environ. 2017;574:1182–208.
30. Ginsberg GL, Balk SJ. Consumer products as sources of chemical exposures to children: case study of triclosan. Curr Opin Pediatr. 2016;28:235–42.
31. Steiling W, Bascompta M, Carthew P, Catalano G, Corea N, D'Haese A, Jackson P, Kromidas L, Meurice P, Rothe H, Singal M. Principle considerations for the risk assessment of sprayed consumer products. Toxicology letters. 2014;227:41–9.

32. Villanueva CM, Kogevinas M, Cordier S, Templeton MR, Vermeulen R, Nuckols JR, Nieuwenhuijsen MJ, Levallois P. Assessing exposure and health consequences of chemicals in drinking water: current state of knowledge and research needs. Environmental health perspectives. 2014;122:213–21.

33. Hernandez AF, Tsatsakis AM. Human exposure to chemical mixtures: Challenges for the integration of toxicology with epidemiology data in risk assessment. Food Chem Toxicol. 2017;103:188–93.

34. Cachada A, da Silva EF, Duarte AC, Pereira R. Risk assessment of urban soils contamination: The particular case of polycyclic aromatic hydrocarbons. Sci Total Environ. 2016;551-552:271–84.

35. Sobus JR, DeWoskin RS, Tan YM, Pleil JD, Phillips MB, George BJ, Christensen K, Schreinemachers DM, Williams MA, Hubal EA, Edwards SW. Uses of NHANES Biomarker Data for Chemical Risk Assessment: Trends, Challenges, and Opportunities. Environmental health perspectives. 2015;123:919–27.

36. Dorne JL. Metabolism, variability and risk assessment. Toxicology. 2010;268:156–64.

37. Valcke M, Krishnan K. Characterization of the human kinetic adjustment factor for the health risk assessment of environmental contaminants. Journal of applied toxicology : JAT. 2014;34:227–40.

38. Tennekes HA, Sanchez-Bayo F. The molecular basis of simple relationships between exposure concentration and toxic effects with time. Toxicology. 2013;309:39–51.

39. OECD. Test No. 453: Combined Chronic Toxicity/Carcinogenicity Studies. OECD Guidelines for the Testing of Chemicals. Section 4: Health Effects. France: OECD Publishing Paris; 2009. http://www.oecd-ilibrary.org/environment/test-no-453-combined-chronic-toxicity-carcinogenicity-studies_9789264071223-en.

40. OECD Test No. 443: Extended One-Generation Reproductive Toxicity Study. OECD Guidelines for the Testing of Chemicals, Section 4: Health Effects. . OECD Publishing Paris, France 2011. http://www.oecd.org/env/test-no-443-extended-one-generation-reproductive-toxicity-study-9789264122550-en.htm.

41. OECD Guideline for the testing of chemicals. Combined Chronic toxicity/carcinogenicity studies. TG 453. 2009.

42. Teitelbaum SL, Li Q, Lambertini L, Belpoggi F, Manservisi F, Falcioni L, Bua L, Silva MJ, Ye X, Calafat AM, Chen J. Paired Serum and Urine Concentrations of Biomarkers of Diethyl Phthalate, Methyl Paraben, and Triclosan in Rats. Environmental health perspectives. 2016;124:39–45.

43. Silvestri F, Bussani R, Giarelli L. Changes in underlying causes of death during 85 years of autopsy practice in Trieste. IARC Sci Publ. 1991;112:3–23.

44. Maltoni C, Ciliberti A, Pinto C, Soffritti M, Belpoggi F, Menarini L. Results of long-term experimental carcinogenicity studies of the effects of gasoline, correlated fuels, and major gasoline aromatics on rats. Annals of the New York Academy of Sciences. 1997;837:15–52.

45. National Toxicology Program.Toxicology and carcinogenesis studies of xylenes (mixed) (cas no. 1330-20-7) in F344/N rats and B6C3F1 mice (gavage studies). https://www.ncbinlmnihgov/pubmed/12732897 1986.

46. Belpoggi F, Soffritti M, Guarino M, Lambertini L, Cevolani D, Maltoni C. Results of long-term experimental studies on the carcinogenicity of ethylene-bis-dithiocarbamate (Mancozeb) in rats. Annals of the New York Academy of Sciences. 2002;982:123–36.

47. Manservisi F, Marquillas CB, Buscaroli A, Huff J, Lauriola M, Mandrioli D, Manservigi M, Panzacchi S, Silbergeld EK, Belpoggi F. An Integrated Experimental Design for the Assessment of Multiple Toxicological End Points in Rat Bioassays. Environmental health perspectives. 2017;125:289–95.

48. Bonassi S, Znaor A, Ceppi M, Lando C, Chang WP, Holland N, Kirsch-Volders M, Zeiger E, Ban S, Barale R, et al. An increased micronucleus frequency in peripheral blood lymphocytes predicts the risk of cancer in humans. Carcinogenesis. 2007;28:625–31.

49. Maluf SW, Erdtmann B. Genomic instability in Down syndrome and Fanconi anemia assessed by micronucleus analysis and single-cell gel electrophoresis. Cancer Genet Cytogenet. 2001;124:71–5.

50. Bonassi S, El-Zein R, Bolognesi C, Fenech M. Micronuclei frequency in peripheral blood lymphocytes and cancer risk: evidence from human studies. Mutagenesis. 2011;26:93–100.

51. Migliore L, Coppede F, Fenech M, Thomas P. Association of micronucleus frequency with neurodegenerative diseases. Mutagenesis. 2011;26:85–92.

52. Andreassi MG, Barale R, Iozzo P, Picano E. The association of micronucleus frequency with obesity, diabetes and cardiovascular disease. Mutagenesis. 2011;26:77–83.

53. Baudhuin LM, Donato LJ, Uphoff TS. How novel molecular diagnostic technologies and biomarkers are revolutionizing genetic testing and patient care. Expert Rev Mol Diagn. 2012;12:25–37.

54. Schwarzenbach H, Hoon DS, Pantel K. Cell-free nucleic acids as biomarkers in cancer patients. Nat Rev Cancer. 2011;11:426–37.

55. Stroun M, Maurice P, Vasioukhin V, Lyautey J, Lederrey C, Lefort F, Rossier A, Chen XQ, Anker P. The origin and mechanism of circulating DNA. Ann N Y Acad Sci. 2000;906:161–8.

56. Mittra I, Nair NK, Mishra PK. Nucleic acids in circulation: are they harmful to the host? Biosci. 2012;37(2):301-12.

57. Chen X, Liang H, Zhang J, Zen K, Zhang CY. Horizontal transfer of microRNAs: molecular mechanisms and clinical applications. Protein & cell. 2012;3:28–37.

58. Schwarzenbach H. Circulating nucleic acids in early diagnosis, prognosis and treatment monitoring: an introduction. Section VII: CNAPS and General Medicine. Holland: Springer Science+Business Media Dordrecht; 2015. p. 143-163.

59. Dong H, Lei J, Ding L, Wen Y, Ju H, Zhang X. MicroRNA: function, detection, and bioanalysis. Chem Rev. 2013;113:6207–33.

60. Reid G, Kirschner MB, van Zandwijk N. Circulating microRNAs: Association with disease and potential use as biomarkers. Crit Rev Oncol Hematol. 2011;80:193–208.

61. Pant S, Hilton H, Burczynski ME. The multifaceted exosome: biogenesis, role in normal and aberrant cellular function, and frontiers for pharmacological and biomarker opportunities. Biochem Pharmacol. 2012;83:1484–94.

62. Zhao L, Liu W, Xiao J, Cao B. The role of exosomes and "exosomal shuttle microRNA" in tumorigenesis and drug resistance. Cancer letters. 2015;356:339–46.

63. Schwarzenbach H. The clinical relevance of circulating, exosomal miRNAs as biomarkers for cancer. Expert Rev Mol Diagn. 2015;15:1159–69.

64. Rozek LS, Dolinoy DC, Sartor MA, Omenn GS. Epigenetics: relevance and implications for public health. Annu Rev Public Health. 2014;35:105–22.

65. Chappell G, Pogribny IP, Guyton KZ, Rusyn I. Epigenetic alterations induced by genotoxic occupational and environmental human chemical carcinogens: A systematic literature review. Mutat Res Rev Mutat Res. 2016;768:27–45.

66. Tran NQV, Miyake K. Neurodevelopmental Disorders and Environmental Toxicants: Epigenetics as an Underlying Mechanism. Int J Genomics. 2017;2017:7526592.

67. Tabish AM, Poels K, Byun HM, Luyts K, Baccarelli AA, Martens J, Kerkhofs S, Seys S, Hoet P, Godderis L. Changes in DNA Methylation in Mouse Lungs after a Single Intra-Tracheal Administration of Nanomaterials. PloS one. 2017;12:e0169886.

68. Oner D, Moisse M, Ghosh M, Duca RC, Poels K, Luyts K, Putzeys E, Cokic SM, Van Landuyt K, Vanoirbeek J, et al. Epigenetic effects of carbon nanotubes in human monocytic cells. Mutagenesis. 2017;32:181–91.

69. Gorrochategui E, Li J, Fullwood NJ, Ying GG, Tian M, Cui L, Shen H, Lacorte S, Tauler R, Martin FL. Diet-sourced carbon-based nanoparticles induce lipid alterations in tissues of zebrafish (Danio rerio) with genomic hypermethylation changes in brain. Mutagenesis. 2017;32:91–103.

70. Ho SM. Environmental epigenetics of asthma: an update. J Allergy Clin Immunol. 2010;126:453–65.

71. Yadav S, Singh M, Yadav R. Organophosphates Induced Alzheimer's Disease: An Epigenetic Aspect. J Clin Epigenet. 2016;2

72. Wang A, Cockburn M, Ly T, Bronstein J, Ritz B. The association between ambient exposure to organophosphates and Parkinson's disease risk. Occup Environ Med. 2014.

73. Fenech M. Cytokinesis-block micronucleus cytome assay. Nat Protoc. 2007;2:1084–104.

74. OECD Guideline for the Testing of Chemicals. In Vitro Mammalian Cell Micronucleus Test (TG 487). 2016.

75. OECD Guideline for the Testing of Chemicals. Mammalian Erythrocyte Micronucleus Test (TG 474). 2016.

76. IAEA. Cytogenetic Dosimetry: Applications in Preparedness for and Response to Radiation Emergencies, in: EPR-Biodosimetry 2011. Vienna: International Atomic Energy Agency; 2011.

77. Special Issue In vivo chemical Genotoxin Exposure and DNA damage in Humans measured using the lymphocyte Cytokinesis-Block Micronucleus Assay Mutat Research Review 2016, 770:1-2016.

78. Nersesyan A, Fenech M, Bolognesi C, Misik M, Setayesh T, Wultsch G, Bonassi S, Thomas P, Knasmuller S. Use of the lymphocyte cytokinesis-block micronucleus assay in occupational biomonitoring of genome damage caused by in vivo exposure to chemical genotoxins: Past, present and future. Mutat Res. 2016;770:1–11.

79. Thomas P, Holland N, Bolognesi C, Kirsch-Volders M, Bonassi S, Zeiger E, Knasmueller S, Fenech M. Buccal micronucleus cytome assay. Nat Protoc. 2009;4:825–37.

80. Bolognesi C, Knasmueller S, Nersesyan A, Thomas P, Fenech M. The HUMNxl scoring criteria for different cell types and nuclear anomalies in the buccal micronucleus cytome assay - an update and expanded photogallery. Mutat Res. 2013;753:100–13.

81. Bolognesi C, Roggieri P, Ropolo M, Thomas P, Hor M, Fenech M, Nersesyan A, Knasmueller S. Buccal micronucleus cytome assay: results of an intra- and inter-laboratory scoring comparison. Mutagenesis. 2015;30:545–55.

82. Bolognesi C, Knasmueller S, Nersesyan A, Roggieri P, Ceppi M, Bruzzone M, Blaszczyk E, Mielzynska-Svach D, Milic M, Bonassi S, et al. Inter-laboratory consistency and variability in the buccal micronucleus cytome assay depends on biomarker scored and laboratory experience: results from the HUMNxl international inter-laboratory scoring exercise. Mutagenesis. 2016.

83. Holland N, Bolognesi C, Kirsch-Volders M, Bonassi S, Zeiger E, Knasmueller S, Fenech M. The micronucleus assay in human buccal cells as a tool for biomonitoring DNA damage: the HUMN project perspective on current status and knowledge gaps. Mutat Res. 2008;659:93–108.

84. Bolognesi C, Bonassi S, Knasmueller S, Fenech M, Bruzzone M, Lando C, Ceppi M. Clinical application of micronucleus test in exfoliated buccal cells: A systematic review and metanalysis. Mutat Res Rev Mutat Res. 2015;766:20–31.

85. Scheepers PB, Bos PM, Konings J, Janssen NAH, Grievink L. Application of biological monitoring for exposure assessment following chemical incidents. A procedure for decision-making. J Expo Sci Environ Epidemiol. 2011;21:247–61.

86. Manno M, Viau C, in-collaboration-with, Cocker J, Colosio C, Lowry L, Mutti A, Nordberg M, Wang S. Biomonitoring for occupational health risk assessment (BOHRA). Toxicol Lett. 2010;192:3–16.

87. Scheepers PTJ, Goën T. Diagnosis. Sci Technol: Monitoring and Prevention of Exposure-related Non-communicable Diseases – Searching for unique signatures; 2017.

88. Edelman P, Osterloh J, Pirkle J, Caudill SP, Grainger J, Jones R, Blount B, Calafat A, Turner W, Feldman D, et al. Biomonitoring of chemical exposure among New York City firefighters responding to the World Trade Center fire and collapse. Environmental health perspectives. 2003;111:1906–11.

89. Boerleider R, Roeleveld N, Scheepers P. Human biological monitoring of mercury for exposure assessment. AIMS Environmental Science. 2017;4:251–76.

90. Bae YS, Kang SW, Seo MS, Baines IC, Tekle E, Chock PB, Rhee SG. Epidermal growth factor (EGF)-induced generation of hydrogen peroxide. Role in EGF receptor-mediated tyrosine phosphorylation. J Biol Chem. 1997;272:217–21.

91. Haddad JJ, Land SC. Redox signaling-mediated regulation of lipopolysaccharide-induced proinflammatory cytokine biosynthesis in alveolar epithelial cells. Antioxid Redox Signal. 2002;4:179–93.

92. Hsu HY, Wen MH. Lipopolysaccharide-mediated reactive oxygen species and signal transduction in the regulation of interleukin-1 gene expression. J Biol Chem. 2002;277:22131–9.

93. Colavitti R, Pani G, Bedogni B, Anzevino R, Borrello S, Waltenberger J, Galeotti T. Reactive oxygen species as downstream mediators of angiogenic signaling by vascular endothelial growth factor receptor-2/KDR. J Biol Chem. 2002;277:3101–8.

94. Junn E, Lee KN, Ju HR, Han SH, Im JY, Kang HS, Lee TH, Bae YS, Ha KS, Lee ZW, et al. Requirement of hydrogen peroxide generation in TGF-beta 1 signal transduction in human lung fibroblast cells: involvement of hydrogen peroxide and Ca2+ in TGF-beta 1-induced IL-6 expression. J Immunol. 2000;165:2190–7.

95. Ovrevik J, Refsnes M, Lag M, Holme JA, Schwarze PE. Activation of Proinflammatory Responses in Cells of the Airway Mucosa by Particulate Matter: Oxidant- and Non-Oxidant-Mediated Triggering Mechanisms. Biomolecules. 2015;5:1399–440.

96. Thannickal VJ, Fanburg BL. Reactive oxygen species in cell signaling. Am J Physiol Lung Cell Mol Physiol. 2000;279:L1005–28.

97. Esposito F, Ammendola R, Faraonio R, Russo T, Cimino F. Redox control of signal transduction, gene expression and cellular senescence. Neurochem Res. 2004;29:617–28.

98. Schieber M, Chandel NS. ROS function in redox signaling and oxidative stress. Curr Biol. 2014;24:R453–62.

99. Sauer H, Wartenberg M, Hescheler J. Reactive oxygen species as intracellular messengers during cell growth and differentiation. Cell Physiol Biochem. 2001;11:173–86.

100. Fisher AB. Redox signaling across cell membranes. Antioxid Redox Signal. 2009;11:1349–56.

101. Barrett EG, Johnston C, Oberdorster G, Finkelstein JN. Silica-induced chemokine expression in alveolar type II cells is mediated by TNF-alpha-induced oxidant stress. Am J Physiol Lung Cell Mol Physiol. 1999;276:L979–88.

102. Totlandsdal AI, Refsnes M, Lag M. Mechanisms involved in ultrafine carbon black-induced release of IL-6 from primary rat epithelial lung cells. Toxicol In Vitro. 2010;24:10–20.

103. Gabelloni ML, Sabbione F, Jancic C, Fuxman Bass J, Keitelman I, Iula L, Oleastro M, Geffner JR, Trevani AS. NADPH oxidase derived reactive oxygen species are involved in human neutrophil IL-1beta secretion but not in inflammasome activation. Eur J Immunol. 2013;43:3324–35.

104. Trifilieff A, Walker C, Keller T, Kottirsch G, Neumann U. Pharmacological profile of PKF242-484 and PKF241-466, novel dual inhibitors of TNF-alpha converting enzyme and matrix metalloproteinases, in models of airway inflammation. Br J Pharmacol. 2002;135:1655–64.

105. Deshpande SS, Angkeow P, Huang J, Ozaki M, Irani K. Rac1 inhibits TNF-alpha-induced endothelial cell apoptosis: dual regulation by reactive oxygen species. Faseb J. 2000;14:1705–14.

106. Murphy C, Stack E, Krivelo S, McPartlin DA, Byrne B, Greef C, Lochhead MJ, Husar G, Devlin S, Elliott CT, O'Kennedy RJ. Detection of the cyanobacterial toxin, microcystin-LR, using a novel recombinant antibody-based optical-planar waveguide platform. Biosensors and Bioelectronics. 2015;67:708–14.

107. Crawley AS, O'Kennedy RJ. The need for effective pancreatic cancer detection and management: a biomarker-based strategy. Expert Review of Molecular Diagnostics. 2015;15:1339–53.

108. Ma H, O'Kennedy RJ. The Purification of Natural and Recombinant Peptide Antibodies by Affinity Chromatographic Strategies. Peptide Antibodies-series Methods in Molecular Biology. 2015;1348:153–65.

109. Loftus JH, Kijanka GS, O'Kennedy R, Loscher CE. Patulin, deoxynivalenol, zearalenone and T-2 toxin affect viability and modulate cytokine secretion in J774A.1 murine macrophages. International Journal of Chemistry. 2016;8:22–32.

110. Gilmartin N, Gião MS, Keevil CW, O'Kennedy RJ. Differential internalin A levels in biofilms of Listeria monocytogenes grown on different surfaces and nutrient conditions. International Journal of Food Microbiology. 2016;219:50–5.

111. Ayyar V, Sushrut A, O'Kennedy R. Coming-of-Age of Antibodies in Cancer Therapeutics. Trends in Pharmacological Sciences. 2016;37:1009–28.

112. O'Reilly JA, Fitzgerald J, Fitzgerald S, Kenny D, Kay EW, O'Kennedy R, Kijanka GS. Diagnostic potential of zinc finger protein-specific autoantibodies and associated linear B-cell epitopes in colorectal cancer. PloS one. 2015;10:e0123469.42.

113. Li H, Hedmer M, Kåredal M, Björk J, Stockfelt L, Tinnerberg H, Albin M, Broberg K. A cross-sectional study of the cardiovascular effects of welding fumes. PLoS one. 2015;10:e0131648.

114. Xu Y, Li H, Hedmer M, Hossain MB, Tinnerberg H, Broberg K, Albin M. Occupational exposure to particles and mitochondrial DNA - relevance for blood pressure. Environmental Health. 2017;6:22.

115. Li H, Hedmer M, Wojdacz T, Hossain MB, Lindh CH, Tinnerberg H, Albin M, Broberg K. Oxidative stress, telomere shortening, and DNA methylation in relation to low-to-moderate occupational exposure to welding fumes. Environment Molecular Mutagenesis. 2015;56:684–93.

116. Hossain MB, Li H, Hedmer M, Tinnerberg H, Albin M, Broberg K. Exposure to welding fumes is associated with hypomethylation of the F2RL3 gene: a cardiovascular disease marker. Occupational Environmental Medicine. 2015;72:845–51.

117. Alhamdow A, Gustavsson P, Rylander L, Jakobsson K, Tinnerberg H, Broberg K. Chimney sweeps in Sweden: a questionnaire-based assessment of long-term changes in work conditions, and current eye and airway symptoms. International Archives of Occupational Environmental Health. 2017;90:207–16.

118. Marie-Desvergne C, Maître A, Bouchard M, Ravanat JL, Viau C. Evaluation of DNA adducts, DNA and RNA oxidative lesions, and 3-hydroxybenzo(a)pyrene as biomarkers of DNA damage in lung following intravenous injection of the parent compound in rats. Chem Res Toxicol. 2010;23:1207–14.

119. Brown TP, Rumsby PC, Capleton AC, Rushton L, Levy LS. Pesticides and Parkinson's disease–is there a link? Environmental health perspectives. 2006;114:156–64.

120. Baldi I, Cantagrel A, Lebailly P, Tison F, Dubroca B, Chrysostome V, Dartigues JF, Brochard P. Association between Parkinson's disease and exposure to pesticides in southwestern France. Neuroepidemiology. 2003;22:305–10.

121. Baldi I, Lebailly P, Mohammed-Brahim B, Letenneur L, Dartigues JF, Brochard P. Neurodegenerative diseases and exposure to pesticides in the elderly. Am J Epidemiol. 2003;157:409–14.

122. Liew Z, Wang A, Bronstein J, Ritz B. Job exposure matrix (JEM)-derived estimates of lifetime occupational pesticide exposure and the risk of Parkinson's disease. Arch Environ Occup Health. 2014;69:241–51.

123. Elbaz A, Clavel J, Rathouz PJ, Moisan F, Galanaud JP, Delemotte B, Alperovitch A, Tzourio C. Professional exposure to pesticides and Parkinson disease. Ann Neurol. 2009;66:494–504.

124. Feldman AL, Johansson AL, Nise G, Gatz M, Pedersen NL, Wirdefeldt K. Occupational exposure in parkinsonian disorders: a 43-year prospective cohort study in men. Parkinsonism Relat Disord. 2011;17:677–82.

125. van der Mark M, Vermeulen R, Nijssen PC, Mulleners WM, Sas AM, van Laar T, Brouwer M, Huss A, Kromhout H. Occupational exposure to pesticides and endotoxin and Parkinson disease in the Netherlands. Occup Environ Med. 2014;71:757–64.

126. Kamel F, Tanner C, Umbach D, Hoppin J, Alavanja M, Blair A, Comyns K, Goldman S, Korell M, Langston J, et al. Pesticide exposure and self-reported Parkinson's disease in the agricultural health study. Am J Epidemiol. 2007;165:364–74.

127. Ritz BR, Paul KC, Bronstein JM. Of Pesticides and Men: a California Story of Genes and Environment in Parkinson's Disease. Curr Environ Health Rep. 2016;3:40–52.

128. Goldberg DW, Wilson JP, Knoblock CA, Ritz B, Cockburn MG. An effective and efficient approach for manually improving geocoded data. Int J Health Geogr. 2008;7:60.

129. Costello S, Cockburn M, Bronstein J, Zhang X, Ritz B. Parkinson's disease and residential exposure to maneb and paraquat from agricultural applications in the central valley of California. Am J Epidemiol. 2009;169:919–26.

130. Wang A, Costello S, Cockburn M, Zhang X, Bronstein J, Ritz B. Parkinson's disease risk from ambient exposure to pesticides. Eur J Epidemiol. 2011;26:547–55.

131. Narayan S, Liew Z, Paul K, Lee PC, Sinsheimer JS, Bronstein JM, Ritz B. Household organophosphorus pesticide use and Parkinson's disease. Int J Epidemiol. 2013;42:1476–85.

132. Gatto NM, Cockburn M, Bronstein J, Manthripragada AD, Ritz B. Well-water consumption and Parkinson's disease in rural California. Environmental health perspectives. 2009;117:1912–8.

133. Fitzmaurice AG, S. L., Rhodes SL, Lulla A, Murphy NP, Lam HA, O'Donnell KC, Barnhill L, Casida JE, Cockburn M, Sagasti A, et al. Aldehyde dehydrogenase inhibition as a pathogenic mechanism in Parkinson disease. Proc Natl Acad Sci U S A. 2013;110:636–41.

134. Paul KC, Sinsheimer JS, Rhodes SL, Cockburn M, Bronstein J, Ritz B. Organophosphate Pesticide Exposures, Nitric Oxide Synthase Gene Variants, and Gene-Pesticide Interactions in a Case-Control Study of Parkinson's Disease, California (USA). Environmental health perspectives. 2016;124:570–7.

135. Rhodes SL, Fitzmaurice AG, Cockburn M, Bronstein JM, Sinsheimer JS, Ritz B. Pesticides that inhibit the ubiquitin-proteasome system: effect measure modification by genetic variation in SKP1 in Parkinsons disease. Environ Res. 2013;126:1–8.

136. Kannarkat GT, Cook DA, Lee JK, Chang J, Chung J, Sandy E, Paul KC, Ritz B, Bronstein J, Factor SA, et al. Common Genetic Variant Association with Altered HLA Expression, Synergy with Pyrethroid Exposure, and Risk for Parkinson's Disease: An Observational and Case-Control Study. NPJ Parkinsons Dis. 2015;1

137. Lee PC, Rhodes SL, Sinsheimer JS, Bronstein J, Ritz B. Functional paraoxonase 1 variants modify the risk of Parkinson's disease due to organophosphate exposure. Environ Int. 2013;56:42–7.

138. Proceedings of the 2nd International DiMoPEx Conference on "Pollution in living and working environments and health", DiMoPEx Working Groups Meeting. Journal of Health and Pollution 2017, 8:in press.

139. Balbus JM, Barouki R, Birnbaum LS, Etzel RA, Gluckman PD Sr, Grandjean P, Hancock C, Hanson MA, Heindel JJ, Hoffman K, et al. Early-life prevention of non-communicable diseases. Lancet. 2013;381:3–4.

140. Bloom D, Cafiero E, Jané-Llopis E, Abrahams-Gessel S, Bloom L, Fathima S, Feigl A, Gaziano T, Mowafi M, Pandya A, et al. The Global Economic Burden of Noncommunicable Diseases. Geneva: World Economic Forum; 2011.

141. Environment and Human Health. Joint EEA-JRC report. EEA Report No 5/2013. Copenhagen: European Environment Agency; 2013.

142. Norman RE, Carpenter DO, Scott J, Brune MN, Sly PD. Environmental exposures: an underrecognized contribution to noncommunicable diseases. Rev Environ Health. 2013;28:59–65.

143. Prüss-Üstün A, Wolf J, Corvalán C, Bos R, Neira M. Preventing disease through healthy environments A global assessment of the burden of disease from environmental risks. Geneva: World Health Organization http://www.appswhoint/iris/bitstream/10665/204585/1/9789241565196_engpdf?ua=1; 2016.

144. Vineis P, Stringhini S, Porta M. The environmental roots of non-communicable diseases (NCDs) and the epigenetic impacts of globalization. Environ Res. 2014;133:424–30.

145. WHO. Ambient air pollution: a global assessment of exposure and burden of disease. Geneva: World Health Organization http://www.appswhoint/iris/bitstream/10665/250141/1/9789241511353-engpdf?ua=1; 2016a.

146. WHO. The public health impacts of chemicals: knowns and unknowns. Geneva: World Health Organization http://www.appswhoint/iris/bitstream/10665/206553/1/WHO_FWC_PHE_EPE1601engpdf; 2016b.

147. WHO Regional Office for Europe. Health 2020: a European policy framework supporting action across government and society for health and well-being. Copenhagen: WHO Regional Office for Europe http://www.eurowhoint/__data/assets/pdf_file/0006/199536/Health2; 2013.

148. WHO Regional Office for Europe. The Minsk Declaration – The Life-course Approach in the Context of Health 2020. Copenhagen: WHO Regional Office for Europe http://www.eurowhoint/__data/assets/pdf_file/0009/289962/The-Minsk-Declaration-EN-rev1pdf?ua=1; 2015a.

149. WHO Regional Office for Europe. Strategic Approach to International Chemicals Management: implementation and priorities in the health sector. Meeting report. Copenhagen: WHO Regional Office for Europe http://www.eurowhoint/__data/assets/pdf_file/0015/303036/SAICM-meeting-report-enpdf?ua=1; 2015b.

150. WHO Regional Office for Europe. Sixth Ministerial Conference on Environment and Health, Copenhagen. http://www.eurowhoint/en/media-centre/events/events/2017/06/sixth-ministerial-conference-on-environment-and-health/read-more 2017a.

151. WHO Regional Office for Europe. Sustainable Development Goals, Copenhagen http://www.eurowhoint/en/health-topics/health-policy/sustainable-development-goals-sdgs 2017b.

152. WHO Regional Office for Europe. Chemical policies and programmes to protect human health and environment in a sustainability perspective. Meeting report, Copenhagen. http://www.eurowhoint/__data/assets/pdf_file/0009/334665/Chemical-safety-meeting-report_new-coverpdf 2017c.

153. WHO Regional Office for Europe. Implementation of the Minamata Convention in the health sector: challenges and opportunities, Copenhagen. http://www.eurowhoint/en/health-topics/environment-and-health/health-impact-assessment/publications/2017/implementation-of-the-minamata-convention-in-the-health-sector-challenges-and-opportunities-2017 2017d.

18

Sulfur dioxide exposure reduces the quantity of CD19+ cells and causes nasal epithelial injury in rats

Ruonan Chai, Hua Xie, Junli Zhang and Zhuang Ma[*] (iD)

Abstract

Background: Reactive airway dysfunction syndrome (RADS), also called irritant-induced asthma, is a type of occupational asthma that can occur within a very short period of latency. The study sought to investigate the influence of sulfur dioxide (SO_2) exposure on CD19+ cells and nasal epithelial injury.

Methods: We investigated the effects of SO_2 on CD19 expression and morphological changes of nasal epithelia in rats. In the study, 20 rats were randomly divided into the SO_2 exposure group that were exposed to 600 ppm SO_2, 2 h/day for consecutive 7 days, and the control group that were exposed to filtered air).

Results: Inhalation of high concentration of SO_2 significantly reduced CD19 expression at both the mRNA transcript and protein levels, and reduced the percentages of $CD19^+$ cells and $CD19^+/CD23^+$ cells in the nasal septum. However, inhalation of high concentration of SO_2 did not affect immunoglobulin (Ig) G, IgA and IgE levels in the serum and nasal septum. More importantly, SO_2 exposure also caused mild structural changes of the nasal septum.

Conclusion: Our results reveal that inhalation of a high concentration of SO_2 reduces CD19 expression and causes structural change of the nasal septum in rats.

Keywords: Reactive airway, Dysfunction syndrome, Asthma, SO_2, CD19

Highlights

- SO_2 inhalation reduced the CD19 expression in nasal septum
- SO_2 exposure decreased the percentage of CD19+ and CD19+/CD23+ cells
- SO2 inhalation does not affect the IgG, IgA and IgE levels

Background

Reactive airway dysfunction syndrome (RADS), also called irritant-induced asthma, is a type of occupational asthma that can occur within a very short period of latency [1]. With intensive studies on the pathogenesis of asthma, a deep insight into RADS has been gained [2]. RADS is characterized clinically by asthma-like symptoms including cough, wheezing, chest tightness,

and breathlessness. The symptoms of RADS usually occur within 24 h after exposure to high amounts of harmful gases [3]. RADS shares no features of immunology and allergy, which is distinct from classic asthma [4]. However, clinical manifestations of both RADS and asthma are very similar and both share common characteristics, especially airway hyperresponsiveness [5]. Therefore, RADS is thought as a type of occupational asthma, or an adult-onset asthma [6]. The exact cause of RADS is not yet known, but the syndrome is considered to be uncommon and recognized in less than one-fifth of workers with "occupational asthma" [7].

Sulfur dioxide (SO_2) emissions are mainly produced from industrial processes, including metal extraction from ores, power plants and refineries. Owing to its rotten-egg odour, sulfur dioxide can be noted at levels between 0.3 and 5 ppm (ppm). Exposure to levels as low as 0.1 to 0.5 ppm can cause bronchoconstriction in humans with asthma. Especially, the influence of exposure to high concentrations of SO_2 for a short time has

* Correspondence: lnuo0111355@sina.com
Department of Respiratory Medicine, General Hospital of Shenyang Military Command, No. 83 Wenhua Road, Shenhe District, Shenyang 110016, China

been documented [8–10]. SO$_2$ accounts for the major proportion of smoke of gunpowder, and its concentration is very high, which might cause respiratory dysfunction syndrome. In addition, SO$_2$ tank leaks or smoke from mine blast can also expose humans to high concentrations of SO$_2$ for a short time.

B-lymphocyte antigen CD19, also known as CD19, is found on the surface of B-cells, a type of white blood cell. CD19 plays a physiological function in establishing intrinsic B cell signaling thresholds through modulating both B cell receptor (BCR)-dependent and independent signaling [11]. CD19 plays an important role in immunoglobulin-induced activation of B cells [12]. CD19 deficiency causes hyporesponsiveness to transmembrane signals, and weak T cell-dependent humoral responses [13]. CD23, also known as Fc epsilon RII, or FcεRII, is important in regulating IgE levels. CD32 is a surface receptor protein, which has a low-affinity for IgG antibodies and down-regulates antibody production in the presence of IgG. Immunoglobulins, including IgG, IgA and IgE, are large, Y-shaped proteins produced by plasma cells to neutralize pathogens such as pathogenic bacteria and viruses. However, the effects of SO$_2$ on CD19 and immunoglobulin expression have not been reported. In this study, we exposed rats to a high concentration of SO$_2$, and determined changes in the percentage of CD19$^+$ cells.

Methods
Animals and reagents
Twenty male Sprague Dawley rats (weighing 180–200 g each) were purchased from Liaoning Changsheng Biotechnology (Shenyang, China). SO$_2$ gas (purity: 99.9%) was purchased from Beijing Ya-nan Gas Scientific and Technology (Beijing, China). Anti-CD19-FITC monoclonal antibody and goat anti-rat IgG, IgA and IgE antibodies were purchased from Abcam Corp. Ltd. (Abcam, UK). Anti-CD32 antibody and goat ABC staining system were purchased from Santa Cruz Biotechnology (Santa Cruz, CA, USA). Rat IgG, IgA and IgE ELISA kit was purchased from eBioscience Corp. (USA). TRIzol reagent was purchased from Takara Corp. (USA). Experiment protocols strictly complied with the Laboratory Animal Administration Rules.

Exposure chamber
SO$_2$ exposure was conducted as previously described with slight modification [14, 15]. The device consists of SO$_2$ source, air pump, intake port, SO$_2$ chamber, SO$_2$ detector and several connective tubes/valves. SO$_2$ was diluted with fresh air in the intake port to yield desired SO$_2$ concentrations. SO$_2$ was delivered to animals via a tube positioned at the upper level of the chamber and distributed homogeneously via a fan in each chamber.

The concentration of SO$_2$ was determined in a real-time manner by SO$_2$ sensor (JSA5-SO$_2$ sensor, Shenzhen Ji-shun-an Technology Co., Ltd., China). The concentration of SO$_2$ in the chamber was selected by adjusting the valve between the intake port and SO$_2$ chamber according to the quantitative value of the SO$_2$ sensor.

Exposure protocol
Twenty rats were randomly divided into the SO$_2$ exposure group and the control group (10 in each group). The rats in the SO$_2$ exposure group were placed into the exposure chamber (600 ppm SO$_2$, 2 h/day) for consecutive 7 days, while rats in the control group were exposed to filtered air in another identical chamber for the same duration. All rats were allowed free access to food and water. After 7-day exposure, the tail vein blood from each rat was taken. The blood was kept at room temperature for 2 h, and clarified by centrifugation to obtain serum. Then, the rats were sacrificed with quick decapitation. The nasal septum was removed and washed with phosphate buffered saline (PBS).

Real time quantitative reverse Transcrption PCR (qRT-PCR)
The nasal septum was collected and total RNA was prepared with Trizol reagent according to the manufacturer's instructions. Real time qRT-PCR was performed using a sequence detection system (ABI PRISM 7000; Applied Biosystems, Life Technologies,Grand Island, NY, USA), with a commercially available kit (SYBR PrimeScriptRT-PCR Kit, TaKaRa Biotechnology). The reactions were performed at least three times independently. The cycle threshold analysis of all samples was set automatically by the ABI PRISM 7000 software. The mRNA expression of the indicated gene was normalized against β-actin. The annealing temperature for β-actin and CD19 was 60 °C.

The sequences of the primers (Sangon, Shanghai, China) used in the study were as follows:

β-actin (211 bp) sense: 5′-CCTCTATGCCAACA CAGTGC-3′, and antisense: 5′-GTACTCCTGCTTGC TGATCC-3′, and CD19 (273 bp) sense: 5′-ATGT GGGTTTGGGGGTCTC-3′, and antisense: 5′-AGGG TCGGTCATTCGCTTC-3′.

Western blotting assays
Western blot analysis was performed of cellular lysates of the nasal septum as described previously [16]. Briefly, proteins were resolved by sodium dodecyl sulfate–polyacrylamidegel electrophoresis (SDS-PAGE, 10% separating, 5% stacking) and transferred to PVDF membranes (Millipore, USA). The membranes were blocked by 5% defat milk in PBS containing 0.1% Tween 20. Thereafter, the membranes were incubated with monoclonal

antibody specific for rat CD19 (dilution 1:5000) at 4 °C overnight. Anti-mouse secondary antibody (dilution 1:5000) was added to membranes and incubated at 37 °C for 45 min. Protein signal was amplified and visualized via chemiluminescence using the ECL detection system and Hyperfilm ECL autoradiography film (Amersham Pharmacia Biotech, Inc.). Protein expression was normalized against β-actin. Images were quantified using the Labworks v3.0.2 image scanning and analysis software (Gel-Pro-Analyzer).

Elisa
The levels of IgG, IgA and IgE in the plasma and nasal septum were measured using commercially available ELISA kit according to the manufacturer's instructions and calculated by generating a standard curve using standard proteins and analyzed using Curve Expert 1.3 Software.

Flow cytometry
The nasal septum was minced and digested with 0.04% collagenase IV in DMEM at 37 °Cfor 1 h. Digested cells were washed with PBS to remove collagenase. The tissues were homogenized and centrifuged. Cells were pooled and suspended in PBS with 1% BSA at a density of 1×10^7 cells/mL. Anti-CD16 and anti-CD32 antibodies were added at a concentration of 1 μg/10^6 cells to block Fc receptors by incubation on ice for 10 min. Cells were washed with PBS and stained with 1 μg anti-CD19-FITC and anti-CD23-PE antibodies at 4°C for 30 min in the dark. The cells were washed again and analyzed by flow cytometry.

Histological analysis
The nasal septum was fixed in 4% formaldehyde. The fixed tissue samples were dehydrated in graded ethanol, embedded in paraffin. Each paraffin block was sectioned into 5-μm-thick slices, which were then dewaxed in xylene, rehydrated in gradient alcohols and rinsed with distilled water. Each section placed on glass slide was stained with hematoxylin and eosin (H&E) and double-blindly evaluated under light microscope by an experienced histologist.

Statistical analysis
All values were expressed as mean ± standard deviation (SD). Data analysis was performed using Student's t test. $P < 0.05$ was considered statistically significant.

Results
SO$_2$ inhalation reduces CD19 expression in the nasal septum
The rats were healthy before the experiment. When exposed to high concentrations of SO$_2$, rats became inactive

and curled together. No obvious symptoms and weight loss were observed after the exposure. The expressions of both CD19 mRNA transcripts and protein were significantly decreased in SO$_2$ exposed rats when compared with the control group (all $P < 0.05$) (Fig. 1a and b).

SO$_2$ exposure significantly decreases the percentage of CD19$^+$ and CD19$^+$/CD23$^+$ cells in the nasal septum
Flow cytometry was applied to determine the percentage of CD19$^+$ and CD19$^+$ CD23$^+$ cells in the nasal septum. The results showed that the proportion of both CD19$^+$ cells (6.49 ± 3.48% vs. 3.71 ± 0.57% $P < 0.05$), and CD19$^+$/CD23$^+$ cells (5.74 ± 3.14% vs. 3.45 ± 0.54%, $P < 0.05$) were significantly decreased after SO$_2$ exposure compared with the control group (Fig. 2a and b).

SO2 inhalation does not affect IgG, IgA and IgE levels in the plasma and nasal septum
Since B lymphocyte plays an important role in activation of antibody production, we measured IgG levels in the plasma and nasal septum after SO$_2$ exposure by ELISA to determine whether antibody production was influenced by the down-regulation of CD19 upon SO$_2$ exposure. However, no differences were observed in IgG, IgA and IgE levels in both the plasma and nasal septum between the two groups (Fig. 3).

Histopathological changes after SO$_2$ exposure
Histopathological studies showed that the structure of nasal septum was damaged and the boundary for different layers was blurry in exposed rats, while the structure of layers in the control group was normal. By contrast, no apparent alveolar hemorrhage and lymphocytes infiltration were observed in both two groups (Fig. 4).

Discussion
In this study, we showed that SO$_2$ exposure not only reduced CD19 expression, but also caused nasal epithelial injury. Considering that SO$_2$ is one of the major components of RADS-related air pollutants, this study might provide important implications for the pathogenesis of RADS.

Irritative chemical gases may firstly cause injury of airway epithelial cells, followed by inflammation, edema and blockage of bronchioles, which are similar to chemical trachitis and bronchitis [17]. RADS has a longer course compared with chemical trachitis and bronchitis. In most cases, lung function in RADS can recover 3–6 months after evacuation of irritating environment. RADS likely progresses into chronic disease, if symptoms persist for more than 6 months [18]. The membrane potential of the cells is altered in high cation condition, whereas changes of membrane potential can elicit the increase of oxygen radicals in cell respiratory burst, which is involved in the inflammatory process [19, 20].

SO_2 is a major composition in air pollutants and is characteristically pungent and suffocating. After exposure, the physiological function of the respiratory system is impaired, accompanied by weakened elasticity of pulmonary alveoli and decreased lung function, which resulted in trachitis, bronchial asthma and emphysema, etc. [21, 22]. In 2012, we obtained a fund to investigate the effect of smoke on the human respiratory system in the battlefield environment. After the analysis of the composition of the smoke, we found that SO_2 was the major component of gunpowder smoke, and the

concentration was very high. Therefore, we designed this experiment to simulate the respiratory dysfunction syndrome caused by smoke inhalation by soldiers or civilians in a war environment and investigate its pathogenesis. In addition, in a peaceful environment, SO_2 tank leaks or smoke from mine blast can also expose humans to high concentrations of SO_2 for a short time. Therefore, the investigation of exposure to high concentration of SO_2 is of practical significance, although 600 ppm is a lethal concentration for humans. CD19 is an important marker of B lymphocytes and plays a key role in B cell signal transduction, activation, differentiation and production of antibody [23]. In this study, the effects of SO_2 exposure on CD19 expression and the percentage of $CD19^+$ cells were investigated after inhalation of high concentration of SO_2. This study revealed an important mechanism underlying SO_2 exposure-induced RADS.

Our results showed that multiple inhalation exposures to high concentration of SO_2 could result in nasal septum injury, but not death in rats. However, potential influence of high concentration of SO_2 on the lungs and bronchoalveolar lavage should be investigated in future study. Additionally, the injury in our study is different from that of bronchial asthma [24]. In classic humoral immunity, bronchial asthma is manifested by increase of

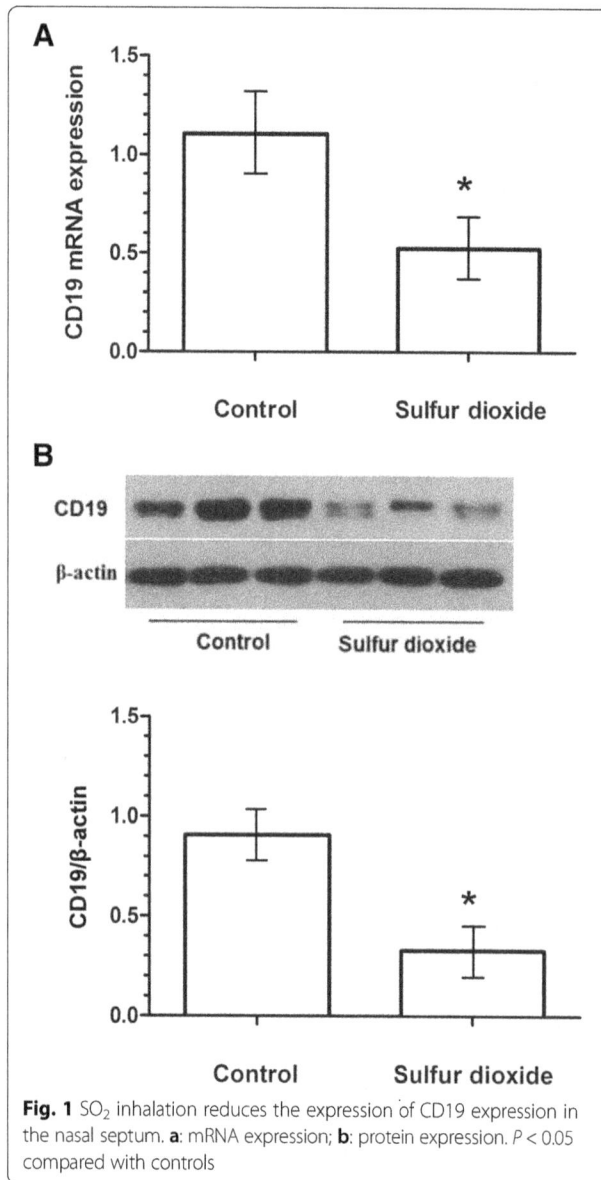

Fig. 1 SO_2 inhalation reduces the expression of CD19 expression in the nasal septum. a: mRNA expression; b: protein expression. $P < 0.05$ compared with controls

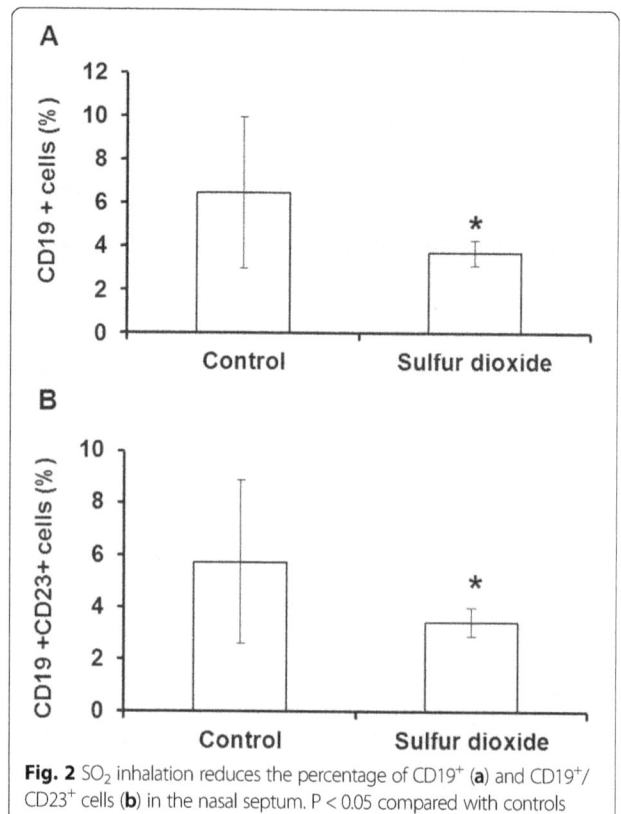

Fig. 2 SO_2 inhalation reduces the percentage of $CD19^+$ (a) and $CD19^+/CD23^+$ cells (b) in the nasal septum. $P < 0.05$ compared with controls

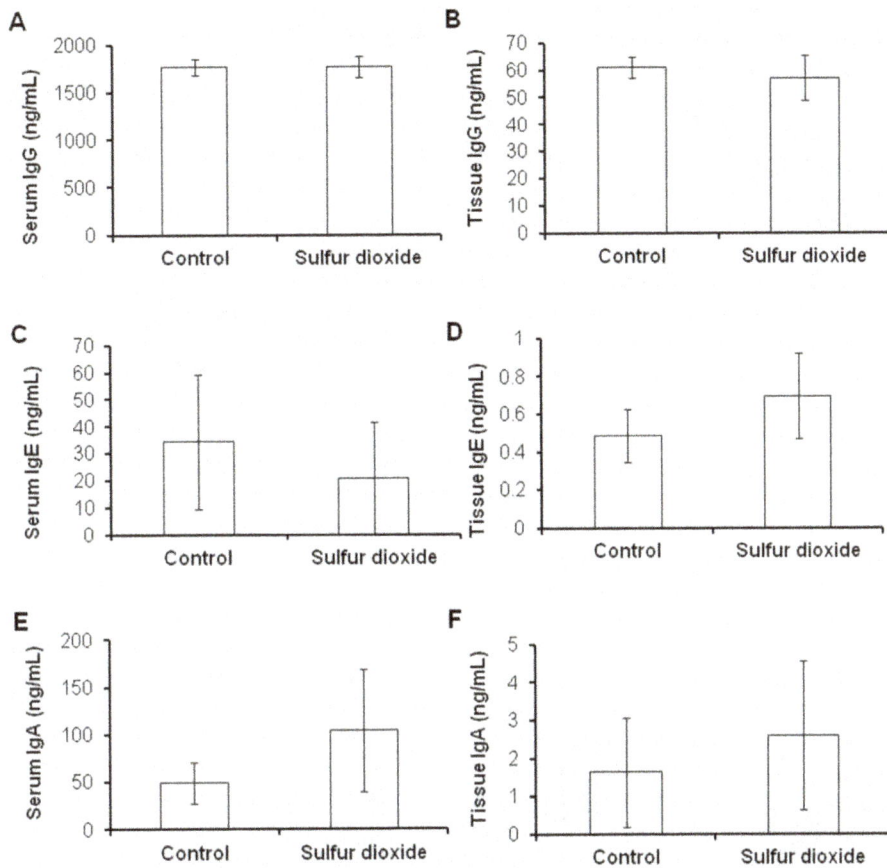

Fig. 3 The representative figure showed that SO$_2$ inhalation did not affect IgG levels in the serum and nasal septum. **a**: IgG level in the serum; **b**: IgG level in the nasal septum; **c**: IgE level in the serum; **d**: IgE level in the nasal septum; **e**: IgA level in the serum; **f**: IgA level in the nasal septum

immunoglobulin (for example IgG) and CD19$^+$ cell counts. Whereas the percentage of CD19$^+$ cells and CD19$^+$/CD23$^+$ cells in nasal mucosa tissues demonstrate a significant decrease compared with the control in our model. Real time qRT-PCR and Western blot analysis further demonstrated a decreased expression of CD19

after inhalation of high concentration of SO$_2$. Moreover, the levels of IgG, IgA and IgE were not influenced. But histopathological studies showed that the structure of the nasal septum appeared blurred.

In summary, multiple SO$_2$ exposures induce structural changes of the nasal septum and down-regulates the

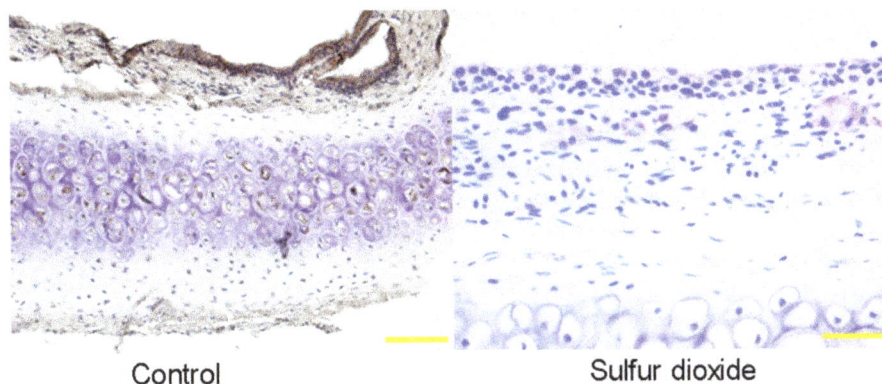

Fig. 4 The structure of the nasal septum of SO$_2$ exposed rats looked blurred, indicating slight structural changes

expression of CD19 in the rat. Further studies are required to explore the molecular mechanism after SO_2 exposure and the role of CD19.

Authors' contributions

RC and ZM contributed to the study design. RC, HX and JZ collected the data and performed data analysis. All authors prepared the manuscript. All authors read and approved the final manuscript.

Competing interests

The authors declare that they have no competing interests.

References

1. Doshi V, Kham N, Kulkarni S, Kapitan K, Henkle J, White P. R-134a (1,1,1,2-Tetrafluoroethane) inhalation induced reactive airways dysfunction syndrome. Am J Therap. 2016;23(3):e969–71.
2. Brooks SM. Then and now reactive airways dysfunction syndrome. J Occup Environ Med. 2016;58:636–7.
3. Shakeri MS, Dick FD, Ayres JG. Which agents cause reactive airways dysfunction syndrome (RADS)? A systematic review. Occup Med. 2008;58:205–11.
4. Murphy DM, O'Byrne PM. Recent advances in the pathophysiology of asthma. Chest. 2010;137:1417–26.
5. Brooks SM, Bernstein IL. Irritant-induced airway disorders. Immunol Allergy Clin. 2011;31:747–68.
6. Muñoz X, Cruz MJ, Bustamante V, Lopez-Campos JL, Barreiro E. Work-related asthma: diagnosis and prognosis of immunological occupational asthma and work-exacerbated asthma. J Invest Allerg Clin. 2014;24:396.
7. SM B. Reactive airways dysfunction syndrome and considerations of irritant-induced asthma. J Occup Environ Med. 2013;55:1118–20.
8. Guarnieri M, Balmes JR. Outdoor air pollution and asthma. Food Chem Toxicol. 1996;34:318.
9. Wang XB, Du JB, Cui H. Sulfur dioxide, a double-faced molecule in mammals. Life Sci. 2014;98:63–7.
10. Charan NB, Myers CG, Lakshminarayan S, Spencer TM. Pulmonary injuries associated with acute sulfur dioxide inhalation. Am Rev Respir Dis. 1979;119:555.
11. Bai X, Huang L, Niu L, Zhang Y, Wang J, Sun X, et al. Mst1 positively regulates B-cell receptor signaling via CD19 transcriptional levels. Blood Adv. 2016;1:219.
12. Poole JA, Mikuls TR, Duryee MJ, Warren KJ, Wyatt TA, Nelson AJ, et al. A role for B cells in organic dust induced lung inflammation. Respir Res. 2017;18:214.
13. Abe M, Wang Z, De CA, Thomson AW. Plasmacytoid dendritic cell precursors induce allogeneic T-cell hyporesponsiveness and prolong heart graft survival. Am J Transpla. 2015;5:1808–19.
14. Bai J, Meng Z. Effects of sulfur dioxide on apoptosis-related gene expressions in lungs from rats. Regul Toxicol Pharmacol. 2005;43:272–9.
15. Li R, Meng Z, Xie J. Effects of sulfur dioxide on the expressions of EGF, EGFR, and COX-2 in airway of asthmatic rats. Arch Environ Con Tox. 2008;54:748–57.
16. Qin G, Meng Z, editors. Effect of Sulfur Dioxide Inhalation on CYP2B1/2 and CYP2E1 in Rat Liver and Lung. Inhal Tox. 2008;581–88.
17. Cooney DJ, Hickey AJ. Cellular response to the deposition of diesel exhaust particle aerosols onto human lung cells grown at the air-liquid interface by inertial impaction. Tox In Vitro. 2011;25:1953–65.
18. Du CL, Wang JD, Chu PC, Guo YL. Acute expanded perlite exposure with persistent reactive airway dysfunction syndrome. Ind Health. 2010;48:119–22.
19. Schreiber R. Ca2+ signaling, intracellular pH and cell volume in cell proliferation. J Membrane Biol. 2005;205:129–37.
20. Xie Y, Zhuang ZX. Chromium(VI)-induced Production of Reactive Oxygen Species, Change of Plasma Membrane Potential and Dissipation of Mitochondria Membrane Potential in Chinese Hamster Lung Cell Cultures. Biomed Environ Sci. 2001;14:199.
21. Winkler T, Suki B. Emergent structure-function relations in emphysema and asthma. Crit Rev Biomed Eng. 2011;39:263–80.
22. Kahana LM, Aronovitch M. Pulmonary surface tension after sulfur dioxide exposure. Am Rev Respir Dis. 1968;98:311–4.
23. Brynjolfsson SF, Mohaddes M, Kärrholm J, Wick MJ. Long-lived plasma cells in human bone marrow can be either CD19+ or CD19. Blood Adv. 2017;1:835–8.
24. Ukena D, Fishman L, Niebling WB. Bronchial asthma: diagnosis and long-term treatment in adults. Dtsch Rztebl Int. 2008;105:385–94.

19

In vitro toxicological evaluation of surgical smoke from human tissue

Jennifer D. Sisler[1], Justine Shaffer[1], Jhy-Charm Soo[2], Ryan F. LeBouf[3], Martin Harper[2,4,5], Yong Qian[1] and Taekhee Lee[2*]

Abstract

Background: Operating room personnel have the potential to be exposed to surgical smoke, the by-product of using electrocautery or laser surgical device, on a daily basis. Surgical smoke is made up of both biological by-products and chemical pollutants that have been shown to cause eye, skin and pulmonary irritation.

Methods: In this study, surgical smoke was collected in real time in cell culture media by using an electrocautery surgical device to cut and coagulate human breast tissues. Airborne particle number concentration and particle distribution were determined by direct reading instruments. Airborne concentration of selected volatile organic compounds (VOCs) were determined by evacuated canisters. Head space analysis was conducted to quantify dissolved VOCs in cell culture medium. Human small airway epithelial cells (SAEC) and RAW 264.7 mouse macrophages (RAW) were exposed to surgical smoke in culture media for 24 h and then assayed for cell viability, lactate dehydrogenase (LDH) and superoxide production.

Results: Our results demonstrated that surgical smoke-generated from human breast tissues induced cytotoxicity and LDH increases in both the SAEC and RAW. However, surgical smoke did not induce superoxide production in the SAEC or RAW.

Conclusion: These data suggest that the surgical smoke is cytotoxic in vitro and support the previously published data that the surgical smoke may be an occupational hazard to healthcare workers.

Keywords: Surgical smoke, Toxicology, Healthcare workers

Background

Approximately 20 million Americans undergo surgery with general anesthesia each year [1]. Nowadays, electrocautery, laser ablation, and ultrasonic scalpel dissection are widely recognized as major advances in surgical technique and are increasingly being used for tissue cutting and hemostasis [2]. Surgical incision and dissection with electrocautery, laser and ultrasonic scalpel are used to cut tissue and decrease bleeding through coagulating small blood vessels. The key feature of these techniques is to heat tissue to high temperatures that burn and rupture cellular membranes and other structures. However, the breakdown of cellular membranes and other tissue structures generates many biological by-products that

mix with chemical compounds used during surgery, which form smoke due to the high temperatures during the surgical procedures. The released surgical smoke contaminates the air with many chemical compounds as by-products of tissue damage, as well as biological materials, including potentially infectious agents [3]. Several studies have found that the complex mixture of surgical smoke contains both chemical pollutants and biological hazards [2, 4–7]. The composition of the surgical smoke varies based upon the type of surgery; however, the following chemical components have been found to be common to most surgeries: acetaldehyde, acrolein, acetonitrile, benzene, hydrogen cyanide (HCN), polyaromatic hydrocarbons (PAHs), styrene, toluene, and xylene [2, 4, 8–11]. Animal studies have shown that rats exposed to smoke from pigskin showed congestive pneumonia, bronchiolitis and emphysema [12] and sheep exposed to smoke from sheep bronchial tissue showed a

* Correspondence: fwc8@cdc.gov
[2]Exposure Assessment Branch, Health Effects Laboratory Division, National Institute for Occupational Safety and Health, Centers for Disease Control and Prevention, 1095 Willowdale Road, Morgantown, West Virginia 26505, USA
Full list of author information is available at the end of the article

decrease of arterial PO$_2$ (hypoxia), depressed tracheal mucus velocity and severe inflammation with dramatic increases of inflammatory cells [13]. A survey showed that operating room nurses reported respiratory problems including nasal congestion, increased coughing, allergies and sinus infections or problems and the prevalence for the nurses was greater than the prevalence in the US [14]. In addition, Health Hazard Evaluations (HHEs) by the National Institute for Occupational Safety and Health (NIOSH) on surgical smoke exposure have been requested repeatedly over the past decades suggesting that OR personnel are experiencing adverse reactions to exposure to surgical smoke [15–19]. Surgical smoke has also been shown to contain several known carcinogenic compounds. NIOSH reported on the mutagenicity of surgical smoke generated in reduction mammoplasty procedures [20]. Recently, it was found that surgical smoke has ultrafine particles that are in the range of 9–81 nm depending on the type and the duration surgery [3, 21]. Ultrafine particles in the surgical smoke have the ability to reach the alveolar region of the lung and cause pulmonary inflammation or disease [22, 23].

Human toxicological response to surgical smoke has not been studied in detail. An in vitro study has shown that surgical smoke collected into cell culture media from cutting porcine liver using an electro-surgical hook knife caused a toxic effect on human breast cancer cells (MCF-7) using the clonogenic assays [24]. Other in vitro studies have shown that electrocautery of cultured retrovirus infected melanoma cells produced airborne viable retrovirus particles and electrocautery of a pellet of melanoma cells released viable melanoma cells [25, 26]. However, another group has shown that tumor ablation with ultrasonically activated scalpel or electrocautery does not release viable airborne cancer cells [27]. Although transmission risk of human virus or cancer cells by inhalation of surgical smoke is not clear, the concerns have been raised that human cancer cells, viruses including human immunodeficiency virus and other pathogens could become airborne through the use of surgical devices [12]. Moreover, the toxicological effects of other biological products and chemical pollutants in surgical smoke have not been fully determined. It is important to better understand the toxicological effects of surgical smoke because surgical smoke could create an occupational hazard to operating room staff. It is important to identify the risk of surgical smoke to guide the installation of the proper protection procedures and devices in surgical rooms. Recently, a survey was performed to determine if the correct engineering controls were being used to protect healthcare workers from exposure to surgical smoke [28]. Their survey concluded that a majority of surgical rooms did not have proper local exhaust ventilation (LEV) because the installation of LEV

in these surgical rooms was not considered in their design. Moreover, those surgical rooms without LEV also did not have respirators and the healthcare workers only used surgical masks [28]. Therefore, the healthcare workers who work in these surgical rooms have no proper protection procedures and devices to prevent the potential exposure to surgical smoke.

While several in vivo and in vitro studies suggest the toxicity of surgical smoke using cultured cells, virus or pig skin, information concerning the toxicological effects of surgical smoke generated from human tissue has been lacking. In this study, the cellular toxicity of surgical smoke of human tissue was assessed. Human breast tissues were cut using an electrocautery surgical device and the surgical smoke was collected in real time into cell culture media, followed by exposure to human small airway epithelial cells (SAEC) and mouse macrophages (RAW). The chemical properties and the in vitro toxicity of surgical smoke generated with real human tissues were analyzed.

Methods
Surgical smoke generation and collection
Fresh human breast tissues obtained from the West Virginia University (WVU) tissue bank were used to generate surgical smoke in unoccupied operating rooms at WVU Ruby Memorial hospitals. The tissues were obtained within 3 h after breast reduction surgeries. Surgical smoke was generated with an electrocautery surgical device (model: ForceFX, Valleylab, Boulder, CO, USA; output power of cut and coagulate was set at 35 watts; cut and coagulation modes mixed use) for 15 min. The smoke was collected with three autoclaved BioSamplers® (SKC Inc., Eighty Four, PA, USA) for each generation and each sampler was loaded with 2 mL of cell medium, either Dulbecco's Modified Eagle Medium (DMEM) or Small Airway Epithelial Cell growth medium (SABM). Inlets of the BioSamplers® were maintained within 5 cm of electrocautery interaction site, as this represents the worst-case situation when OR personnel lean in over the patient during surgery. Samples were collected at 12.5 l/min over 15 mins to collect the smoke visually observed from the interaction site. A total of 24 surgical smoke generations (each 15 mins generation) were conducted in 6 different sampling sessions. A total of 33 samples, and 39 samples, were collected using BioSamplers® loaded with DMEM and SABM, respectively, along with 33 background samples (air sampling with the BioSamplers® was conducted without generation of surgical smoke for each cell medium) and 11 field blank samples (no sampling).

Air sampling and sample analysis
Direct reading instrument measurement
Particle number concentration and particle distribution were measured in real time with direct reading

instruments. The number concentration of particles in the size range of 0.01–1.0 μm were measured using a condensation particle counter (CPC, model 3007, TSI Inc., Shoreview, MN, USA) every second. The particle size distribution of ultrafine particles was measured by a Scanning Mobility Particle Sizer (SMPS, model 3034, TSI Inc., size range from 10 to 414 nm) or Nanoscan SMPS nanoparticle sizer (Model 3910, TSI Inc., size range from 11.5 to 365.2 nm), but not for all of the generations due to instruments availability.

Scanning electron microscope analysis

A field emission scanning electron microscope (SEM; model S-4800-2, Hitachi High Technologies America Inc.) was utilized to characterize airborne particles collected in cell medium. Surgical smoke sample collected in the DMEM media sample was filtered onto a polycarbonate filter (pore size 0.45 μm, 25-mm diameter) and desiccated and sputter-coated with gold and platinum. SEM analysis for the SABM media could not be conducted because the media was too dense to be filtered.

VOCs sampling and analysis

Volatile organic compounds were collected using evacuated canisters following NIOSH draft canister method for VOCs in air [29]. Area sampling was conducted using 6 L (SilicoCan, Restek Corporation, Bellefonte, PA, USA) or 600 mL (Silonite® miniCans with Micro-QT Valves, Entech Instrument Inc., Simi Valley, CA, USA) canisters. Critical orifice (Restek Corporation) or sapphire restrictors (Restek Corporation) were utilized to maintain flow rates of the passively sampling evacuated canisters. The flow rates of 6 L and 600 mL of the canisters were 100 or 35 cm^3/min, respectively. A grab sampling technique of filling canisters within 1 min was utilized to collect VOCs within 5 cm from electrocautery interaction site. Area sampling technique was used in sampling #1, #2 and #3 and grab sampling technique was in sampling #4, #5 and #6. The air samples were analyzed using a preconcentrator (7200, Entech Instrument Inc.) and gas chromatography-mass spectrometry (Agilent Technologies, Inc., Santa Clara, CA, USA) system in accordance with the methodology presented in a recently published method validation study [29, 30]. The study quantified VOCs associated with healthcare settings including: α-pinene, acetone, benzene, chloroform, ethanol, ethyl benzene, hexane, isopropyl alcohol, d-limonene, m, p-xylene, methyl methacrylate, methylene chloride, o-xylene, and toluene. Three additional VOCs were added to the target list for this study: acetaldehyde, acetonitrile, and styrene. Other VOCs were qualitatively identified by comparing their mass spectra to the NIST 2008 Mass Spectral Library. They were included if the quality factor of comparison was greater than 90%.

Head space analysis

In order to quantify dissolved VOCs in the cell media, head space analysis was conducted although it is not a direct measurement of the cell medium. One mL sample from each blank and the DMEM and SABM containing surgical smoke was transferred into a sealed 40 mL amber volatile organic analysis vial and allowed to rest for 24 h at room temperature (21 °C) in the laboratory. Then 2 mL of headspace air was transferred to a 450 mL canister and pressurized to approximately 1.5 times of atmospheric pressure. Using the canister analysis system, the concentrations were calculated in parts per billion (ppb) of analytes in the headspace. VOCs concentration from the blank of each medium was subtracted from the surgical smoke samples. Two samples were collected for each cell medium in sampling #4 and #6.

Cell culture–human small airway epithelial cells

Dr. Tom K. Hei at Columbia University (New York, NY, USA) provided the human small airway epithelial cell lines (SAEC) and these were cultured as previously described [31]. Briefly, the SAEC were maintained in serum free SABM with the following supplements: bovine pituitary extract, hydrocortisone, human epidermal growth factor, epinephrine, transferrin, insulin, retinoic, triiodothyronine, gentimicin amphotericin-B, and bovine serum free albumin-fatty acid free which are all provided as a bullet kit from the manufacturer (Lonza Inc., Allendale, NJ, USA). The SAEC were plated at the appropriate density and allowed to fully attach for 24 h at which point the media was changed. At 48 h after seating the cells, the media was changed to SABM free of supplements. For the last 24 h of the assay, the surgical smoke SABM was added to the SAEC before being assayed.

Cell culture–RAW 264.7 mouse macrophage

Mouse macrophage cells RAW 264.7 (RAW) were purchased from American Type Culture Collection (ATCC) (Manassas, VA, USA) and were maintained following source company guidelines. The RAW cells are cultured in DMEM with L-glutamine (Lonza, Allendale, NJ, USA) with the following supplements: 10% feta bovine serum (FBS) (Flowery Branch, GA, USA) and 5% penicillin/streptomycin (Lonza, Allendale, NJ, USA). RAW cells were plated at the correct density for each experiment and after 24 h were treated with the surgical smoke-DMEM for an additional 24 h before assayed.

Cytotoxicity of surgical smoke in vitro

SAEC were plated at 1.5×10^4 cells per well and the RAW cells were plated at 1.0×10^4 cells per well (BD Biosciences, San Jose, CA, USA). Changes in cellular proliferation after a 24 h treatment with surgical smoke were assayed using the 3-(4,5-dimethylthiazol-2-yl)-5-(3-

carboxymethoxyphenyl)-2-(4-sulfophenyl)-2H-tetrazolium (MTS) assay (Cell Titer 96 ° Aqueous One Solution Cell Proliferation Assay kit (Promega, Madison, WI, USA) following the manufacturer's guidelines.

Lactate dehydrogenase production in vitro after treatment with surgical smoke

To measure the membrane integrity of the SAEC or RAW cells, 1.5×10^4 SAEC and 1.0×10^4 RAW per well were plated in 96 well plates and assayed after a 24 h treatment with surgical smoke using the CytoTox-ONE™ Homogeneous Membrane Integrity Assay (Promega, Madison, WI, USA) following the manufacturer's protocol.

Reactive oxygen species (ROS) production after treatment with surgical smoke

SAEC and RAW were plated at 1.5×10^4 and 1.0×10^4 cells per well in a 96 well plate, respectively. For the last thirty minutes of a 24 h treatment with surgical smoke, the cells were dosed with 5 µM 2′,7′-dichlorofluorescin diacetate (DCFDA) (Life Technologies, Carlsbad, CA) in dimethyl sulfoxide (DMSO). The plate was then read at 492 nm and 517 nm wavelengths in a microplate reader to analyze the ROS production.

Results

Airborne particles and VOCs concentrations of surgical smoke

The generation rate of the smoke may be different not only from real surgeries but also between each 15 min generation. It was technically difficult to quantify collected particles and dissolved VOCs in cell medium; therefore, airborne particles and VOCs concentrations during generations were reported together with head space analysis of VOC samples dissolved in cell culture media, which approximates real human exposure in healthcare environment.

Average particle number concentrations in operating room background (30 min) and each surgical smoke generation (15 min) measured by a condensation particle counter (particle size range 0.01–1.0 µm) for each sampling are shown in Fig. 1. The average background particle concentration ranged from 1 to 1600 particles/cm³. Due to a malfunction of the CPC, particle concentrations in sampling #5 were not obtained. The average particle number concentrations ranged from 900 (Generation #1 in Sampling #1) to 54,000 (Generation #2 in Sampling #4) particles/cm³. Ratios of average of 15 min surgical smoke generation to average of background particle number concentration ranged from 2 (sampling #2 and #5) to 5200 (sampling #1; high ratio due to low background concentration ≈ 1 particle/cm³). An example of the particle size distributions in Sampling #6 is shown in Fig. 2. Average and standard deviation of the count median diameters was 92 ± 1.7 nm. Background particle distribution was significantly different from particle distributions of all generations ($p < 0.05$) and generation #3 and #4 showed significant difference in accordance with a two-way ANOVA using Tukey's Studentized Range test (SAS Ver. 9.4, SAS Institute Inc., Cary NC).Qualitative SEM analysis was conducted with samples from filtered DMEM media sample and an example of a particle is shown in Fig. 3 along with un-calibrated elemental counts by energy-dispersive x-ray spectrometer. The particles were amorphous shape and had similar X-ray element distributions. Airborne particles in the micrometer size-range were observed but particles in nanometer sizes that

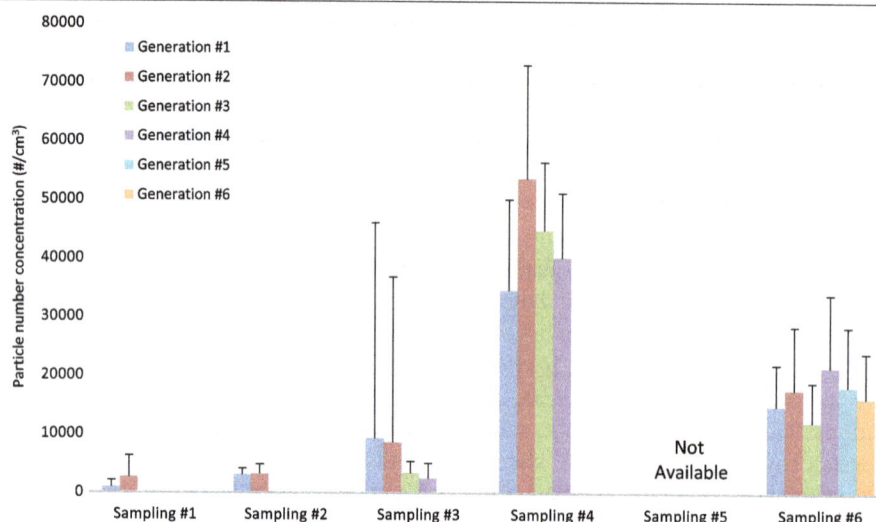

Fig. 1 Average and standard deviation of particle number concentration in each surgical smoke generation (15 min) measured by a condensation particle counter (particle size range 0.01–1.0 µm)

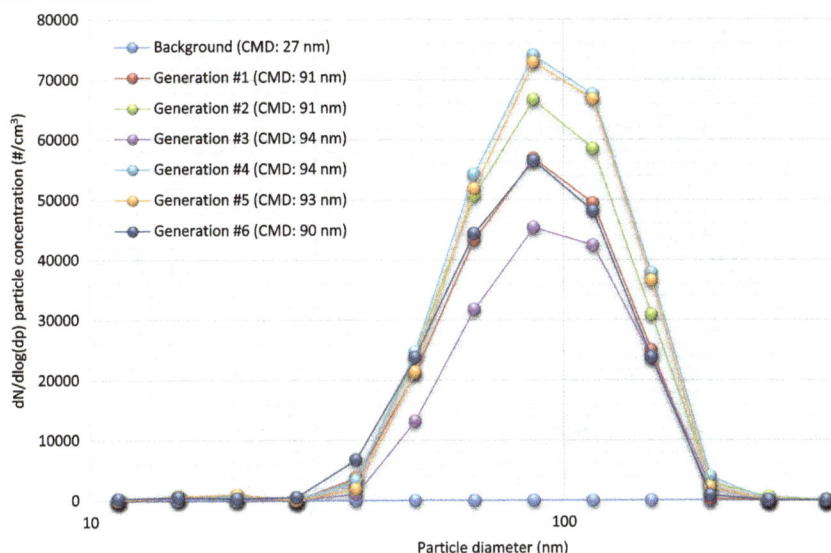

Fig. 2 Particle size distribution of surgical smoke measured with a Nanoscan Scanning Mobility Particle Sizer nanoparticle sizer (Sampling #6). CMD is counter median diameter

were detected with direct reading instruments were not identified.

Average concentrations ($\mu g/m^3$; average of all canister samples ($n = 36$), area and grab sampling, from each sampling session) of VOCs sampled with evacuated canisters for each sampling are shown in Table 1 along with average background concentrations. Higher concentrations of VOCs were found with grab sampling than area sampling. All targeted 17 different VOCs were detected in most of sampling sessions. Higher concentration of the VOCs were found in sampling with surgical smoke compared to background concentration. Acetaldehyde, ethanol and isopropyl alcohol were predominantly detected in every sample with high concentrations (up to 14,000 $\mu g/m^3$ of isopropyl alcohol) compared to other VOCs. Tentatively identified VOCs found in background air sampling with the NIST 2008 Mass Spectral Library(quality factor > 90%) were propene, 2-propanol, 2-propanone, 3-buten-2-one, acetone, acetonitrile, butane 2,2-dimethyl-, ethanol, isoflurane, pentane 2-methyl-, phenol, sevoflurane. Tentatively identified VOCs found in air sampling with surgical smoke generation were 1-propene, 2-methyl-; 1 butanal, 3-methyl-; 1 butanal, 2-methyl-; propene; propyne; 1,4-pentadiene; 1,3-butadiene, 2-methyl-; 2-propenenitrile; 1,3-butadiene; 1-buten-3-yne, 2-methyl-; 1-hexene; 1-heptene; *trans*-1-butyl-2-methylcyclopropane; 2-butenenitrile; 3-butenenitrile; pyridine; pyrrole; propanal, 2-methyl-; 1,3-pentadiene; 1,3-cyclopentadiene; cyclopentene; 2-propenal; *cis*-1-butyl-2-methyl-cyclopropane; cyclopropane, 1-ethyl-2-heptyl-; cyclopropane, ethylidene-; pentane; 2-methyl-1-butene; 1-

decanol; 2,3-pentadiene; 4-methyl-1,3-pentadiene; 1-pentene, 2-methyl-; 1-methylcyclopropene; 1,3-pentadiene, (E)-; 1H-pyrrole.

Head space analysis results are shown in Table 2. Less VOCs were detected by the head space analysis compared to canister sample analysis due to different solubility and volatility of the VOCs while some VOCs were higher concentrations with large variation.

Cytotoxicity of surgical smoke

It has been suggested that surgical smoke is toxic both in vitro and in vivo [12, 24]. Because the surgical smoke has ultrafine particles, the pulmonary alveolar region could potentially be affected; therefore, cytotoxicity was measured in human small airway epithelial cells (SAEC). Macrophage cells are the first line of defense against any foreign material that enters the body; therefore it is of importance to measure the cytotoxicity of RAW cells. SAEC and RAW cells were dosed with surgical smoke collected into the respective media or a background or field blank sample control using an MTS assay. Surgical smoke caused approximately 25% cell death in the SAEC and 40% in the RAW cells compared to background and field blank (Fig. 4). Both of these changes were statistically significant ($p < 0.05$) when compared to either the background or field blank samples. This would suggest that the cell death seen is due to the surgical smoke generated from the human breast tissue. Taken together this data would suggest that the surgical smoke is more cytotoxic to the RAW cells when compared to the SAEC cells.

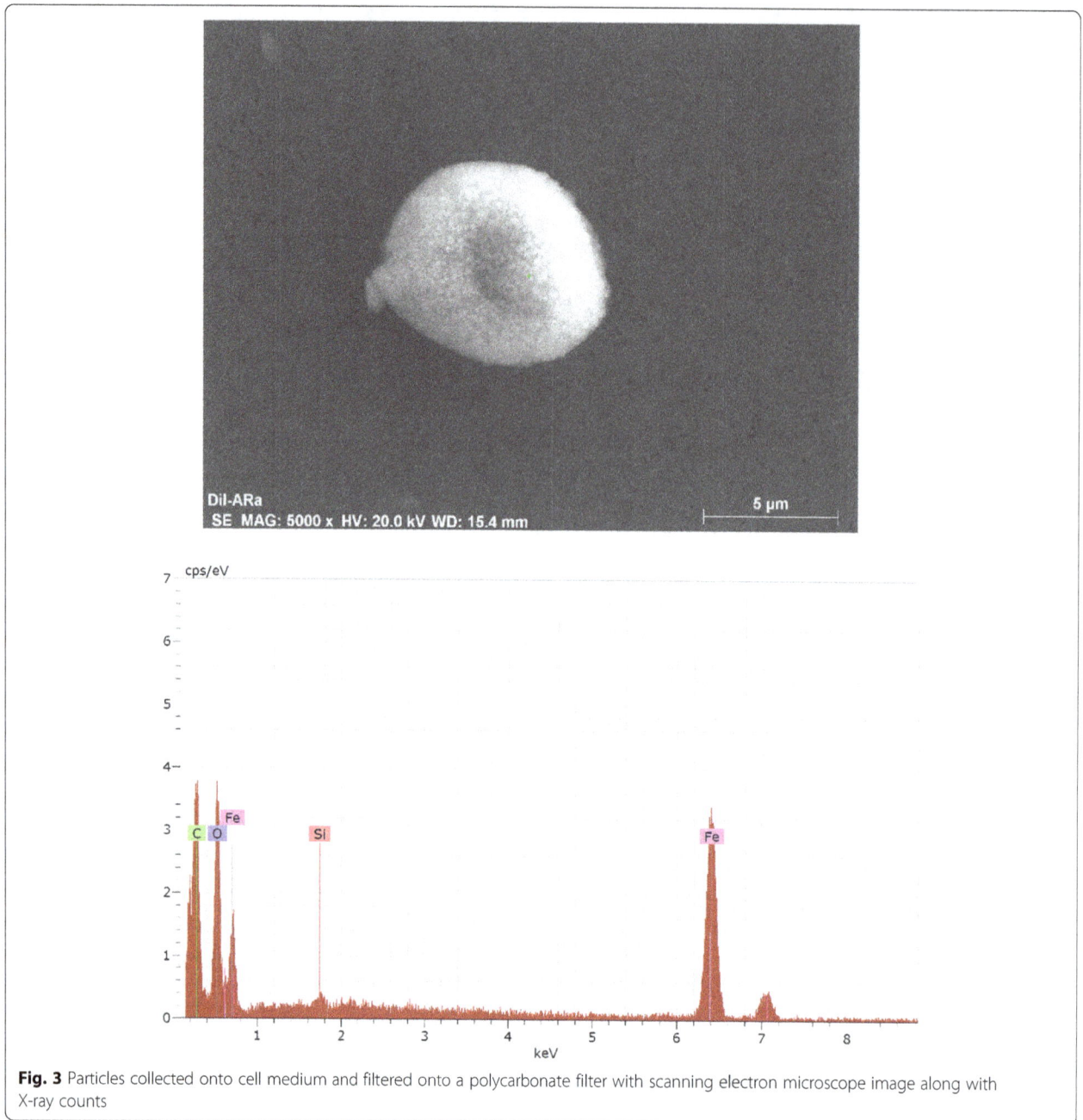

Fig. 3 Particles collected onto cell medium and filtered onto a polycarbonate filter with scanning electron microscope image along with X-ray counts

Production of lactate dehydrogenase (LDH) by surgical smoke

Ultrafine particles have been shown to induce the production of lactate dehydrogenase (LDH) which is a measurement of cellular membrane damage [32, 33]. To analyze the integrity of the cellular membrane, lactate dehydrogenase (LDH) levels released into the cell culture media after a 24 h treatment of surgical smoke were analyzed. Figure 5 shows that both SAEC and RAW cells produced significantly higher levels of LDH after a 24 h dose of surgical smoke compared to both the background and field blank samples. This would suggest that

the surgical smoke caused membrane damage in both the SAEC and RAW cells.

Production of ROS by surgical smoke

ROS production has been shown to be a key mechanism to lead to cytotoxicity both in vitro and in vivo [34, 35]. Therefore, it was of interest to determine if surgical smoke induced the production of ROS. To determine if ROS was produced, 5 μM DCFDA was added to the SAEC and RAW cells for the last 30 min of a 24 h exposure of surgical smoke. If free radicals are present, DCFDA is oxidized and cleaved into DCF which fluoresces. As shown in

Table 1 Average concentrations (μg/m³) of volatile organic compounds from surgical smoke generation

	REL (μg/m3)	Background	Sampling #1	Sampling #2	Sampling #3	Sampling #4	Sampling #5	Sampling #6
Acetaldehyde	lowest feasible	12	13	17	1200	940	630	2100
Acetone	590,000	21	30	41	38	150	81	170
acetonitrile	34,000	5	1	12	440	410	130	570
α-pinene	–	4	–	–	5	4	5	9
Benzene	3190	2	1	–	120	560	220	130
Chloroform	9780	–	–	–	–	–	10	–
d-Limonene	–	7	–	11	10	12	10	18
Ethanol	1,900,000	450	37	1200	290	810	230	1100
Ethylbenzene	435,000	2	–	5	51	39	15	23
Isopropyl Alcohol	980,000	870	110	1000	380	1900	400	14,000
m,p-Xylene	435,000	3	4	4	21	13	10	3
Methyl methacrylate	410,000	4	–	–	8	–	11	–
Methylene chloride	lowest feasible	–	–	–	–	–	7	–
n-Hexane	180,000	3	–	–	22	85	42	33
o-Xylene	435,000	0	6	–	4	6	6	2
Styrene	215,000	–	–	–	91	49	17	31
Toluene	375,000	4	4	6	90	190	72	99

-: below detection limit or not detected
REL: Recommended exposure limits from National Institute for Occupational Safety and Health

Table 2 Volatile organic compounds concentrations from head space analysis

Volatile Organic Compounds	REL (μg/m³)	Dulbecco's Modified Eagle Medium (μg/m³)		Small Airway Epithelial Cell growth medium (μg/m³)	
		Test 1	Test 2	Test 1	Test 2
Acetaldehyde	lowest feasible	1700	4000	1700	2900
Acetone	590,000	*	*	540	*
Acetonitrile	34,000	420	–	440	–
alpha-Pinene	–	–	–	–	–
Benzene	3190	–	160	31	260
Chloroform	9780	–	–	–	–
D-Limonene	–	–	–	–	–
Ethanol	1,900,000	*	*	490	5800
Ethylbenzene	435,000	*	–	700	98
Isopropyl Alcohol	980,000	25,000	47,000	4400	37,000
m,p-Xylene	435,000	*	–	550	140
Methyl Methacrylate	410,000	–	–	–	–
Methylene Chloride	lowest feasible	–	–	–	–
n-Hexane	180,000	–	–	–	–
o-Xylene	435,000	–	–	–	–
Styrene	215,000	–	–	–	–
Toluene	375,000	*	–	66	110

-: below detection limit or not detected
*: the concentration from surgical smoke is smaller than blank cell medium
REL: Recommended exposure limits from National Institute for Occupational Safety and Health

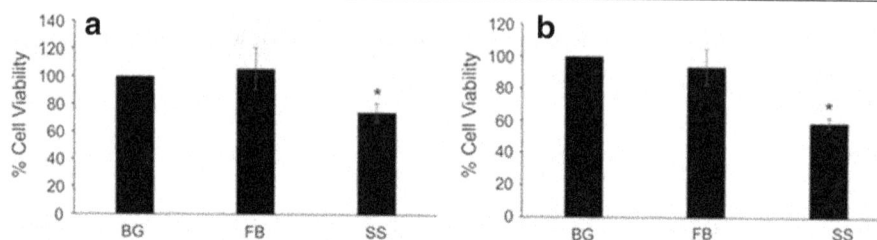

Fig. 4 Surgical Smoke Induced Cytotoxicity. (**a**) SAEC and (**b**) RAW were dosed with surgical smoke for 24 h and then cytotoxicity was measured using an MTS assay. The t-test was applied. Values represent mean ± standard error. $n = 4$ independent biological replicates. * indicates $p < 0.05$ compared to field blank (FB)

Fig. 6, neither SAEC nor RAW cells shown significant increases in ROS production compared to the background or field blanks. This would suggest that the molecular mechanism leading to the cytotoxicity seen by the MTS and LDH assay is independent to superoxide radicals. While there was a trend that SAEC cells did produce ROS compared to the controls, it was not significant and would need further analysis to determine if it was a true induction.

Discussion

The levels of smoke generated in this study most likely represent the worst possible case of exposure, when OR personnel lean in over the patient during surgery, which is likely only for brief periods of time during the workday. Particle concentrations measured with direct reading instruments were comparable to previous studies. Average particle number concentrations measured with a CPC in six different surgeries without local exhaust ventilation (LEV) control ranged from 74 to 12,200 particles/cm^3 with a range of 2–490,000 particles/cm^3 [36]. Ragde et al. reported ultrafine particle exposure levels in five different surgeries when LEV was utilized and a maximum peak level was 272,000 particles/cm^3 while average levels were between 300 and 3900 particles/cm^3 [3]. The average particle number concentration from the present study ranged from 900 to 54,000 particles/cm^3. Elmashae et al. (2018) simulated OR facility to assess surgical smoke (from lamb muscle tissue) exposure of

unprotected OR workers and reported that peaks of the particle size distribution were between 60 and 150 nm, which is consistent with the present study (count median diameters 92 ± 1.7 nm; Fig. 2) [37]. The differences in particle concentrations between the studies might be attributable to surgery type, tissue types, power level of electrocautery, ventilation rate of the operation room, surgeon's technique, utilizing LEV system, etc. Personal VOC exposure levels from full-shift sampling were lower than the concentrations found during the 15 min or 1 mins sampling of the present study because the majority of a workers' shift would not involve electrocauterization. For instance, LeBouf et al. [29] reported VOCs exposure levels in 14 occupations of healthcare workers and personal exposure levels (µg/m^3) of surgical technologists (geometric mean) were 1031 (ethanol), 1077 (isopropyl alcohol), 0.98 (benzene), 112 (toluene), < 0.16 (ethylbenzene), 1.8 (m,p-xylene), < 0.19 (o-xylene), 72 (acetone), 0.14 (hexane), < 0.17 (methyl methacrylate), 3.1 (methylene chloride), 0.18 (chloroform). Relatively high levels of ethanol and isopropanol are to be expected in hospital settings and were also noted in our background results.

Large number concentration of ultrafine particles measured by direct reading instrument were not identified by SEM analysis in this study. A companion study compared airborne particle and VOCs levels with and without LEV controls and utilized the same procedure and human tissues as the present study to generate the

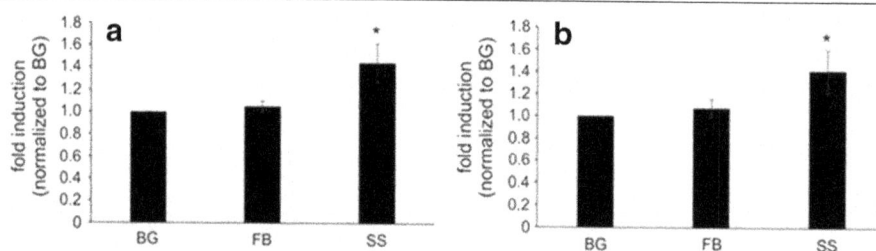

Fig. 5 Surgical Smoke Induced Lactate Dehydrogenase. (**a**) SAEC and (**b**) RAW cells were dosed with surgical smoke for 24 h and analyzed for the production of LDH. The t-test was applied. Values represent mean ± standard error. n = 4 independent biological replicates. * indicates $p < 0.05$ compared to field blank (FB)

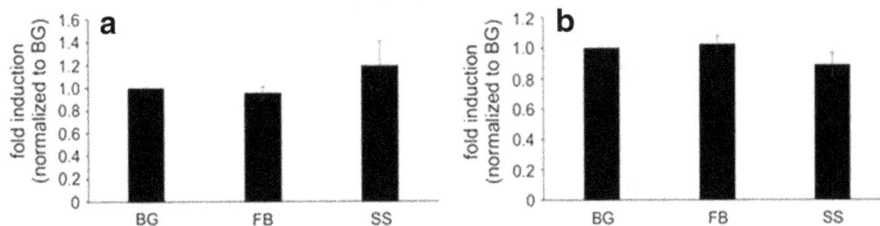

Fig. 6 ROS Induced by Surgical Smoke. (**a**) SAEC and (**b**) RAW dosed cells were analyzed for DCFDA after a 24 h treatment with surgical smoke. The t-test was applied. Values represent mean ± standard error. n = 4 independent biological replicates

surgical smoke [38]. The study conducted qualitative scanning electron microscope (SEM) analysis using an inhalable sampler (IOM sampler) to detect airborne surgical smoke particles along with elemental counts by energy-dispersive x-ray. The finding from that study was comparable to the present study. The particles were amorphous in shape and had similar elemental distribution. Airborne particles in micrometer sizes were observed in 45 samples but ultrafine particles were not identified. Most of the airborne particles appeared to be water or steam from cellular fluid from adipose tissues as previously noted [5, 39]. Kunachak and Sobhon reported SEM images of smoke particles generated with a carbon dioxide laser from papillomatous tissue and particles sizes ranged from 0.5 to 27 μm [39]. Particles smaller than 500 nm were not found.

The results of the MTS assays in this study suggest that the surgical smoke is cytotoxic to both the SAEC and RAW cell lines, but to varying degrees. One possible reason for the difference seen in the levels of cytotoxic effect on the cell lines is because the molecular mechanisms related to cell death in each cell line are different. To explain the cytotoxic effects of the surgical smoke in SAEC and RAW, LDH was measured and shown to be elevated in both the SAEC and RAW which correlates with the MTS assay. This data would suggest that the surgical smoke is a potential health hazard to individuals during surgery, which correlates with previously published data [24]. The cytotoxicity could be related to the exposure to the VOCs dissolved in the culture media listed in Tables 1 and 2 or it could possibly be due to the surgical smoke collected in the culture media. The results of Tables 1 and 2 demonstrated that all the concentrations of the VOCs are below the NIOSH RELs. Thus, it is possible that the VOCs may not play a major role in the surgical smoke-induced cellular toxicity. To clarify this point, additional studies will need to be performed to separate the particles and VOCs. In the present study, concentrations of airborne VOCs have been determined (Table 1) whereas the exact concentrations of the VOCs in cell culture medium have not determined. The head space analysis was applied to indirectly measure the concentrations of the dissolved VOCs in the cell culture

medium. Therefore, it is possible that some disparities might exist between our measured concentrations of VOCs and the real concentrations in the cell culture medium due to the different solubility and the rate of evaporation of each VOC. In the future, the direct measurement of the VOC concentration in the cell culture medium needs to be developed to identify the contribution of the VOCs in surgical smoke-induced cellular toxicity.

Oxidative stress can mediate molecular mechanisms of cytotoxicity in particulate exposure [35]. Oxidative stress is a term that encompasses superoxide radicals (O_2^-), hydrogen peroxide (H_2O_2), hydroxyl radical (^-OH) and peroxynitrite ($ONOO^-$) [34]. To determine if oxidative stress played a role in the cytotoxicity that is seen in the SAEC and RAW after treatment with surgical smoke, DCFDA was used to measure ROS production. Based upon the results, ROS production was not elevated in either the SAEC or RAW suggesting the cytotoxicity seen from surgical smoke is independent of ROS production. To investigate other possible mechanisms, further experiments would be needed. Ultrafine particles are also deposited in the nasal airways and this may be worth further investigation given the reporting of sinonasal symptoms [14].

Conclusions
This study collected surgical smoke (particulate and VOCs) into cell culture media in a real-time exposure setting that allowed for characterization of the particles and analysis of the VOCs released into the air, and the analysis of the toxic effects of the smoke in an in vitro model. The results indicate that the surgical smoke is toxic in both the SAEC and RAW although to varying degrees. This data again is consistent with previously published data. To fully understand the toxic effect of the surgical smoke, further experiments would need to be performed in vitro to determine if the particles or the VOCs (or the combination) are the cause of the identified cytotoxicity and also to perform in vivo testing.

Abbreviations
CPC: condensation particle counter; DCFDA: 2',7'-dichlorofluorescin diacetate; DMEM: Dulbecco's Modified Eagle Medium; DMSO: Dimethyl sulfoxide;

FBS: fetal bovine serum; HCN: hydrogen cyanide; HHEs: Health Hazard Evaluations; IOM: Institute of Occupational Medicine; LDH: Lactate dehydrogenase; LEV: Local exhaust ventilation; MTS: 3-(4,5-dimethylthiazol-2-yl)-5-(3-carboxymethoxyphenyl)-2-(4-sulfophenyl)-2H-tetrazolium; NIOSH: National Institute for Occupational Safety and Health; PAHs: Polyaromatic hydrocarbons; ppb: Parts per billion; RAW: RAW 264.7 mouse macrophages; ROS: Reactive oxygen species; SABM: Small Airway Epithelial Cell growth medium; SAEC: Small airway epithelial cells; SEM: Scanning electron microscope; SMPS: Scanning mobility particle sizer; VOCs: Volatile organic compounds; WVU: West Virginia University

Acknowledgements
Special thanks to Dr. Debra Novak, RN who provided insight and expertise and National Personal Protective Technology Laboratory and WVU Ruby Memorial hospital for supporting the project.

Funding
National Institute for Occupational Safety and Health, Project #927ZLEN: Evaluation of Surgical Smoke Exposures in Medical Facilities.

Disclaimer
The findings and conclusions in this report are those of the authors and do not necessarily represent the views of the National Institute for Occupational Safety and Health, Centers for Disease Control and Prevention.

Authors' contributions
JSisler, JShaffer and YQ were involved in the design of the toxicology study, the toxicological assays and the preparation of the manuscript. TL, JCS, RLeBouf and MH were involved in air sampling, collection of surgical smoke, VOCs analysis and preparation of the manuscript. All authors read and approved the final manuscript.

Authors' information
The authors are biologist and research industrial hygienist at the Centers for Disease Control and Prevention/National Institute for Occupational Safety and Health.

Competing interests
The authors declare that they have no competing interests.

Author details
[1]Pathology and Physiology Research Branch, Health Effects Laboratory Division, National Institute for Occupational Safety and Health, Centers for Disease Control and Prevention, 1095 Willowdale Road, Morgantown, West Virginia 26505, USA. [2]Exposure Assessment Branch, Health Effects Laboratory Division, National Institute for Occupational Safety and Health, Centers for Disease Control and Prevention, 1095 Willowdale Road, Morgantown, West Virginia 26505, USA. [3]Field Study Branch, Respiratory Health Division, National Institute for Occupational Safety and Health, Centers for Disease Control and Prevention, 1095 Willowdale Road, Morgantown, West Virginia 26505, USA. [4]Zefon International, Inc., 5350 SW 1st Lane, Ocala, FL, USA. [5]Department of Environmental Engineering Sciences, University of Florida, Gainesville, FL, USA.

References
1. Roan S. Even when surgery is over, sedation's risks could linger. Death rates are higher for months afterward, studies find. Los Angeles Times: Doctors search for a reason; 2005.
2. Bigony L. Risks associated with exposure to surgical smoke plume: a review of the literature. AORN J. 2007;86(6):1013–20. quiz 1021-4
3. Ragde SF, Jorgensen RB, Foreland S. Characterisation of exposure to ultrafine particles from surgical smoke by use of a fast mobility particle sizer. Ann Occup Hyg. 2016;60(7):860–74.
4. Barrett WL, Garber SM. Surgical smoke: a review of the literature. Is this just a lot of hot air. Surg Endosc. 2003;17(6):979–87.
5. Gonzalez-Bayon L, Gonzalez-Moreno S, Ortega-Perez G. Safety considerations for operating room personnel during hyperthermic intraoperative intraperitoneal chemotherapy perfusion. Eur J Surg Oncol. 2006;32(6):619–24.
6. Al Sahaf OS, Vega-Carrascal I, Cunningham FO, McGrath JP, Bloomfield FJ. Chemical composition of smoke produced by high-frequency electrosurgery. Ir J Med Sci. 2007;176(3):229–32.
7. Hill DS, O'Neill JK, Powell RJ, Oliver DW. Surgical smoke - a health hazard in the operating theatre: a study to quantify exposure and a survey of the use of smoke extractor systems in UK plastic surgery units. J Plast Reconstr Aesthet Surg. 2012;65(7):911–6.
8. Ortolano GA, Cervia JS, Canonica FP. Surgical smoke- a concern for infection control practitioners., in managing. Infect Control. 2009:48–54.
9. Pierce JS, Lacey SE, Lippert JF, Lopez R, Franke JE. Laser-generated air contaminants from medical laser applications: a state-of-the-science review of exposure characterization, health effects, and control. J Occup Environ Hyg. 2011;8(7):447–66.
10. Pierce JS, Lacey SE, Lippert JF, Lopez R, Franke JE, Colvard MD. An assessment of the occupational hazards related to medical lasers. J Occup Environ Med. 2011;53(11):1302–9.
11. Ulmer BC. The hazards of surgical smoke. AORN J. 2008;87(4):721–34. quiz 735-8
12. Baggish MS, Elbakry M. The effects of laser smoke on the lungs of rats. Am J Obstet Gynecol. 1987;156(5):1260–5.
13. Freitag L, Chapman GA, Sielczak M, Ahmed A, Russin D. Laser smoke effect on the bronchial system. Lasers Surg Med. 1987;7(3):283–8.
14. Ball K. Compliance with surgical smoke evacuation guidelines: implications for practice. AORN J. 2010;92(2):142–9.
15. King B, McCullough J. Health hazard evaluation report HETA #2001-0066-3019. NIOSH. 2006;
16. King B, McCullough J. Health hazard evaluation report HETA #2000-0402-3021. NIOSH. 2006;
17. King B, McCullough J. Health hazard evaluation report HETA #2001-0030-3020. NIOSH. 2006;
18. Moss EC, Bryant C, Stewart J, Whong WZ, Fleeger A, Gunter BJ. Health hazard evaluation report HETA 88-101-2008. NIOSH. 1990;
19. Bryant CJ, Gorman R, Stewart J, Whong Z. Health hazard evaluation report HETA-85-126-1932. NIOSH. 1985;
20. Gatti JE, Bryant CJ, Noone RB, Murphy JB. The mutagenicity of electrocautery smoke. Plast Reconstr Surg. 1992;89(5):781–4. discussion 785-6
21. Eshleman EJ, LeBlanc M, Rokoff LB, Xu Y, Hu R, Lee K, et al. Occupational exposures and determinants of ultrafine particle concentrations during laser hair removal procedures. Environ Health. 2017;16(1):30.
22. Daigle CC, Chalupa DC, Gibb FR, Morrow PE, Oberdorster G, Utell MJ, et al. Ultrafine particle deposition in humans during rest and exercise. Inhal Toxicol. 2003;15(6):539–52.
23. Chalupa DC, Morrow PE, Oberdorster G, Utell MJ, Frampton MW. Ultrafine particle deposition in subjects with asthma. Environ Health Perspect. 2004; 112(8):879–82.
24. Hensman C, Newman EL, Shimi SM, Cuschieri A. Cytotoxicity of electro-surgical smoke produced in an anoxic environment. Am J Surg. 1998; 175(3):240–1.
25. Ziegler BL, Thomas CA, Meier T, Muller R, Fliedner TM, Weber L. Generation of infectious retrovirus aerosol through medical laser irradiation. Lasers Surg Med. 1998;22(1):37–41.
26. Fletcher JN, Mew D, DesCoteaux JG. Dissemination of melanoma cells within electrocautery plume. Am J Surg. 1999;178(1):57–9.
27. Nduka CC, Poland N, Kennedy M, Dye J, Darzi A. Does the ultrasonically activated scalpel release viable airborne cancer cells? Surg Endosc. 1998; 12(8):1031–4.

.

28. Steege AL, Boiano JM, Sweeney MH. Secondhand smoke in the operating room? Precautionary practices lacking for surgical smoke. Am J Ind Med. 2016;59(11):1020–31.

29. LeBouf RF, Stefaniak AB, Virji MA. Validation of evacuated canisters for sampling volatile organic compounds in healthcare settings. J Environ Monit. 2012;14(3):977–83.

30. LeBouf RF, Virji MA, Saito R, Henneberger PK, Simcox N, Stefaniak AB. Exposure to volatile organic compounds in healthcare settings. Occup Environ Med. 2014;71(9):642–50.

31. Piao CQ, Liu L, Zhao YL, Balajee AS, Suzuki M, Hei TK. Immortalization of human small airway epithelial cells by ectopic expression of telomerase. Carcinogenesis. 2005;26(4):725–31.

32. Lu S, Zhang W, Zhang R, Liu P, Wang Q, Shang Y, et al. Comparison of cellular toxicity caused by ambient ultrafine particles and engineered metal oxide nanoparticles. Part Fibre Toxicol. 2015;12:5.

33. Thomson EM, Breznan D, Karthikeyan S, MacKinnon-Roy C, Charland JP, Dabek-Zlotorzynska E, et al. Cytotoxic and inflammatory potential of size-fractionated particulate matter collected repeatedly within a small urban area. Part Fibre Toxicol. 2015;12:24.

34. Qian Y, Castranova V, Shi X. New perspectives in arsenic-induced cell signal transduction. J Inorg Biochem. 2003;96(2–3):271–8.

35. Xia T, Kovochich M, Nel A. The role of reactive oxygen species and oxidative stress in mediating particulate matter injury. Clin Occup Environ Med. 2006; 5(4):817–36.

36. Bruske-Hohlfeld I, Preissler G, Jauch KW, Pitz M, Nowak D, Peters A, et al. Surgical smoke and ultrafine particles. J Occup Med Toxicol. 2008;3:31.

37. Elmashae Y, Richard HK, Yermakov M, Reponen T, Grinshpun SA. Surgical smoke simulation study: physical characterization and respiratory protection. Aerosol Sci Technol. 2018;52(1):38–45.

38. Lee T, Soo JC, LeBouf RF, Burns D, Schwegler-Berry D, Kashon M et al. Surgical smoke control with local exhaust ventilation: Experimental study. J Occup Environ Hyg. 2018;15(4):341–50.

39. Kunachak S, Sobhon P. The potential alveolar hazard of carbon dioxide laser-induced smoke. J Med Assoc Thail. 1998;81(4):278–82.

20

Occupational infection and needle stick injury among clinical laboratory workers in Al-Madinah city

Omar F. Khabour[1,2]* iD, Khalil H. Al Ali[1] and Waleed H. Mahallawi[1]

Abstract

Background: Clinical laboratory workers face biohazard such as needlestick injury and occupational infection on a daily basis. In this study, we examined self-reported frequency of occupational infection and needlestick injury among the clinical laboratory workers in Al- Madinah, Saudi Arabia.

Methods: A total of 234 clinical laboratory workers were recruited from private and government health sectors to answer a self-administered questionnaire that was prepared to achieve the aims of the study.

Results: The results showed that approximately 33% of the sample had an experienced occupational infection while 24% had experienced a needlestick injury. Approximately, 49% reported that they always recap needle after use, whereas 15% reported doing that most of the times. Occupational infection, needlestick injury and recapping needles after use were associated with lack of training on biosafety ($P < 0.05$).

Conclusion: The frequency of occupational infection and needlestick injury among clinical laboratory workers in Al-Madinah is high. Interventions related to biosafety and infection control and the use of needlestick prevention devices might be useful in lowering such frequency.

Keywords: Biosafety, Clinical laboratory, Al-Madinah, Occupational infection, Needlestick

Background

Clinical laboratory workers are subjected daily to occupational hazards that include infections from biological samples and contaminated equipment [1]. For example, literature showed that workers at clinical laboratory are at increased risk of acquiring viral infections such as hepatitis viruses (HBV and HCV), human immunodeficiency viruses (HIV), Middle East Respiratory Syndrome (MERS-CoV), and others [2, 3]. In addition, bacterial occupational infection has been shown to be high among clinical laboratory workers and other health care providers [4–6]. For example, in a study that was conducted in the United Kingdom, clinical laboratory workers were at about seven times higher risk of acquiring tuberculosis infection in reference to the general population [7].

One of the major sources of infection among health care professionals is needlestick injuries [8, 9]. According to the literature, needlestick injury is responsible for the majority of hepatitis and HIV infections among health care professionals. In addition, the majority of these infections occur in developing countries [10]. Analysis of needlestick injuries showed that injuries could happen during all steps of needle use procedures [8]. However recapping of the needle, work load and lack of training, and not following safety precautions are among major risk factors [11–13]. Requiring workers to follow procedures and practices related to infection control, injury prevention and the use of protective equipment can significantly reduce infections and needlestick injury [14, 15].

The aim of the current study is to investigate self-reported frequency of occupational infection and needlestick injury among the clinical laboratory workers in Al- Madinah. In addition, factors that are associated with these incidences were also examined.

---

* Correspondence: ofkhabour@taibahu.edu.sa
[1]Department of Clinical Laboratory Sciences, Taibah University, Al-Madinah 41477, Saudi Arabia
[2]Department of Medical Laboratory Sciences, Jordan University of Science and Technology, Irbid, Jordan

AL-Madinah city, the second holiest site in Islam after Mecca, receives more than 10 million pilgrims each year, who come from all the world. The city provides health services to pilgrims and residents through 10 major hospitals and several medical centers. The considerable diversity of patients and heavy load highlight the importance of adopting good practices and safety protection measures to limit the spread of diseases in the city. Therefore, this study was designed to examine the self-reported occurrence of needlestick injuries, safety practices (i.e. recapping), and occupational infection among laboratory workers in Al-Madinah. The results of the current study can be used for interventions that target the enhancement of biosafety measures among Al-Madinah clinical laboratory workers.

Methods

Study participants

A survey-based study design was adapted to investigate the incidence and factors associated with needlestick injury and occupational infection among clinical laboratory workers in Al-Madinah city. Al-Madinah is the second holy city after Mecca in Saudi Arabia that host the Prophet's Mosque. According to the Statistics Directorate, the population of Al-Madinah is estimated to be close to 1.5 million. The city receives more than 10 million pilgrims each year who came from most world countries.

Clinical laboratory staff from the majority of Al-Madinah clinics (eight private and ten governmental) was invited to be part of the study. Details about the purpose of the study and assurance of confidentiality were presented to participants as part of the recruitment procedure. About 405 participants were invited to fill out the questionnaire among which 234 agreed to participate (58%). The questionnaire was anonymous and self-administered and required about 5–8 min to fill out. This anonymity was a requirement that ensured no possible risks for the participants. To ensure confidentiality, the research team has removed the IP addresses from the data spreadsheet after completion of the recruitment process. The study was approved by the Institutional Review Board of the Faculty of Applied Medical Sciences (ID number: MLT 2016–23).

Study instrument

The questionnaire was prepared from previous studies that examined needlestick injury, occupation safety and factors associated with their incidence [16–18]. The questionnaire comprised of 20 items that were presented with a choice of answers. The instrument was subjected to several revisions after comments were received from colleagues at the Department of Medical Laboratory Sciences and a pilot study that involved 20 staff from diagnostic clinical labs. The questionnaire was divided into three parts. The first part gathered information about participants' age, gender, experience, prior training on biosafety, specialty, academic degree and place of work. The second part focused on needlestick injury and related behaviors such as covering needle after use (re-sheathing or re-capping). In this part, the participants were asked if they have experienced a needlestick injury during their career period. In addition, the participant was asked about frequency of re-capping needles after use. The third part focused on occupational infection and knowledge about disinfection procedures and infection routes. Participants were asked if they have

Table 1 General characteristics of participants

Variable	Category	Number of subjects	Percentage
Age	18–30	135	57.7%
	31–40	70	29.9%
	> 40	29	12.4%
Gender	Male	147	62.8%
	Female	87	37.2%
Social position	Married	130	55.6%
	Single	96	41.0%
	Divorced/widowed	8	3.4%
Place of work	Governmental clinics	132	56.4%
	Private clinics	102	43.6%
Academic degree	College degrez	30	12.8%
	Bachelor degree	167	71.4%
	Graduate degree	37	15.8%
Academic Field	Laboratory Sciences	174	74.4%
	Applied Biology	25	10.7%
	Health Science	19	8.1%
	Others	16	6.8%
Assigned work	Clinical chemistry	71	30.3%
	Hematology	99	42.3%
	Histology/pathology	27	11.5%
	Microbiology/Immunology	37	15.8%
Years of experience	≤ 3	91	38.9%
	4–6	64	27.4%
	7–10	50	21.4%
	> 10	28	12.0%
Position	Residency	50	21.4%
	Technician	141	60.3%
	Lab director	18	7.7%
	Consultant	25	10.7%
Training on Biosafety	Yes	152	65.0%
	No	82	35.0%

experienced an occupational infection, which was defined as acquiring bacterial or viral infection from work place during their career period. Participants filled the questionnaire electronically using google forms.

Statistical analysis

The SPSS software was used to analyze the data, which was presented as frequencies and number of participants in each category. Chi square test, Fisher Exact test and odd ratios with 95% confidence intervals were used to correlate demographic variables with needlestick and occupational infection. The P value of significance was set at 0.05 threshold.

Results

A total of 234 medical laboratory workers was recruited to participate in the study. The majority (Table 1) of participants were young (57.7%, age range: 18–30), males (62.8%), married (55.6%), belong to governmental clinics (56.4%), bachelor degree holder (71.4%), have a specialty in clinical laboratory sciences (74.4%), works as technicians (60.3%) and received training on laboratory safety (65%). About 40% have less than 3 years of experience, whereas 27.4% have between 4 and 6 years of experience (Table 1). The sample is well distributed according different branches of laboratory sciences that include clinical chemistry (30.3%), hematology (42.3%), histology (11.5%) and microbiology/immunology (15.8%). All

Table 2 Incidence of needle stick injuries among participants

Variable	Category	(Yes) Had needle stick injuries	(NO) Had needle stick injuries	Odd ratio	95% confidence interval	P. value
Age	18–30	32 (57.2%)	103 (57.9%)	–	–	
	31–40	18 (32.1%)	52 (29.2%)	1.123	0.60–2.09	0.714
	> 40	6 (10.7%)	23 (12.9%)	0.864	0.35–2.08	0.739
Gender	Male	39 (69.6%)	108 (60.7%)	–	–	
	Female	17 (30.4%)	70 (39.3%)	0.672	0.37–1.20	0.181
Social status	Married	34 (60.7%)	96 (53.9%)	–	–	
	Single	18 (32.1%)	78 (43.8%)	0.643	0.36–1.15	0.139
	Divorced/widowed	4 (7.1%)	4 (2.2%)	3.098	0.62–15.5	0.167
Place of work	Governmental clinics	25 (44.6%)	107 (60.1%)	–	–	
	Private clinics	31 (55.4%)	71 (39.9%)	1.833	1.04–3.21	0.034
Academic degree	College degree	8 (14.3%)	22 (12.4%)	–	–	
	Bachelor degree	38 (67.9%)	129 (72.5%)	0.798	0.34–1.84	0.598
	Graduate degree	10 (17.9%)	27 (15.2%)	1.020	0.36–2.88	0.957
Academic Field	Laboratory Sciences	40 (71.4%)	134 (75.3%)	–	–	
	Applied Biology	9 (16.1%)	16 (9.0%)	1.877	0.77–4.52	0.159
	Health Science	6 (10.7%)	13 (7.3%)	1.452	0.55–3.81	0.449
	Others	1 (1.8%)	15 (8.4%)	0.261	0.05–1.28	0.099
Assigned work	Clinical chemistry	15 (26.8%)	55 (30.9%)	–	–	
	Hematology	22 (39.3%)	77 (43.3%)	1.041	0.53–2.04	0.906
	Histology/pathology	8 (14.3%)	19 (10.7%)	1.460	0.56–3.75	0.431
	Microbiology/Immunology	10 (17.9%)	27 (15.2%)	1.377	0.58–3.24	0.464
Years of experience	≤ 3	16 (28.6%)	75 (42.1%)	–	–	
	4–6	18 (32.1%)	46 (25.8%)	1.782	0.88–3.59	0.106
	7–10	17 (30.4%)	33 (18.5%)	2.286	0.92–4.81	0.062
	> 10	4 (7.1%)	24 (13.5%)	0.724	0.26–2.01	0.536
Position	Residency	14 (25.0%)	36 (20.2%)	–	–	
	Technician	32 (57.1%)	109 (61.2%)	0.747	0.37–1.49	0.408
	Lab director	7 (12.5%)	(6.2%)11	1.733	0.56–5.37	0.341
	Consultant	3 (5.4%)	22 (12.4%)	0.333	0.10–1.10	0.072
Training on Biosafety	Yes	29 (51.8%)	123 (69.1%)	–	–	
	No	(48.2%) 27	(30.9%) 55	2.054	1.15–3.66	0.014

participants were vaccinated against HBV as this a requirement by health law in Saudi Arabia before employment in medical laboratories.

The results showed that about 24% of the sample had experienced a needlestick injury. The results showed that the needlestick injury was associated with private clinics ($P < 0.05$) and lack of training on biosafety (Table 2). The participants were asked about capping needle directly after use. Approximately, 49% reported that they always do that, whereas 15% reported doing that most of the times (Table 3). Recapping needle after use, was associated with governmental clinics ($P < 0.01$), technician/residency staff ($P < 0.01$) and lack of training ($P < 0.05$, Table 3). Table 4 shows the incidence of

occupational infection among participants. The incidence was about 33% and it was associated with college degrees ($P < 0.05$) and training on biosafety ($P < 0.05$, Table 4).

Figure 1 shows the awareness of participants about disinfection procedures and infection routes. The results showed that the majority of participants reported excellent to very good awareness levels (> 80%).

Discussions
In this study, the incidence of occupational infection and needlestick injury among clinical laboratory workers in Al-Madinah city was investigated.

Table 3 Covering needle directly after use as reported by participants expressed as number of participants (%)

Variable	Category	Always	Most Times	Neutral	Sometimes	Never	P. value
Age	18–30	76 (61.3)	21 (61.8)	26 (48.1)	6 (50.0)	6 (60.0)	0.770
	31–40	35 (28.2)	8 (23.5)	18 (33.3)	6 (50.0)	3 (30.0)	
	> 40	13 (10.6)	5 (14.7)	9 (16.7)	0 (0.0)	1 (10.0)	
Gender	Male	80 (64.55)	18 (52.9)	36 (66.7)	8 (66.7)	5 (50.0)	0.610
	Female	44 (35.5)	16 (47.1)	18 (33.3)	4 (33.3)	5 (50.0)	
Social status	Married	73 (58.9)	18 (52.9)	27 (50.0)	7 (58.3)	5 (50.0)	0.804
	Single	46 (37.1)	16 (47.1)	24 (44.4)	5 (41.7)	5 (50.0)	
	Divorced/widowed	5 (4.0)	0 (0.0)	3 (5.6)	0 (0.0)	0 (0.0)	
Place of work	Governmental clinics	79 (63.7)	18 (52.9)	21 (38.9)	5 (41.7)	9 (90.0)	0.004
	Private clinics	45 (36.3)	16 (47.1)	33 (61.1)	7 (58.3)	1 (10.0)	
Academic degree	College degree	16 (12.9)	7 (20.6)	4 (7.4)	3 (25.0)	0 (0.0)	0.066
	Bachelor degree	88 (71.0)	26 (76.5)	41 (75.9)	6 (50.0)	6 (60.0)	
	Graduate degree	20 (16.1)	1 (2.9)	9 (16.7)	3 (25.8)	4 (40.0)	
Academic Field	Laboratory Sciences	87 (70.2)	24 (70.6)	46 (85.2)	10 (83.3)	7 (70.0)	0.631
	Applied Biology	14 (11.3)	4 (11.8)	4 (7.4)	1 (8.3)	2 (20.0)	
	Health Science	10 (8.1)	4 (11.8)	3 (5.6)	1 (8.3)	1 (10.0)	
	Others	13 (10.5)	2 (5.9)	1 (1.9)	0 (0.0)	0 (0.0)	
Assigned work	Clinical chemistry	37 (29.8)	9 (26.5)	15 (27.8)	7 (58.3)	3 (30.0)	0.658
	Hematology	50 (40.3)	17 (50.0)	25 (46.3)	3 (25.0)	4 (40.0)	
	Histology/pathology	14 (11.3)	6 (17.6)	4 (7.4)	2 (16.7)	1 (10.0)	
	Microbiology/ Immunology	23 (18.5)	2 (5.9)	10 (18.5)	0 (0.0)	2 (20.0)	
Years of experience	≤ 3	54 (43.5)	17 (50.0)	12 (22.2)	4 (33.3)	4 (40.0)	0.365
	4–6	31 (25.0)	6 (17.6)	18 (33.3)	5 (41.7)	4 (40.0)	
	7–10	23 (18.5)	8 (23.5)	16 (29.6)	3 (25.0)	0 (0.0)	
	> 10	15 (12.1)	3 (8.8)	8 (14.8)	0 (0.0)	2 (20.0)	
Position	Residency	32 (25.8)	8 (23.5)	10 (18.5)	0 (0.0)	0 (0.0)	0.001
	Technician	74 (59.7)	19 (55.9)	37 (68.5)	6 (50.0)	5 (50.0)	
	Lab director	9 (7.3)	4 (11.8)	3 (5.6)	0 (0.0)	2 (20.0)	
	Consultant	9 (7.3)	3 (8.8)	4 (7.4)	6 (50.0)	3 (30.0)	
Training on biosafety	Yes	69 (55.6)	24 (70.6)	46 (85.2)	7 (58.3)	6 (60.0)	0.024
	No	55 (44.4)	10 (29.4)	8 (14.8)	5 (41.7)	4 (40.0)	

Table 4 Incidence of occupational infection among participants

Variable	Category	Yes	No	Odd ratio	95% confidence interval	P. value
Age	18–30	47 (60.2%)	88 (56.4%)	–	–	
	31–40	23 (29.5%)	47 (30.1%)	0.933	0.50–1.74	0.828
	> 40	8 (10.3%)	21 (13.5%)	0.666	0.27–1.62	
Gender	Male	47 (60.2%)	100 (64.1%)	–	–	
	Female	31 (39.7%)	56 (35.9%)	1.185	0.66–2.09	0.560
Social status	Married	43 (55.1%)	87 (55.8%)	–	–	
	Single	29 (37.2%)	67 (42.9%)	0.876	0.49–1.55	0.652
	Divorced/widowed	6 (7.7%)	2 (1.3%)	7.12	0.84–59.86	0.070
Place of work	Governmental clinics	43 (55.1%)	89 (57.1%)	–	–	
	Private clinics	35 (44.9%)	67 (42.9%)	1.084	0.620–1.895	0.775
Academic degree	College degree	17 (21.8%)	13 (8.3%)	–	–	
	Bachelor degree	50 (64.1%)	117 (75.0%)	0.310	0.12–0.74	0.009
	Graduate degree	11 (14.1%)	26 (16.7%)	0.318	0.10–0.93	0.037
Academic Field	Laboratory Sciences	56 (71.8%)	118 (75.6%)	–	–	
	Applied Biology	12 (15.4%)	13 (8.3%)	1.97	0.79–4.94	0.144
	Health Science	4 (5.1%)	15 (9.6%)	0.527	0.17–1.61	0.264
	Others	6 (7.7%)	10 (6.4%)	1.206	0.41–3.49	0.729
Assigned work	Clinical chemistry	29 (37.2%)	42 (26.9%)	–	–	
	Hematology	28 (35.9%)	71 (45.5%)	0.571	0.29–1.10	0.096
	Histology/pathology	8 (10.3%)	19 (12.2%)	0.608	0.22–1.61	0.317
	Microbiology/ Immunology	13 (16.7%)	24 (15.4%)	0.827	0.35–1.94	0.662
Years of experience	≤ 3	33 (42.3%)	58 (37.2%)	–	–	
	4–6	18 (23.1%)	46 (29.5%)	0.675	0.33–1.36	0.272
	7–10	15 (19.2%)	35 (22.4%)	0.760	0.35–1.62	0.478
	> 10	11 (14.1%)	17 (10.9%)	1.23	0.48–3.10	0.656
Position	Residency	19 (24.4%)	31 (19.9%)	–	–	
	Technician	47 (60.3%)	94 (60.3%)	1.400	0.57–3.39	0.457
	Lab director	5 (6.4%)	13 (8.3%)	0.750	0.24–2.29	0.613
	Consultant	7 (9.0%)	18 (11.5%)	0.751	0.29–1.91	0.546
Training on Biosafety	Yes	42 (53.8%)	110 (70.5%)	–	–	
	No	36 (46.2%)	46 (29.5%)	2.085	1.16–3.74	0.013

With respect to the self-reported frequency of needlestick injury, approximately 24% of the sample had such experience during their career period. This rate is comparable to what was reported in some previous studies [16–18]. For example, an incidence rate of 22.4% sharp injuries over a period of 12 months was reported in a cross-sectional study that was conducted in Dominican Republic [16]. In an Egyptian cross-sectional interview-based study, about 36% of participants reported exposure to at least 1 needlestick injury during the past 3 months [18]. However, higher frequencies (63–73%) were reported in cross-sectional survey-based studies that were conducted in Bosnia [19] and Afghanistan [20] and include the whole career period.

Needlestick injuries reported in this study could be due to what was reported by the participants that they always (49%) recap needle after use, whereas 15% reported doing that most of the times. Recapping needle after use was associated technician/residency staff and lack of training. In a Poland study, 64% of respondents occasionally recap needles after injections [21]. In Morocco, 51% reported recapping needles after use [22]. In a review that was conducted by De Carli and colleagues [8], issues related to management of sharp disposals, needle recapping, and the transfer of sampled blood from syringes into tubes account for the majority of needlestick injuries. Thus, behavior of medical staff plays an important in sharp injuries [23]. Needlestick and sharp injuries can be prevented by

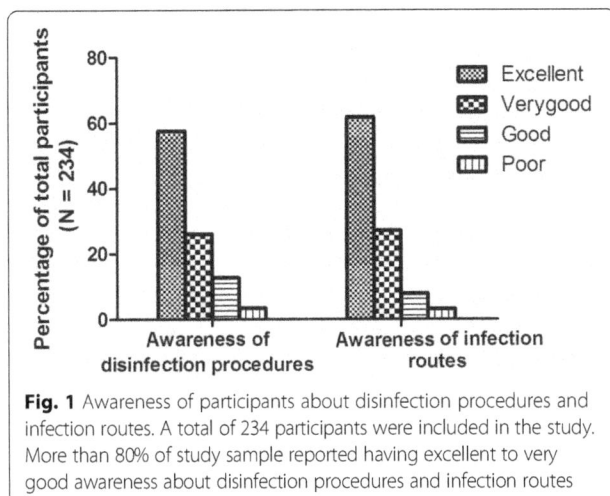

Fig. 1 Awareness of participants about disinfection procedures and infection routes. A total of 234 participants were included in the study. More than 80% of study sample reported having excellent to very good awareness about disinfection procedures and infection routes

applying educational and biosafety training programs and needle protective devices [24, 25]. The finding of the present study that needlestick injuries were strongly associated with the lack of training on biosafety and private clinics confirmed the importance of education in reducing sharp injuries in medical laboratories. Finally, the results showed that needledstick injuries were less frequent in governmental clinics and recapping was performed more frequently. Thus, additional factors seem to contribute to needlestick injury, such as workloads and adherence to safety guidelines that are expected to differ in governmental and private clinics. More studies are required to determine the exact factors that contribute to the observed high frequency of needlestick injury among Al-Madinah clinical laboratory workers.

The results showed that approximately 33% of participants experienced occupational infection during their career period. Previous studies have shown increased risk of clinical laboratory workers to diverse types of infection from their work places [26] that include blood borne pathogens (HBV, HCV, HIV), respiratory illnesses (MERS-CoV, influenza viruses, Tuberculosis) [27] and skin infections [28]. In a cross-sectional survey study that was conducted in clinics from 10 Moroccan cities, 58.9% of the subjects underwent at least one occupational blood exposure [22]. The results showed an association between occupational infection and college degree holders and training on biosafety.

The results showed that > 80% of the sample reported very-good to excellent knowledge regarding infection routes and disinfection procedures. Thus, other factors apart from education are likely to play a role in determining incorrect behaviors such as the adherence to infection control guidelines. However, the association between needlestick injury and occupational infection with lack of training on biosafety highlights the importance of training in reducing such biohazards. Previous studies have

pointed to the effectiveness of the adherence to infection control guidelines, use of injury prevention devices and biosafety educational programs in the prevention of occupational infection and injury [29, 30].

In this cross-sectional study, we asked the participants if they have ever experienced needlestick injury or occupational infection. To have a better assessment of the current situation, conduction of a longitudinal study is strongly recommended where the incidence of such biohazards can be accurately measured. Inclusion of more questions in the assessment such as how often the participants perform phlebotomy and whether they use needlestick prevention devices are strongly recommended. Other limitations include the validity of key measures such as recall bias and social desirability related to recapping practices, selection bias and the data were not adjusted for confounder factors.

In conclusion, the frequency occupational infection and needlestick injury among clinical laboratory workers in Al-Madinah was relatively high as self-reported by participants. Strict implementation of biohazard guidelines in the health care settings and the use of needlestick prevention devices are recommended to reduce the risk of occupational health infections.

Acknowledgments
Authors would like to thank the Clinical Laboratory Sciences Department at Taibah University for their support.

Funding
Taibah University.

Authors' contributions
All authors (OK, KA and WM) contributed to study design, data collection and data analysis/interpretations. OK prepared the first draft of the manuscript and Dr. KA and WM revised the first draft of the manuscript and finalized it. All authors read and approved the final manuscript.

Competing interests
The authors declare that they have no competing interests.

References
1. Nathavitharana RR, Bond P, Dramowski A, et al. Agents of change: the role of healthcare workers in the prevention of nosocomial and occupational tuberculosis. Presse Med. 2017;46:e53–62.
2. Pedrosa PB, Cardoso TA. Viral infections in workers in hospital and research laboratory settings: a comparative review of infection modes and respective biosafety aspects. Int J Infect Dis. 2011;15:e366–76.
3. Tarantola A, Abiteboul D, Rachline A. Infection risks following accidental exposure to blood or body fluids in health care workers: a review of pathogens transmitted in published cases. Am J Infect Control. 2006;34:367–75.
4. Auta A, Adewuyi EO, Tor-Anyiin A, et al. Health-care workers' occupational exposures to body fluids in 21 countries in Africa: systematic review and meta-analysis. Bull World Health Organ. 2017;95:831–41F.

5. Baron EJ, Miller JM. Bacterial and fungal infections among diagnostic laboratory workers: evaluating the risks. Diagn Microbiol Infect Dis. 2008;60:241–6.

6. Joshi R, Reingold AL, Menzies D, Pai M. Tuberculosis among health-care workers in low- and middle-income countries: a systematic review. PLoS Med. 2006;3:e494.

7. Tormey WP, O'Hagan C. Cerebrospinal fluid protein and glucose examinations and tuberculosis:will laboratory safety regulations force a change of practice? Biochem Med (Zagreb). 2015;25:359–62.

8. De Carli G, Abiteboul D, Puro V. The importance of implementing safe sharps practices in the laboratory setting in Europe. Biochem Med (Zagreb). 2014;24:45–56.

9. Marini MA, Giangregorio M, Kraskinski JC. Complying with the occupational safety and health Administration's Bloodborne pathogens standard: implementing needleless systems and intravenous safety devices. Pediatr Emerg Care. 2004;20:209–14.

10. Sabermoghaddam M, Sarbaz M, Lashkardoost H, et al. Incidence of occupational exposure to blood and body fluids and measures taken by health care workers before and after exposure in regional hospitals of a developing country: a multicenter study. Am J Infect Control. 2015; 43:1137–8.

11. Gabriel J. Reducing needlestick and sharps injuries among healthcare workers. Nurs Stand. 2009;23:41–4.

12. Matsubara C, Sakisaka K, Sychareun V, Phensavanh A, Ali M. Prevalence and risk factors of needle stick and sharp injury among tertiary hospital workers, Vientiane, Lao PDR. J Occup Health. 2017;59:581–5.

13. Motaarefi H, Mahmoudi H, Mohammadi E, Hasanpour-Dehkordi A. Factors associated with Needlestick injuries in health care occupations: a systematic review. J Clin Diagn Res. 2016;10:IE01–4.

14. Glenngard AH, Persson U. Costs associated with sharps injuries in the Swedish health care setting and potential cost savings from needle-stick prevention devices with needle and syringe. Scand J Infect Dis. 2009;41: 296–302.

15. Tarigan LH, Cifuentes M, Quinn M, Kriebel D. Prevention of needle-stick injuries in healthcare facilities: a meta-analysis. Infect Control Hosp Epidemiol. 2015;36:823–9.

16. Moro PL, Moore A, Balcacer P, et al. Epidemiology of needlesticks and other sharps injuries and injection safety practices in the Dominican Republic. Am J Infect Control. 2007;35:552–9.

17. Qazi AR, Siddiqui FA, Faridi S, et al. Comparison of awareness about precautions for needle stick injuries: a survey among health care workers at a tertiary care center in Pakistan. Patient Saf Surg. 2016;10:19.

18. Talaat M, Kandeel A, El-Shoubary W, et al. Occupational exposure to needlestick injuries and hepatitis B vaccination coverage among health care workers in Egypt. Am J Infect Control. 2003;31:469–74.

19. Musa S, Peek-Asa C, Young T, Jovanovic N. Needle stick injuries, sharp injuries and other occupational exposures to blood and body fluids among health care workers in a general hospital in Sarajevo, Bosnia and Herzegovina. Int J Occup Saf Health. 2014;4:31–7.

20. Salehi AS, Garner P. Occupational injury history and universal precautions awareness: a survey in Kabul hospital staff. BMC Infect Dis. 2010;10:19.

21. Rogowska-Szadkowska D, Stanislawowicz M, Chlabicz S. Risk of needle stick injuries in health care workers: bad habits (recapping needles) last long. Przegl Epidemiol. 2010;64:293–5.

22. Laraqui O, Laraqui S, Tripodi D, et al. Assessing knowledge, attitude, and practice on occupational blood exposure in caregiving facilities, in Morocco. Med Mal Infect. 2008;38:658–66.

23. Castella A, Vallino A, Argentero PA, Zotti CM. Preventability of percutaneous injuries in healthcare workers: a year-long survey in Italy. J Hosp Infect. 2003; 55:290–4.

24. Adams D. Needlestick and sharps injuries: practice update. Nurs Stand. 2012; 26:49–57. quiz 58

25. Wilburn SQ. Needlestick and sharps injury prevention. Online J Issues Nurs. 2004;9:5.

26. Wei Q, Li XY, Wang L, et al. Preliminary studies on pathogenic microorganisms laboratory-acquired infections cases in recent years and its control strategies. Zhnghua Shi Yan He Lin Chuang Bing Du Xue Za Zhi. 2011;25:390–2.

27. Chughtai AA, Seale H, Dung TC, et al. Compliance with the use of medical and cloth masks among healthcare Workers in Vietnam. Ann Occup Hyg. 2016;60:619–30.

28. Duman Y, Yakupogullari Y, Otlu B, Tekerekoglu MS. Laboratory-acquired skin infections in a clinical microbiologist: is wearing only gloves really safe? Am J Infect Control. 2016;44:935–7.

29. Rice BD, Tomkins SE, Ncube FM. Sharp truth: health care workers remain at risk of bloodborne infection. Occup Med (Lond). 2015;65:210–4.

30. Trim JC, Elliott TS. A review of sharps injuries and preventative strategies. J Hosp Infect. 2003;53:237–42.

21

Epworth sleepiness scale in medical residents: quality of sleep and its relationship to quality of life

Yehia Z. Alami[1], Beesan T. Ghanim[1] and Sa'ed H. Zyoud[2,3*]

Abstract

Background: Resident doctors are continuously exposed to prolonged working hours and night shifts, making them susceptible to the many physical, psychological, and cognitive side effects of sleep deprivation, which may affect their quality of life. Therefore, this study aimed to determine the prevalence of sleep penury in resident doctors and to assess the association between self-apprehended sleepiness and quality of life.

Methods: A cross-sectional study was carried out in the governmental hospitals in the North of the West Bank between May 2017 and September 2017. Doctors enrolled in residency programmes completed questionnaires about general, sociodemographic, and sleep characteristics. The doctors completed the Arabic Version of the Epworth Sleepiness Scale (ArESS) to assess subjective daytime sleepiness and the RAND 36-item short-form health survey (SF-36) to determine quality of life.

Results: A total of 101 participants were enrolled. Daytime sleepiness was observed in 37.6% ($n = 38$) of the participants with an ESS score of ≥10. There was a notable negative correlation between the ESS and quality of health index in the physical composition ($r = -0.351$, $p < 0.001$) demonstrated in the following four subscales: the physical functioning ($p < 0.001$), role limitations due to physical health ($p = 0.045$), body pain ($p = 0.036$), and general health ($p < 0.001$) components of the SF-36 scale. Females and residents of the centre region had poorer mental quality ($p = 0.006$ and 0.020, respectively).

Conclusions: More than one third of the resident doctors suffer from daytime sleepiness according to the ESS. This was proven to significantly affect several aspects of their quality of life, including physical function and health, body pain, and general health. Sleep deprivation and improvement of quality of life require health promotion actions among medical residents.

Keywords: Residents, Epworth, Sleepiness, Quality of life, SF-36

Background

According to many articles, sleep deprivation affects many physiological and psychological aspects of one's life [1–3]. Sleep deprivation affects episodic memory as well as self-awareness and responsibility [3–5]. Sleep loss also severely affects the emotional memory in its contextual and non-contextual aspects [6]. Neuronal apoptosis using adrenergic receptors can be triggered due to the deprivation of rapid eye movement (REM) sleep component [7], as well as induce anxiolytic-like effects by dopaminergic influences [8]. According to De Bernardi Rodrigues et al., sleep deprivation is associated with decreased sensitivity to insulin and centripetal distribution of fat in adolescence [9].

One of the many professions that is continuously exposed to prolonged periods of sleep deprivation is that of a resident doctor. The prolonged working hours of resident physicians make them vulnerable to the consequences of sleep penury, which affects their task performance and quality of life [10]. The residents' poor

---
* Correspondence: saedzyoud@yahoo.com; saedzyoud@najah.edu
[2]Poison Control and Drug Information Center (PCDIC), College of Medicine and Health Sciences, An-Najah National University, Nablus 44839, Palestine
[3]Department of Clinical and Community Pharmacy, Department of Pharmacy, College of Medicine and Health Sciences, An-Najah National University, Nablus 44839, Palestine
Full list of author information is available at the end of the article

sleep quality is associated with increased body mass index (BMI), poorer lipid profile, poor quality of food consumed, and increase in waist circumference [11]. The nature of this poor sleep may also affect the residents psychologically by making them depressed, anxious, and insomnious [12–14]. Immune function has also been studied in relation to poor sleep quality, indicating the probability of inflammatory responses, triggered by short sleep duration, producing metabolic, respiratory, and cardiovascular diseases. In addition, it has been reported that poor sleep might cause elevated C-reactive protein levels, an inflammatory marker for cardiovascular diseases [10, 15].

Several studies have demonstrated how sleep deprivation negatively impacts one's well-being in general and how it negatively influences resident doctors specifically [3, 5, 10, 12–14, 16, 17]. However, to our knowledge, little is known about the effects of daytime sleepiness on residents' health [16]. Although limited studies have been conducted and published about sleep habits and problems among Palestinian university students [18, 19], Palestinian patients diagnosed with cancer [20], and the Palestinian population [21], no studies have been conducted to focus on the relationship between self-reported sleepiness, as surrogate marker of poor sleep, and quality of life in resident doctors in Palestine. Therefore, the purposes of this investigation are to determine the prevalence of self-reported sleepiness in resident doctors and to assess the association between sleepiness and their quality of life. The significance of this study may be reflected in the rules and policies of the Ministry of Health by proposing new working hours, changing on-call guidelines and duties, strengthening the on-call team, improving sleeping places to promote better sleep hygiene, offering free times for taking naps [16, 22], providing stress-relieving activities, and adopting rewarding programmes i.e. providing extra money and increasing residents' days-off to galvanise the resident physicians.

Methods
Study design and population
A cross-sectional study design was employed to achieve the research objectives. The study took place amongst a group of health care practitioners, as it included resident doctors who are training in different specialities. Resident doctors who are general practitioners were excluded because they are not in the medical training (residency) programme.

Setting
The data were collected from governmental hospitals in three cities in the North of the West Bank (Jenin, Nablus, and Tulkarm). These hospitals are the sites of the

medical training programme for the resident doctors in North of the West Bank.

Sample size and sampling technique
The estimated number of resident doctors licensed by the Palestinian Medical Association who worked at the surveyed hospitals was around 130. Accordingly, the Raosoft sample size calculator was used to perceive the sample size [23] by keeping an indicator percentage of 0.50, a margin of error of 5%, and a confidence interval of 95%. The calculated sample size was 98. Between May 2017 and September 2017, we enrolled a convenience sample of 126 resident doctors.

Data collection
The doctors completed surveys about their sociodemographic, general, and sleep characteristics. Sociodemographic and general characteristics included age, sex, marital status, governorates they come from in the West Bank (north, central, south), who they live with (with family or not), BMI and change in weight during residency, presence of chronic diseases, place of graduation, working department, number of residency years, and years of work experience. Sleep characteristics included questions about sleeping hours on days with and without shifts, caffeine intake, smoking, use of sleeping pills, time to fall asleep, and waking up during sleep.

Instruments
Physicians were asked to complete two instruments: the Arabic Version of the Epworth sleepiness scale (ArESS) to assess the quality of sleep and the RAND 36-item short-form health survey (SF-36).

Arabic Version of the Epworth sleepiness scale (ArESS)
The Epworth Sleepiness Scale (ESS) was developed to assess sleepiness during daytime. The ESS questionnaire consists of eight questions about daily situations that can induce sleepiness. Each question has the lowest score of 0 ('no chance of falling asleep') to 3 ('high chance of falling asleep'). The score ranges can sum up to 24 and are categorised as normal (ESS < 10) or positive for daytime sleepiness (ESS ≥ 10) [24]. We used the ArESS, which has been validated and is reliable to be used in populations that are Arabic-speaking [25]. Permission to use the ArESS was given by Professor Hamdan Al-Jahdali via e-mail correspondence. There is a high level of internal consistency within the ArESS in our study, as measured by Cronbach's alpha (0.749).

RAND 36-item short-form health survey (SF-36)
This survey was employed to discern the general quality of life based on the previous one month's experiences [26]. It consists of 36 items divided into subscales, each

Table 1 Sociodemographic and general characteristics

Variables	n (%)
Age (per years)	
≤ 28	60(59.4)
> 28	41(40.6)
Sex	
Male	86(85.1)
Female	15(14.9)
Marital status	
Married	48(47.5)
Unmarried	53(52.5)
Governorate [a]	
North	79(78.2)
Central	5(5.0)
South	17(16.8)
Living with family	
Yes	79(78.2)
No	22(21.8)
Body mass index [b]	
Underweight/normal	39(38.6)
Overweight	50(49.5)
Obese	12(11.9)
Weight change during residency	
Increased	39(38.6)
Decreased	27(26.7)
No change	35(34.7)
Chronic diseases	
Hypertension	3(3.0)
Place of graduation [c]	
Local	28(27.7)
Regional	52(51.5)
Western	21(20.8)
Working department	
General surgery	23(22.8)
Internal medicine	11(10.9)
Paediatrics	22(21.8)
Gynecology and obstetrics	14(13.9)
Anaesthesia	11(10.9)
Radiology	7(6.9)
Orthopaedics	13(12.9)
Residency years (per years)	
≤ 1	37(36.6)
> 1	64(63.4)

Table 1 Sociodemographic and general characteristics (Continued)

Variables	n (%)
Years of experience (per years)	
≤ 2	33(32.7)
3–4	41(40.6)
> 4	27(26.7)

n frequency, SD standard deviation, % percentage
[a] Governorates: North (Jenin, Nablus, Tulkarm, Qalqilya, Salfit, Tubas), Central (Jerusalem, Ramallah), South (Bethlehem, Hebron)
[b] Body mass index: Underweight/normal (≤24), overweight (> 24 – < 30), obese (≥30)
[c] Place of graduation: Local (Palestine), regional (Arab-world countries other than Palestine), western (remaining countries worldwide)

with its own score: physical functioning (PF), role limitations due to physical health (RP), bodily pain (BP), general health (GH), role limitations due to emotional problems (RE), vitality/energy and fatigue (VT), mental health (MH), social functioning (SF), and health change in the past year (HC). We categorised the first four components to yield the physical composite score and the latter four components to produce the mental composite score as Zhu et al. reported [27]. The scores varied between 0 and 100; the higher score, the better the quality of life is [28]. We used the Arabic model of the inquiry, which is valid and reliable [29]. Cronbach's alpha for all subscales of the SF-36 for our study exceed alpha of 0.70. Face and content validity of the final version of instrument was discussed and evaluated by a panel of three researchers who are expert in research related to sleep and QOL for assessing the organization, appropriateness meaning of terms, clinical terminology, completeness, and logical sequence of the statements.

Table 2 36-Item Short Form Health Survey (SF-36)

Variables	Mean ± SD
Physical functioning	80.2 ± 22.3
Role limitations due to physical health	61.9 ± 38.2
Role limitations due to emotional problems	45.9 ± 42.9
Energy/fatigue	39.6 ± 16.7
Emotional well-being	50.6 ± 18.8
Social functioning	49.9 ± 24.7
Pain	68.7 ± 22.7
General health	61.0 ± 17.2
Health change	42.1 ± 19.7
PCS	67.9 ± 19.9
MCS	46.4 ± 19.6
Average total	55.5 ± 16.4

n frequency, SD standard deviation, % percentage, PCS physical composite score, MCS mental composite score

Table 3 PCS and MCS according to sociodemographic and general characteristics

	n (%)	PCS Median [Q1–Q3]	p value [d]	MCS Median [Q1–Q3]	p value [d]
Age (per years)					
≤ 28	60 (59.4)	70.4[50.2–87.4]	0.849 [e]	41.0[28.3–61.9]	0.424 [e]
> 28	41(40.6)	72.0[52.5–85.0]		44.3[33.0–65.5]	
Sex					
Male	86 (85.1)	71.6[51.7–87.1]	0.369 [e]	45.3[32.2–64.6]	**0.006** [e]
Female	15 (14.9)	62.0[49.5–80.0]		28.0[20.3–41.5]	
Marital status					
Married	48(47.5)	57.5[48.9–87.1]	0.570 [e]	41.5[31.3–62.6]	0.957 [e]
Unmarried	53(52.5)	72.0[52.3–86.0]		44.0[28.1–64.0]	
Governorate [a]					
North	79(78.2)	72.0[52.5–85.8]		42.0[28.3–62.0]	**0.020** [f]
Central	5(5.0)	48.3[36.6–82.9]		24.0[17.4–37.5]	
South	17(16.8)	70.0[46.9–89.8]	0.512 [f]	59.0[35.3–70.1]	
Living with family					
Yes	79(78.2)	72.0[52.0–87.0]	0.103 [e]	44.8[28.3–65.3]	0.248 [e]
No	22(21.8)	58.5[45.9–77.5]		39.0[28.4–49.9]	
Body mass index [b]					
Underweight/normal	39(38.6)	70.8[51.3–88.3]	0.368 [f]	41.5[27.0–64.5]	0.899 [f]
Overweight	50(49.5)	73.5[52.5–86.6]		42.6[32.1–63.1]	
Obese	12(11.9)	56.3[47.4–78.0]		43.6[31.8–61.9]	
Weight change during residency					
Increased	39(38.6)	72.5[49.5–88.3]	0.238 [f]	49.5[32.0–67.3]	0.147 [f]
Decreased	27(26.7)	59.5[48.3–80.8]		36.3[26.3–59.0]	
No change	35(34.7)	72.0[52.5–88.8]		44.8[32.0–65.3]	
Place of graduation [c]					
Local	28(27.7)	70.0[51.6–86.7]	0.085 [f]	41.4[26.4–57.6]	0.130 [f]
Regional	52(51.5)	64.4[47.1–82.8]		40.4[28.3–64.1]	
Western	21(20.8)	82.5[62.6–90.4]		51.3[40.4–68.9]	
Working department					
General surgery	23(22.8)	62.5[50.0–86.3]	0.156 [f]	38.3[26.0–53.8]	0.585 [f]
Internal medicine	11(10.9)	87.0[60.8–90.0]		54.0[32.0–73.0]	
Paediatrics	22(21.8)	59.1[48.4–78.4]		43.4[30.9–58.4]	
Gynecology and obstetrics	14(13.9)	69.8[47.5–80.6]		35.9[27.8–65.6]	
Anaesthesia	11(10.9)	85.8[74.5–95.0]		49.5[40.8–64.8]	
Radiology	7(6.9)	72.0[52.5–83.3]		38.5[26.3–72.8]	
Orthopaedics	13(12.9)	70.8[52.3–89.4]		48.8[35.4–67.0]	
Residency years (per years)					
≤ 1	37(36.6)	72.0[50.4–88.1]		47.8[30.8–65.0]	0.196 [e]
> 1	64(63.4)	68.8[51.3–85.0]	0.617 [e]	41.0[28.3–58.1]	
Years of experience (per years)					
≤ 2	33(32.7)	72.0[51.0–88.1]		54.0[30.8–66.3]	0.149 [f]
3–4	41(40.6)	60.8[49.1–82.5]	0.116 [f]	40.0[28.3–53.5]	
> 4	27(26.7)	75.8[52.5–88.8]		41.0[27.8–71.0]	

n frequency, *%* percentage, *PCS* physical composite score, *MCS* mental composite score
[a] Governorates: North (Jenin, Nablus, Tulkarm, Qalqilya, Salfit, Tubas), Central (Jerusalem, Ramallah), South (Bethlehem, Hebron)
[b] Body mass index: Underweight/normal (≤24), overweight (> 24 – < 30), obese (≥30)
[c] Place of graduation: Local (Palestine), regional (Arab-world countries other than Palestine), western (remaining countries worldwide)
[d] The *p*-value is bold where it is less than the significance level cut-off of 0.05
[e] Statistical significance of differences calculated using the Mann–Whitney U test
[f] Statistical significance of differences calculated using the Kruskal–Wallis test

Table 4 Sleep characteristics

Variables	n (%)
Smoking	40(39.6)
Caffeine use	95(94.1)
Coffee (per ml)	
None	20(19.8)
Up to 100	8(7.9)
Up to 200	22(21.8)
Up to 300	31(30.7)
More than 300	20(19.8)
Tea (per ml)	
None	34(33.7)
Up to 100	33(32.7)
Up to 200	18(17.8)
Up to 300	11(10.9)
More than 300	5(5.0)
Energy drinks (per ml)	
None	87(86.1)
Up to 100	6(5.9)
Up to 200	3(3.0)
Up to 300	5(5.0)
Caffeine at night (times per week)	
None	34(33.7)
Once or twice	29(28.7)
Three to four	16(15.8)
More than four	22(21.8)
Non-shift sleep hours	
≤ 4 h	5(5.0)
4–6 h	61(60.4)
≥ 6 h	35(34.7)
Shift sleep hours	
≤ 4 h	85(84.1)
4–6 h	14(13.9)
≥ 6 h	2(2.0)
Sleeping pills use	4(4.0)
Time taken to fall asleep	
≤ 10mins	27(26.7)
10–30 min	35(34.7)
30–60 min	28(27.7)
> 60mins	11(10.9)
Waking up during sleep	73(72.3)
Wake up to eat	17(16.8)
Wake up due to noise	59(58.4)
Sleep walking	0(0.0)
Nightmares	51(50.5)

Table 4 Sleep characteristics (Continued)

Variables	n (%)
Epworth Sleepiness Scale	
< 10	63(62.4)
≥ 10	38(37.6)

Ethical approval

All rules of conduct were authorised by the Institutional Review Boards (IRB) before initiation of this study, and permission to interview the medical residents was granted by the local health authorities.

Statistical analysis

All statistical analyses for our data were performed using the Statistical Package for Social Sciences version 15 (SPSS Inc., Chicago, IL, USA). Continuous data are presented as mean ± standard deviation (SD) or median (Q1–Q3; interquartile range) or frequency (percentage) for categorical variables. Data were tested for normality using the Kolmogorov–Smirnov test. In comparing two groups, we used Mann–Whitney U tests, and for comparing more than two groups, we used Kruskal–Wallis tests. We assessed the correlation between ESS and SF-36 domains using the Pearson's correlation coefficient; p values < 0.05 were considered significant. Internal consistency reliability for all scales was assessed using Cronbach's alpha.

Results

The characteristics of the resident doctors

Overall, 126 questionnaire were distributed, 112 (88.8%) were returned, 101 (80.1%) were accepted, and 11 (8.7%) were rejected for incompleteness ($n = 8$) or for respondents being general practitioners ($n = 3$). Of the 101 participants, 86 were male (85.1%) and 15 were female (14.9%), with a mean age of 28.5 ± 2.5. Table 1 shows the sociodemographic and general characteristics of the participants.

Health-related quality of life in the participant residents

The means of the SF-36 subscales were calculated in Table 2, and the results, as shown in Additional file 1: Table S1 and Table S2, indicate a statistically significant difference in all of the subscale components with different variables at $p < 0.05$ except for mental health, which showed no significance. As for physical functioning, there is significance with the years of experience ($p = 0.032$). Role physical was significant in residents living with their family ($p = 0.043$). Role emotional shows significance with the residents' governorates ($p = 0.042$), years of residency ($p = 0.004$), and years of experience ($p = 0.010$). Vitality has significance with gender ($p = 0.019$), age ($p = 0.016$), marital status ($p = 0.021$), and

Table 5 Epworth Sleepiness Scale according to sociodemographic and general characteristics

Variables	n (%)	ESS Median [Q1–Q3]	P value [d]
Age (per years)			
≤ 28	60(59.4)	9.0[5.0–11.0]	0.670 [e]
> 28	41(40.6)	8.0[6.5–11.0]	
Sex			
Male	86(85.1)	8.5[6.0–11.0]	0.958 [e]
Female	15(14.9)	9.0[4.0–12.0]	
Marital status			
Married	48(47.5)	9.0[6.3–12.0]	0.067 [e]
Unmarried	53(52.5)	8.0[5.0–11.0]	
Governorate [a]			
North	79(78.2)	9.0[6.0–11.0]	0.861[f]
Central	5(5.0)	10.0[5.5–13.5]	
South	17(16.8)	8.0[5.5–13.5]	
Living with family			
Yes	79(78.2)	8.0[5.0–11.0]	0.063 [e]
No	22(21.8)	10.0[7.0–12.3]	
Body mass index [b]			
Underweight/normal	39(38.6)	8.0[5.0–11.0]	0.110 [f]
Overweight	50(49.5)	9.0[7.0–12.0]	
Obese	12(11.9)	7.0[4.5–11.8]	
Weight change during residency			
Increased	39(38.6)	9.0[6.0–12.0]	0.300 [f]
Decreased	27(26.7)	9.0[6.0–12.0]	
No change	35(34.7)	7.0[5.0–11.0]	
Place of graduation [c]			
Local	28(27.7)	9.0[7.0–11.0]	0.650 [f]
Regional	52(51.5)	8.5[6.0–11.0]	
Western	21(20.8)	7.0[4.0–11.5]	
Working department			
General surgery	23(22.8)	9.0[7.0–13.0]	0.755 [f]
Internal medicine	11(10.9)	8.0[4.0–9.0]	
Paediatrics	22(21.8)	8.5[6.3–11.3]	
Gynecology and obstetrics	14(13.9)	9.0[7.0–10.3]	
Anaesthesia	11(10.9)	5.0[4.0–13.0]	
Radiology	7(6.9)	8.0[5.0–11.0]	
Orthopaedics	13(12.9)	9.0[4.0–11.5]	
Residency years (per years)			
≤ 1	37(36.6)	8.0[4.0–11.0]	0.064 [e]
> 1	64(63.4)	9.0[7.0–11.0]	

Table 5 Epworth Sleepiness Scale according to sociodemographic and general characteristics *(Continued)*

Variables	n (%)	ESS Median [Q1–Q3]	P value [d]
Years of experience (per years)			
≤ 2	33(32.7)	8.0[4.0–10.0]	0.243 [f]
3–4	41(40.6)	9.0[6.5–12.0]	
> 4	27(26.7)	9.0[6.0–12.0]	

n frequency, *%* percentage, *ESS* Epworth Sleepiness Scale
[a] Governorates: North (Jenin, Nablus, Tulkarm, Qalqilya, Salfit, Tubas), Central (Jerusalem, Ramallah), South (Bethlehem, Hebron)
[b] Body mass index: Underweight/normal (≤24), overweight (> 24 – < 30), obese (≥30)
[c] Place of graduation: Local (Palestine), regional (Arab-world countries other than Palestine), western (remaining countries worldwide)
[d] The *p*-value is bold where it is less than the significance level cut-off of 0.05
[e] Statistical significance of differences calculated using the Mann–Whitney U test
[f] Statistical significance of differences calculated using the Kruskal–Wallis test

place of graduation ($p = 0.004$). Social functioning is significant with gender ($p = 0.006$) and place of graduation ($p = 0.049$). Body pain is associated with change in weight during residency ($p = 0.039$) and the country of graduation ($p = 0.005$). General health is affected by the country of graduation ($p = 0.022$) and years of experience ($p = 0.044$). Health change is affected by weight change during residency ($p = 0.023$). On the other hand, as Table 3 shows, the mental composite score (MCS) was significant with gender ($p = 0.006$) and the governorates of the residents ($p = 0.020$); the physical composite score (PCS) had no apparent significance.

The sleep characteristics of the resident doctors

The sleep features of the participants are detailed in Table 4. The ESS median is 9, and a score of ≥10 indicating daytime sleepiness is observed in 38 (37.6%) participants. The ESS is compared with sociodemographic and general characteristics to yield no significant association between them, as shown in Table 5. In comparing the ESS with the sleep characteristics, the only significant difference present is in having nightmares ($p = 0.004$), as Table 6 elaborates.

Quality of health and sleepiness

There is a significant correlation between sleepiness and quality of health among the residents as provided by the negative correlation between the ESS and the SF-36 scores of the physical functioning ($r = -0.397$, $p < 0.001$), role limitations due to physical health ($r = -0.200$, $p = 0.045$), body pain ($r = -0.209$, $p = 0.036$), general health ($r = -0.392$, $p < 0.001$), and health change ($r = -0.199$, $p = 0.046$) subscales, as shown in Additional file 1: Table S2. There are also significant positive correlations between the subscales of the SF-36 themselves as proved in Additional file 1: Table S2. This is also manifested in

Table 6 Epworth Sleepiness Scale according to sleep characteristics

Variables	n (%)	ESS Median [Q1–Q3]	P value [a]
Smoking			
Yes	40(39.6)	9.0[5.3–11.8]	0.728 [b]
No	61(60.4)	8.0[6.0–11.0]	
Coffee (per ml)			
None	20(19.8)	7.5[6.3–9.8]	0.222 [c]
Up to 100	8(7.9)	9.0[8.0–13.0]	
Up to 200	22(21.8)	8.5[6.5–12.0]	
Up to 300	31(31.7)	9.0[7.0–12.0]	
More than 300	20(19.8)	5.5[3.3–10.8]	
Tea (per ml)			
None	34(33.7)	8.0[4.0–11.3]	0.145 [c]
Up to 100	33(32.7)	9.0[7.0–12.0]	
Up to 200	18(17.8)	8.0[4.3–11.3]	
Up to 300	11(10.9)	8.0[7.0–13.0]	
More than 300	5(5.0)	4.0[3.0–7.5]	
Energy drinks (per ml)			
None	87(86.1)	9.0[6.0–11.0]	0.661 [c]
Up to 100	6(5.9)	8.0[3.5–14.3]	
Up to 200	3(3.0)	8.0[7.0–8.5]	
Up to 300	5(5.0)	7.0[2.0–10.0]	
Caffeine at night (times per week)			
No	34(33.7)	8.0[7.0–11.3]	0.371 [c]
Once or twice	29(28.7)	8.0[5.0–12.0]	
Three to four	16(15.8)	9.0[7.5–11.0]	
More than four	22(21.8)	7.0[4.0–10.3]	
Non-shift sleep hours			
≤4 h	5(5.0)	11.0[7.5–14.0]	0.297 [c]
4–6 h	61(60.4)	9.0[6.0–11.0]	
≥6 h	35(34.7)	8.0[4.0–10.0]	
Shift sleep hours			
≤4 h	85(84.1)	8.0[6.0–11.0]	0.568 [c]
4-6 h	14(13.9)	9.0[4.8–12.5]	
≥6 h	2(2.0)	6.5[5.0–8.0]	
Sleeping pill use			
Yes	4(4.0)	13.5[4.0–15.5]	0.196 [b]
No	97(96.0)	8.0[6.0–11.0]	
Time taken to fall asleep			
≤ 10mins	27(26.7)	9.0[7.0–11.0]	0.275 [c]
10–30 min	35(34.7)	8.0[6.0–11.0]	
30–60 min	28(27.7)	8.0[6.0–12.0]	
> 60mins	11(10.9)	6.0[2.0–9.0]	

Table 6 Epworth Sleepiness Scale according to sleep characteristics *(Continued)*

Variables	n (%)	ESS Median [Q1–Q3]	P value [a]
Waking up during sleep			
Yes	73(72.3)	9.0[6.0–11.0]	0.741 [b]
No	28(27.7)	8.5[4.8–12.8]	
Wake up to eat			
Yes	17(16.8)	9.0[7.0–12.0]	0.492 [b]
No	84(83.2)	8.5[5.3–11.0]	
Wake up due to noise			
Yes	59(58.4)	9.0[5.0–11.0]	0.953 [b]
No	42(41.6)	8.5[7.0–12.0]	
Nightmares			
Yes	51(50.5)	9.0[8.0–12.0]	**0.004** [b]
No	50(49.5)	7.0[4.0–10.3]	

n frequency, *SD* standard deviation, *%* percentage, *ml* millilitres, *h* hours, *mins* minutes
[a] The p-value is bold where it is less than the significance level cut-off of 0.05
[b] Statistical significance of differences calculated using the Mann–Whitney U test
[c] Statistical significance of differences calculated using the Kruskal–Wallis test

correlating the ESS and PCS, as there is a significant negative correlation between them ($r = -0.351$, $p < 0.001$), unlike the ESS and MCS, where no significant correlation is present ($r = -0.097$, $p = 0.334$).

Discussion

This study aimed to assess the residents' sleepiness and their quality of life. Few studies have linked those two categories, and no such study has been conducted in Palestine. Hereby, valid Arabic models of both the SF-36 and the ESS were used to fulfill the purpose of this study [25, 30]. The data gave the impression that medical residents may have reduced quality of both physical and mental health, but the results of this study were unanticipated regarding physical impairment. Our population may have had associations in some of the physical subscales with certain sociodemographic and general characteristics, but the PCS was unable to demonstrate so. Contrary to the insignificant result of the PCS in our study, a poor lipid profile and harmful lifestyle were exhibited among residents in Pikovsky et al. study, which may be reflected in their physical health [10]. This inconsistency may be due to the large number of residents in the same department and an unequal work load among them at the above-mentioned hospitals.

Regarding the participants' mental health, the MCS manifested a poorer mental status in residents coming from the central region (Ramallah and Jerusalem) and in female participants. Distance plays a role in this case, as residents from the central region usually do not take dormitories, unlike the southern population, according to Belayachi et al. [31].

Female doctors are more prone to mental health liability compared to male doctors, as indicated by Sundquist and Johansson [32].

Concerning the sleepiness of the participants, 38 (37.6%) were sleepy by scoring 10 or more on the ESS, but, contrary to our expectation, having nightmares is surprisingly the only single factor between both the sociodemographic and sleep features to yield a significant relationship with the ESS. To support our result, Paul et al. elaborated that nightmares are associated with significantly decreased quality of sleep [33]. A systematic review by Bolster and Rourke found that in seven studies concerning shift hours, restriction had no influence on the residents' well-being, which could explain why there was no association between working hours and the ESS [34].

In the current study, correlating sleepiness with quality of life showed that daytime sleepiness leads to poor physical composite but, surprisingly, has an insignificant effect on the mental aspect according to the MCS. This finding is contrary to previous studies that suggested a worsening individual mood, depressive symptoms, and emotional exhaustion [17, 31].

Although this study is the first study of its kind to investigate the quality of life among resident doctors and their quality of sleep, several limitations that should be noted. First, the current study was limited by involving just the north of West Bank governmental hospitals i.e. Nablus, Jenin and Tulkarm, which led to a small sampling size, preventing generalisation. Second, being a cross-sectional type of study also made it difficult to know whether our outcome was affected prior to the residency period. Additionally, as a cross-sectional design was used, a causal relationship was difficult to infer. Third, the small number of female practitioners in the residency programmes is another drawback. Fourth, possibility that the scales were inaccurately filled in as they are self-reporting scales. Fifth, the exclusion of ophthalmology, otolaryngology, and emergency wards due to scarcity of residents also raised the susceptibility of bias. Sixth, ESS has low efficiency when used in evaluating sleepiness in general populations such as in our study [35, 36]. Finally, we did not use standardized and validated questionnaires to evaluate sleep quality and quantity; moreover sleep deprivation is evaluated only on number of hours of sleep and not by sleep logs or actigraphy. In this way none information is collected about possible co-occurrence of sleep disorders (e.g. snoring, obstructive sleep apnea, insomnia, restless legs syndrome etc) which may influence daytime sleepiness.

Conclusions

This paper has examined independently the qualities of life and sleep of West Bank medical residents working in the northern hospitals as well as the relationship between them. It appeared that female residents and those from the central region had poorer quality of life in the mental aspect. The paper also indicated increased sleepiness in participants who experience nightmares. Moreover, this study identified that daytime sleepiness impacts the residents physically, leading to a decreased quality of life. Daytime sleepiness and improvement of quality of life require health promotion actions among medical residents. Therefore, there is a definite need to enhance current policies regarding the residency programme schedule and, if needed, to further restrict working hours, and increasing the number of residents during each shift. One of the practical implications that can be made to ameliorate the residents' well-being is to promote better sleep hygiene by providing time and comfortable rooms for a nap, and stress-relief activities.

Abbreviations

ArESS: Arabic Version of the Epworth Sleepiness Scale; BMI: Body mass index; BP: Bodily pain; ESS: Epworth sleepiness scale; GH: General health; HC: Health change in the past year; IRB: Institutional review board; MCS: Mental composite score; MH: Mental health; PCS: Physical composite score; PF: Physical functioning; Q1–Q3: Interquartile range; RE: Role limitations due to emotional problems; REM: Rapid eye movement; RP: Role limitations due to physical health; SD: Standard deviation; SF: Social functioning; SF-36: 36-Item Short Form Health Survey; SPSS: Statistical Package for Social Sciences; VT: Vitality/energy and fatigue

Acknowledgments

Not applicable.

Authors' contributions

YA, and BG collected data, performed the analysis and wrote the draft manuscript. Searched the literature, and drafted the manuscript. SZ conceptualised and designed the study, coordinated, supervised, advised on data analysis and reviewed the manuscript, and assisted in the final write-up of the manuscript. All authors read and approved the final manuscript.

Competing interests

The authors declare that they have no competing interests.

Author details

[1]Department of Medicine, College of Medicine and Health Sciences, An-Najah National University, Nablus 44839, Palestine. [2]Poison Control and Drug Information Center (PCDIC), College of Medicine and Health Sciences, An-Najah National University, Nablus 44839, Palestine. [3]Department of Clinical and Community Pharmacy, Department of Pharmacy, College of Medicine and Health Sciences, An-Najah National University, Nablus 44839, Palestine.

References

1. Saxena AD, George CF. Sleep and motor performance in on-call internal medicine residents. Sleep. 2005;28(11):1386–91.

2. Ayalon RD, Friedman F Jr. The effect of sleep deprivation on fine motor coordination in obstetrics and gynecology residents. Am J Obstet Gynecol. 2008;199(5):576. e1–5

3. Hamui-Sutton L, Barragan-Perez V, Fuentes-Garcia R, Monsalvo-Obregon EC, Fouilloux-Morales C. Sleep deprivation effects on cognitive, psychomotor skills and its relationship with personal characteristics of resident doctors. Cir Cir. 2013;81(4):317–27.

4. Wang L, Chen Y, Yao Y, Pan Y, Sun Y. Sleep deprivation disturbed regional brain activity in healthy subjects: evidence from a functional magnetic resonance-imaging study. Neuropsychiatr Dis Treat. 2016;12:801–7.

5. Kim HJ, Kim JH, Park KD, Choi KG, Lee HW. A survey of sleep deprivation patterns and their effects on cognitive functions of residents and interns in Korea. Sleep Med. 2011;12(4):390–6.

6. Tempesta D, Socci V, Coppo M, Dello Ioio G, Nepa V, De Gennaro L, et al. The effect of sleep deprivation on the encoding of contextual and non-contextual aspects of emotional memory. Neurobiol Learn Mem. 2016;131:9–17.

7. Somarajan BI, Khanday MA, Mallick BN. Rapid eye movement sleep deprivation induces neuronal apoptosis by noradrenaline acting on Alpha1 adrenoceptor and by triggering mitochondrial intrinsic pathway. Front Neurol. 2016;7:25.

8. Noseda AC, Targa AD, Rodrigues LS, Aurich MF, Lima MM. REM sleep deprivation promotes a dopaminergic influence in the striatal MT2 anxiolytic-like effects. Sleep Sci. 2016;9(1):47–54.

9. De Bernardi Rodrigues AM, da Silva Cde C, Vasques AC, Camilo DF, Barreiro F, Cassani RS, et al. Association of Sleep Deprivation with Reduction in insulin sensitivity as assessed by the hyperglycemic clamp technique in adolescents. JAMA Pediatr. 2016;170(5):487–94.

10. Pikovsky O, Oron M, Shiyovich A, Perry ZH, Nesher L. The impact of sleep deprivation on sleepiness, risk factors and professional performance in medical residents. Isr Med Assoc J. 2013;15(12):739–44.

11. Mota MC, Waterhouse J, De-Souza DA, Rossato LT, Silva CM, Araujo MB, et al. Sleep pattern is associated with adipokine levels and nutritional markers in resident physicians. Chronobiol Int. 2014;31(10):1130–8.

12. Johnson EO, Roth T, Breslau N. The association of insomnia with anxiety disorders and depression: exploration of the direction of risk. J Psychiatr Res. 2006;40(8):700–8.

13. Al-Maddah EM, Al-Dabal BK, Khalil MS. Prevalence of sleep deprivation and relation with depressive symptoms among medical residents in king Fahd university hospital, Saudi Arabia. Sultan Qaboos Univ Med J. 2015;15(1):e78–84.

14. Min AA, Sbarra DA, Keim SM. Sleep disturbances predict prospective declines in resident physicians' psychological well-being. Med Educ Online. 2015;20:28530.

15. Meier-Ewert HK, Ridker PM, Rifai N, Regan MM, Price NJ, Dinges DF, et al. Effect of sleep loss on C-reactive protein, an inflammatory marker of cardiovascular risk. J Am Coll Cardiol. 2004;43(4):678–83.

16. Belayachi J, Benjelloun O, Madani N, Abidi K, Dendane T, Zeggwagh AA, et al. Self-perceived sleepiness in emergency training physicians: prevalence and relationship with quality of life. J Occup Med Toxicol. 2013;8(1):24.

17. Wali SO, Qutah K, Abushanab L, Basamh R, Abushanab J, Krayem A. Effect of on-call-related sleep deprivation on physicians' mood and alertness. Ann Thorac Med. 2013;8(1):22–7.

18. Sweileh WM, Ali IA, Sawalha AF, Abu-Taha AS, Zyoud SH, Al-Jabi SW. Sleep habits and sleep problems among Palestinian students. Child Adolesc Psychiatry Ment Health. 2011;5(1):25.

19. Sweileh WM, Ali I, Sawalha AF, Abu-Tah AS, Zyoud SH, Al-Jabi SW. Gender differences in sleep habits and sleep-related problems in Arab Palestinian university students. Int J Disabil Hum Dev. 2012;11(3):289–93.

20. Dreidi MM, Hamdan-Mansour AM. Pain, sleep disturbance, and quality of life among Palestinian patients diagnosed with Cancer. J Cancer Educ. 2016;31(4):796–803.

21. El-Kharoubi AR. Sleep disorders and excessive daytime sleepiness in the Palestinian population. Neurosciences (Riyadh). 2004;9(1):46–8.

22. McDonald J, Potyk D, Fischer D, Parmenter B, Lillis T, Tompkins L, et al. Napping on the night shift: a study of sleep, performance, and learning in physicians-in-training. J Grad Med Educ. 2013;5(4):634–8.

23. Raosoft. Sample Size Calculator. http://www.raosoft.com/samplesize.html. Accessed 20 Apr 2014.

24. Johns MW. Reliability and factor analysis of the Epworth sleepiness scale. Sleep. 1992;15(4):376–81.

25. Ahmed AE, Fatani A, Al-Harbi A, Al-Shimemeri A, Ali YZ, Baharoon S, et al. Validation of the Arabic version of the Epworth sleepiness scale. J Epidemiol Glob Health. 2014;4(4):297–302.

26. Hays RD, Sherbourne CD, Mazel RM. The RAND 36-item health survey 1.0. Health Econ. 1993;2(3):217–27.

27. Zhu YX, Li T, Fan SR, Liu XP, Liang YH, Liu P. Health-related quality of life as measured with the short-form 36 (SF-36) questionnaire in patients with recurrent vulvovaginal candidiasis. Health Qual Life Outcomes. 2016;14(1):65.

28. Ware JE Jr, Sherbourne CD. The MOS 36-item short-form health survey (SF-36). I Conceptual framework and item selection. Med Care. 1992;30(6):473–83.

29. Coons SJ, Alabdulmohsin SA, Draugalis JR, Hays RD. Reliability of an Arabic version of the RAND-36 health survey and its equivalence to the US-English version. Med Care. 1998;36(3):428–32.

30. Guermazi M, Allouch C, Yahia M, Huissa TB, Ghorbel S, Damak J, et al. Translation in Arabic, adaptation and validation of the SF-36 health survey for use in Tunisia. Ann Phys Rehabil Med. 2012;55(6):388–403.

31. Belayachi J, Rkain I, Rkain H, Madani N, Amlaiky F, Zekraoui A, et al. Burnout syndrome in Moroccan training resident: impact on quality of life. Iran J Public Health. 2016;45(2):260–2.

32. Sundquist J, Johansson SE. Impaired health status, and mental health, lower vitality and social functioning in women general practitioners in Sweden. A cross-sectional survey. Scand J Prim Health Care. 1999;17(2):81–6.

33. Paul F, Schredl M, Alpers GW. Nightmares affect the experience of sleep quality but not sleep architecture: an ambulatory polysomnographic study. Borderline Personal Disord Emot Dysregul. 2015;2:3.

34. Bolster L, Rourke L. The effect of restricting Residents' duty hours on patient safety, resident well-being, and resident education: an updated systematic review. J Grad Med Educ. 2015;7(3):349–63.

35. Baiardi S, La Morgia C, Sciamanna L, Gerosa A, Cirignotta F, Mondini S. Is the Epworth sleepiness scale a useful tool for screening excessive daytime sleepiness in commercial drivers? Accid Anal Prev. 2018;110:187–9.

36. Kendzerska TB, Smith PM, Brignardello-Petersen R, Leung RS, Tomlinson GA. Evaluation of the measurement properties of the Epworth sleepiness scale: a systematic review. Sleep Med Rev. 2014;18(4):321–31.

22

Food offerings on board and dietary intake of European and Kiribati seafarers - cross-sectional data from the seafarer nutrition study

Birgit-Christiane Zyriax[1*], Robert von Katzler[2], Bettina Jagemann[3], Joachim Westenhoefer[4], Hans-Joachim Jensen[2], Volker Harth[2] and Marcus Oldenburg[2]

Abstract

Background: Overweight and cardiovascular risk factors are a common phenomenon in seafarers. According to internal observation particularly crew members from the Pacific Island State of Kiribati are exposed to a high risk. However, in mixed crews, cultural background plays an important role, influencing food choice, and the actual risk.

Methods: The Seafarer Nutrition Study (SeaNut study) compared dietary factors in 48 Kiribati and 33 European male seafarers recruited from four merchant ships with a high level of Kiribati manning within a German shipping company. Analysis encompassed the assessment of dietary quality on board, satisfaction with prepared dishes, and individual food intake obtained from 24-h recalls in comparison with nutritional recommendations.

Results: The overall supply of meat, fat and eggs was more than double, whereas the proportions of fruits, vegetables, dairy products and cereals were much lower than recommended. Based on the reported food choices, both groups, but notably Kiribati seafarers, did not reach reference values as to macronutrient, micronutrient and fiber intake. In addition, satisfaction with the meals served, food preferences and knowledge about a healthy diet varied markedly between Kiribati and Europeans.

Conclusions: The present analysis of the SeaNut study revealed the necessity of future health intervention programs, including the quality of the food supply as well as information about a healthy diet and adequate food selection. In mixed crews, culture-specific differences should be considered, in order to facilitate the long-term success of interventions.

Trial registration: German Clinical Trials Registry DRKS00010819 retrospectively. Registered 18 July 2016 (www. germanctr.de).

Keywords: Seafarer, Kiribati, Diet, Food offerings, Food choice, Anthropometry

Background

Previous research indicates that seafarers on merchant ships are exposed to a high risk of overweight and cardiovascular disease due to specific work conditions [1]. Obesity not only increases the risk of cardiovascular events but also affects physical performance in daily duties and safety of operations and may become a problem in cases of acute complications without adequate access to professional medical service [2, 3]. Restricted food choice, limited leisure time possibilities, and smoking in addition to psychosocial stress and homesickness, characterize the specific workplace conditions, and the risk appears to increase with increasing duration of employment at sea [4–6]. However, according to an internal report of a German shipping company particularly crew members from the Pacific Island State of Kiribati are affected by a substantial weight gain

* Correspondence: bzyriax@uke.de
[1]Preventive Medicine and Nutrition, Institute for Health Services Research in Dermatology and Nursing (IVDP), University Medical Center Hamburg-Eppendorf, Martinistr. 52 - Bldg. O56 – D-20246, Hamburg, Germany
Full list of author information is available at the end of the article

during their stay on board. Currently more than 60,000 seafarers are employed on German vessels with a share of at least 2% from this very small Pacific Island. In Germany, there are some shipping companies with a high proportion of Kiribati seafarers as these employees are known to be very experienced in seafaring and medical fit for sea service. The social-economic status of Kiribati seamen is generally low, corresponding with their often low-rank position on board as non-officers.

Predominantly limited opportunities to select a healthy, balanced diet for several months on board may contribute to the high prevalence of overweight and associated cardiovascular risk factors among seafarers [1, 2]. Due to the stressful working conditions, eating is an important daily pleasure. A survey of two Danish shipping companies in a homogeneous collective reported a higher frequency of overeating as well as a higher intake of cakes, sweets and sugared beverages on board compared with the home setting [7]. In addition, previous research indicates that the traditional diet on board seems to be meat-oriented, while the consumption of fresh fruits and vegetables is rather low [8, 9].

Overall, research providing a detailed assessment of food offerings on board, as well as satisfaction with prepared meals and individual food choice in multi-ethnic crews is limited. This prompted us to investigate the Seafarer Nutrition Study (SeaNut) to analyze food quantity and quality on merchant vessels in relation to current recommendations and to compare individual nutrition intake, food preferences and satisfaction of European and Kiribati seafarers in order to identify unhealthy dietary habits.

Methods
Design and recruitment
The SeaNut study is a cross-sectional study comparing dietary and lifestyle factors, anthropometric parameters in seafarers of European origin with those from Kiribati, a Pacific island group. Between April and August 2014, over a course of more than 100 days a total of 81 male seafarers, 33 from European countries (i.a. 18 from Germany, 9 from Poland) and 48 Kiribati, were recruited from four merchant ships of a German shipping company during the sea voyage. Since the shipping company tries to assign groups of seafarers of the same origin on their ships, 4 vessels with a particular high number of Kiribati were identified for examination. The study protocol was approved by the Ethics committee of Medical Association Hamburg and conducted according to the principles of the Declaration of Helsinki. Written informed consent was obtained from all participants.

Data collection
All interviews and physical examinations were taken on board of the ships and conducted in English, the official language on board and performed by the same previously trained physician.

Assessment of demographic and clinical data
Information about demographic characteristics, occupation, medication use, and family history of cardiovascular disease was obtained using questionnaires. Body height and weight were measured during the ship's stay in port. Body mass index (BMI) was calculated as BMI = (weight, kg)/(height, m)^2. Overweight was defined as a BMI $\geq$ 25 kg/m^2, while a BMI $\geq$ 30 kg/m^2 was considered as obesity. To assess the weight development of the Kiribati crew members up to the current shipboard examination, information about weight and height from their prior medical fitness tests ashore were obtained. Waist circumference (WC) was measured halfway between the lower rib margin and the iliac crest. A waist circumference > 94 cm was defined as central obesity, however cut-off values referred to Europeans as no reference-values were available for Kiribati in the literature.

Assessment of food offerings on board and individual satisfaction
To assess the quality and quantity of the diet on board, the preparation and the composition of the three main courses per day were analyzed on every ship on seven consecutive days, taken into account recipes and the proportional distribution of relevant food groups. Meal components were weighted and a 'standard plate' representing the average offering on board was calculated and photographed. Since special nutritional guidelines for seafarers and particularly reference values for Kiribati are lacking the analysis mainly comprised the proportional intake of six relevant food groups representing a healthy balanced diet according to nutritional recommendations: Cereals and potatoes (33%), vegetables and salads (23%), dairy products (17%), fruits (14%), meat, processed meat, eggs and fish (11%), and finally, fat and oils (2%) (Fig. 1) [10]. Apart from an additional pan with freely available rice the food provision for officers and non-officers did not differ aboard the four examined vessels.

Regarding the daily food offerings on board, during a structured interview all seafarers were asked about their satisfaction (single choice question: "Are you satisfied with the supply of food you have on board?"), individual wishes and suggestions (multiple choice question: "Imagine you could make changes related to the food on board. Please check from the following list the items which you would change."), and in addition their knowledge about a healthy diet (single choice question: "Did you feel well-informed about- healthy food?" Yes-No). These questions were analyzed on a group basis, comparing European vs. Kiribati seafarers [11].

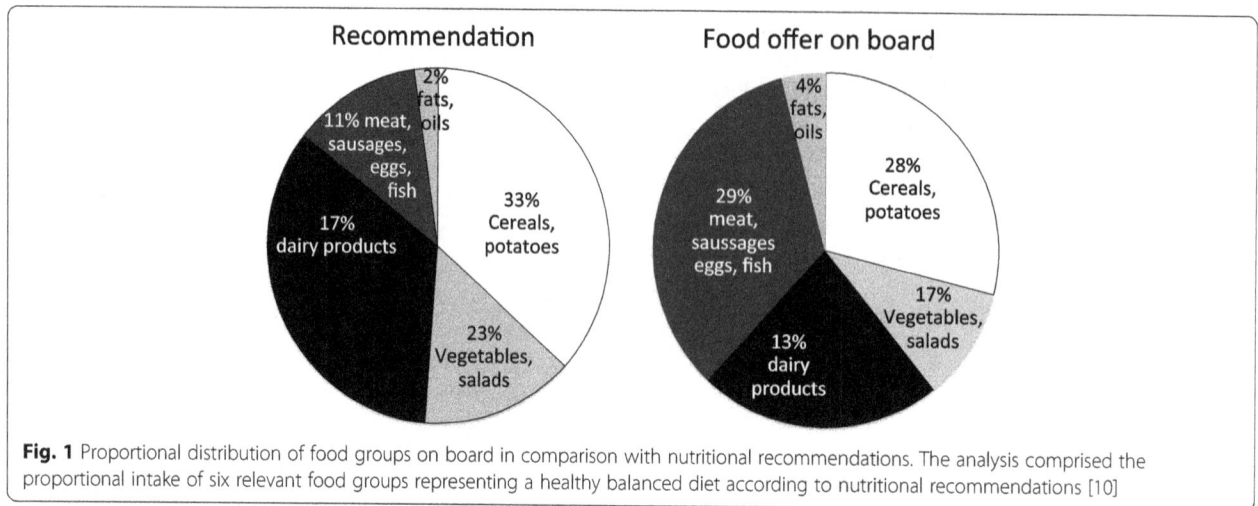

Fig. 1 Proportional distribution of food groups on board in comparison with nutritional recommendations. The analysis comprised the proportional intake of six relevant food groups representing a healthy balanced diet according to nutritional recommendations [10]

Assessment of individual food intake

Individual nutrition intake was obtained by the 24-h dietary recall method, an instrument, that is widely used in surveys and cross-sectional and cohort studies. As an open instrument the tool is suited for the assessment of dietary intake independent of cultural background [12]. This retrospective method consists of recalling and quantifying the intake of all foods and beverages consumed in the 24-h period prior to the interview and is therefore not influenced by shift work. The data were collected via face-to-face interview. The above described "standard-plate" was used as a supporting instrument to improve the assessment of dietary intake by considering portion size. Nutrition assessment followed a standardized protocol [13]. On the average, three non-consecutive 24-h recalls per person were applied (range 2–5). The results were compared with the recommendations of the German, Swiss, and Austrian Nutrition Societies [14], because information about nutrition requirements of the Kiribati population are lacking. Food records from 39 Kiribati and 24 European seafarers were available. In order to achieve a high data quality, the assessed food intake was only used from seafarers with at least two 24-h recalls available. Unfortunately several participants gave only one 24-h recall and were consequently not included. For the evaluation of the nutrition data, the OptiDiet Basic Software version 5.1 was used, which includes 15,000 foods (food items) based on the German food composition database BLS version 3.01 [15].

Statistical analysis

Baseline characteristics of the two groups (Kiribati and European) are reported as median (min-max) for continuous data or percentages for categorical data and compared using Mann–Whitney U-tests or likelihood ratio chi-square tests, as appropriate. In cases of a smaller number of incidents, Fisher's exact-test was used. P-values below 0.05 were considered to indicate

statistically significant results. Statistical analyses were performed using SPSS version 20 (IBM Corporation, New York, NY).

Results

Baseline characteristics

Median age did not differ between Kiribati and European crew members (Table 1). Most of the seafarers were married. However, more Kiribati than Europeans reported having one or more child. Occupational position differed significantly. None of the Kiribati but two-thirds of the European seafarers were employed as officers (11 nautical officers, 7 technical officers, 15 engine-room ratings, 48 deck ratings). Among Kiribati, 58% were assigned as deck ratings, 27% as engine-room ratings and 15% as galley

Table 1 Baseline characteristics of the population

Variables	Europeans $n=33$	Kiribati $n=48$	Significance P-value
Age (years)	33 (20–60)	38 (23–64)	ns [b]
Family status			
Married (%)	67	77	ns [a]
≥ 1 child (%)	46	81	0.001 [a]
Occupational status			
Officer (%)	67	0	< 0.001 [c]
Non-officer (%)	33	100	
Body mass index (kg/m²)	25.4 (18.3–35.0)	30.1 (21.1–40.5)	< 0.001 [b]
Waist circumference (cm)	93.0 (75–115)	97 (74–125)	0.045 [b]
Current smokers (%)	47	56	ns [a]

Values are given as percentage, or median (min-max)
[a]P-value of chi-square test
[b]P-value of Mann–Whitney U-test
[c]P-value of Fisher's exact-test

personnel. In view of the rather small sample size of the study, the occupational status was not included in further analysis. Compared with Europeans, median BMI and waist circumference were significantly higher in the Kiribati (Table 1). Kiribati were more often characterized by a higher prevalence of smoking. However, the results failed to show significance (Table 1). No differences of demographic or nutrition-related data were observed between the ships.

Food offerings on board and individual satisfaction

To assess the quality of the diet offered on board, the composition of the "standard-plate" was compared with nutritional recommendations [10]. The analysis clearly showed that the amounts of meat, processed meat and eggs were approximately triple, while the amount of fats and oils was double the recommendation (Fig. 1). Only once a week fish was offered on board. In contrast, the proportions of offered fruits, vegetables and salads as well as those of dairy products, cereals, and potatoes were below the recommendations (Fig. 1).

Information about individual satisfaction with the food offers on board and food preferences varied markedly depending on cultural background (Fig. 2). While half of Kiribati desired more fish, none of the European seafarers did. More Europeans reported that they would appreciate a better trained cook. However, statements common to both groups focused on a greater variety of food, the preparation of more vegetables and salads, less fatty food and the availability of free mineral water.

The majority of the crew reported that job satisfaction depends on the quality of food offered (Kiribati: 61%; Europeans: 55%). However, only 24% of Kiribati and 30% of Europeans rated the taste of the food as good. Interestingly, 67% of Kiribati and 72% of European seafarers would appreciate consuming a healthier diet on board, but only 54% of Kiribati and 85% of the Europeans felt properly informed about balanced nutrition ($p = 0.005$). Fewer Kiribati agreed with the statement that the

preparation of dishes considered culture-specific preferences (data not shown). Both groups reported receiving sufficient food on board (Kiribati: 94%; Europeans: 88%), yet 42% of Europeans and 21% of Kiribati stored food in their cabins ($p = 0.042$; mainly confectionery, fruits and nuts). Notably more Kiribati than Europeans were affected by stomach aches (36% vs 9%; $p = 0.008$) and diarrhea (15% vs 3%; ns) after meals.

Intake of energy and macronutrients

Daily food intake depends on the offerings on board. However, personal decisions about the amount of food consumed and individual food preferences are possible. Based on the evaluation of the 24-h recalls a higher intake of energy, fat protein and carbohydrates was calculated for Kiribati seafarers, whereas less alcohol consumption was reported (Table 2). With regard to relative energy consumption only the percentage of protein intake differed between Kiribati and European crew members (20% vs 17%). On the average total carbohydrate and fiber intake was lower than recommended in both groups: 75% of Europeans and 87% of Kiribati reported a carbohydrate intake below 50% of total energy consumption. Furthermore, 92% of European and 100% of Kiribati seafarers did not reach the reference value of 30 g fiber per day. In contrast, mean sugar intake (sucrose) was higher than recommended, regardless of cultural background. In addition, Kiribati as well as European seafarers consumed high amounts of fat, particularly saturated fat and cholesterol (Table 2): 67% of Europeans and 92% of Kiribati reported a fat intake above 30% of total energy consumption, while cholesterol intake in 88% of European and all Kiribati seafarers was above the reference value of 300 mg per day. Saturated fat intake in Kiribati as well as in Europeans contributed to 15% of total calorie

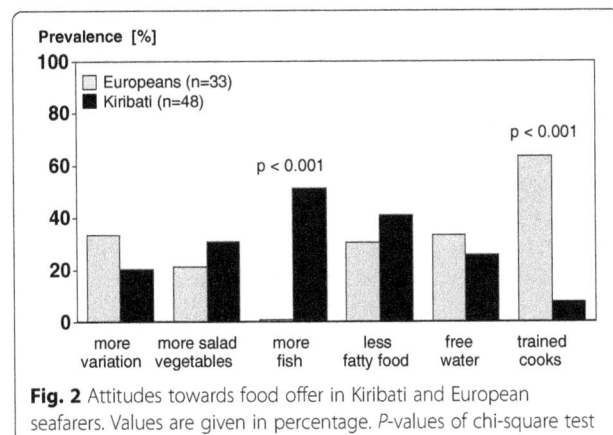

Fig. 2 Attitudes towards food offer in Kiribati and European seafarers. Values are given in percentage. *P*-values of chi-square test

Table 2 Self-reported energy and macronutrient intake of European and Kiribati seafarers

Intake per day	Europeans n = 24	Kiribati n = 39	Significance P-value
Energy (kcal)	3,094 (2,008–3,920)	3,315 (2,541–4,253)	0.017
Protein (g)	123.3 (61–180)	161.2 (116–205)	0.001
Carbohydrates (g)	311 (222–432)	357 (193–512)	0.006
Saccharose (g)	59.8 (23.8–140.6)	73.7 (6.1–215.2)	ns
Fiber (g)	21.5 (11.2–38.2)	17.1 (10.8–28.4)	< 0.001
Fat (g)	117.1 (68.7–207.8)	135.9 (75.0–208.1)	0.015
Saturated fat (g)	54.6 (26.8–91.3)	57.3 (22.5–97.4)	0.089
n-6 fatty acids (g)	13.6 (5.2–31.0)	18.6 (10.5–30.9)	0.002
n-3 fatty acids (g)	2.3 (1.3–5.3)	2.4 (1.2–5.0)	ns
Cholesterol (mg)	507 (206–1185)	871 (396–1533)	< 0.001
Alcohol (g)	13.1 (0.1–52.3)	0.5 (0.01–700)	< 0.001
Water (l)	3.0 (1.5–4.9)	2.5 (1.5–4.1)	0.008

Values are given as median (min-max). P-value of Mann–Whitney U-test intake, which is more than double the recommended < 7% of energy intake according to the guidelines of the American Heart Association [16]. In contrast, the intake of polyunsaturated fat, particularly fatty acids of omega-3 origin (e.g., fish, nuts, rapeseed oil) was low, which was also reflected by an unfavorable omega-6 to omega-3 quotient above the recommended ratio of 1.5 (data not shown).

Intake of vitamins and minerals

Evaluation of micronutrient intake showed that mean daily intake of folic acid was significantly lower in Kiribati than in Europeans (0.24 (0.13–0.38) mg vs 0.30 (0.14–0.41) mg, whereas mean ingestion of iodine did not differ (Kiribati: 0.12 (0.05–0.20) mg; European: 0.10 (0.05–0.16) mg; ns). However, mean dietary intake of both micronutrients was obviously below the recommendation in both groups (folic acid: 0.30 mg/day; iodine: 0.2 mg/day) [13]. In addition, except for vitamin B12, a considerable portion of seafarers did not reach the recommended threshold (Fig. 3). None of the crew members fulfilled the recommendation as to vitamin D intake. Interestingly, despite exposure to sunlight (UVB), 54% of Kiribati and 76% of Europeans were characterized by vitamin D plasma levels below 20 ng/dl (data not shown). Regarding salt consumption, daily sodium intake of all seafarers exceeded the recommendation of < 2.3 g corresponding to < 6 g salt per day [14, 16]. Besides the intake of micronutrients from food, European seafarers but none of the Kiribati reported using supplements containing vitamins (27%) or minerals (24%). However, evaluation of the obtained data is difficult as various products were reported.

Discussion

To our knowledge this is the first comprehensive investigation assessing food quality, satisfaction with on-board food availability and individual food choice in European and Kiribati seafarers. Taking into account the six

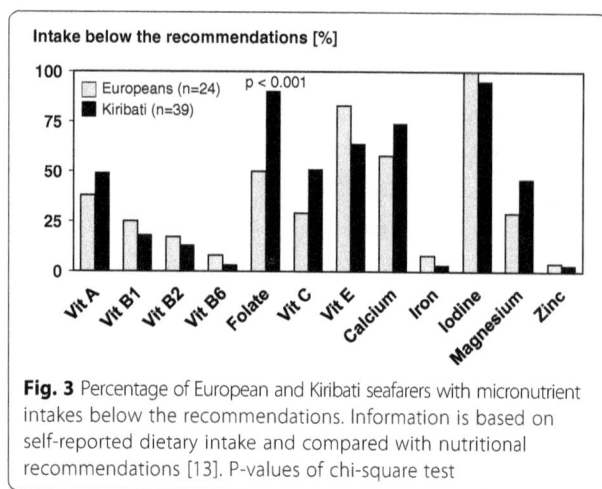

Fig. 3 Percentage of European and Kiribati seafarers with micronutrient intakes below the recommendations. Information is based on self-reported dietary intake and compared with nutritional recommendations [13]. P-values of chi-square test

relevant food groups that characterize a healthy diet, one principal finding of the SeaNut study was that the overall food supply on board did not meet nutritional recommendations. However, although both ethnic groups received the same food offerings, individual food choice revealed that the observed mismatch was more pronounced in Kiribati concerning to folate and by trend to vitamin C, calcium and magnesium (Fig. 3). In addition, satisfaction with prepared dishes, individual food preferences, and knowledge about a healthy diet varied markedly between Kiribati and Europeans. Therefore, in mixed crews effective health programs targeting food offerings and individual food choice on board should consider cultural background, which may facilitate or hinder the implementation and long-term success of interventions.

Food supply and food choice

According to the present analysis, the diet on board was more meat-, and fat-oriented, while fewer fruits, vegetables, dairy products, cereals and potatoes were offered. These findings are largely supported by previous research [7, 9]. According to a Polish study, the energy intake of crew members substantially exceeded the recommended daily level [8]. Based on Danish research, obesity represents a major public health issue among seafarers, and there is a call for corporate action to address its increasing rates [2, 17]. Interestingly, in the SeaNut study, the preferential selection of energy-dense food concomitant with a strikingly high intake of calories, saturated fat, cholesterol, sugar, salt, and less fiber was common, but predominantly observed in the Kiribati. In fact, overall, Kiribati seafarers were more satisfied with the food supply and reported consuming more food during their stay on board than at home. Historically, Pacific Islanders were not overweight and consumed more fish. However, dietary patterns in the Federal States of Micronesia have shifted. Processed food rich in saturated fat and refined carbohydrates imported mostly from the U.S. contributed to the global rise in obesity [18–20].

According to an internal observation from a previous study the total energy expenditure per day depends on the occupational position (2.880 kcal nautical officers, 3.563 kcal ratings deck and 3.389 kcal engine room personnel) (unpublished data). These data indicate strenuous physical tasks especially for ratings as mainly represented by Kiribati in this study. In spite of this physical effort, Kiribati were characterized by substantial weight gain on board and a much higher BMI and waist circumference in comparison with Europeans. In addition, dietary habits have a major impact on coronary heart disease independent of, and additive to, that of conventional risk factors, which underscores the importance of nutritional interventions on board [21].

Job satisfaction depends on the quality of the food supply

Of course, food is an important pleasure of the day, and overeating has been described previously as a common phenomenon in seafarers due to specific workplace conditions [7, 22]. Stressful conditions such as shift work, long working hours, less sleep and irregular meal times influence appetite, emotional eating, and food choice. Consequently, a higher amount of energy-dense, fat- and sugar-rich food is preferred [23]. In addition, stress exaggerates diet-induced obesity through neuropeptide Y, leading to the accumulation of abdominal fat [24]. In fact, compared with Europeans, Kiribati were more often identified as having a higher stress level, but the difference was not significant (data not shown). Another relevant determinant of obesity is the socioeconomic condition, e.g., the fact that Kiribati hold lower-ranked positions [25]. However, according to a previous report, a higher frequency of overeating on board did neither depend on professional status nor workplace [22]. Hence, in terms of obesity, cultural background and genetic aspects, which cannot be excluded, appear to play an important role [25, 26]. Recently, a cross-sectional study of another Pacific island society indicated a nutritional transition toward more imported and processed foods and a more sedentary lifestyle associated with a higher prevalence of the metabolic syndrome [27]. Still, more information about eating behaviors of non-Europeans, particularly Kiribati is required.

A more balanced diet on board is favored

Interestingly, despite their cultural differences, most Kiribati and European seafarers reported that they would appreciate a more balanced diet on board. In line with this statement, both groups asked for the preparation of more vegetables and salads, fewer fatty foods, the availability of free mineral water, and actions to be taken to improve food quality on board. As a consequence of the limited supply of fresh fruits, vegetables, legumes, potatoes, and cereals a consistent number of crew members fail to meet the recommended daily intake of micronutrients such as folate and vitamin C, as well as magnesium. Calcium deficiency reflects the rather low consumption of dairy products by the crew. Certainly, with regard to the high prevalence rate of lactose intolerance in Polynesian populations, calcium sources such as vegetables (e.g., broccoli, cabbage) and calcium-rich mineral water should be considered [28]. Carbohydrate intolerance may also explain in part the higher prevalence of gastrointestinal disorders in Kiribati seafarers compared with Europeans. Nevertheless, it might be necessary to provide improved logistics (e.g. larger fresh food supply aboard ships, more frequent deliveries, larger refrigeration rooms) to accommodate the need for more fresh and healthy food.

Challenges in promoting a healthy diet on board

Despite favoring a more balanced diet, Kiribati felt less informed about the criteria for good nutrition and were not able to assess whether the prepared meals included a variety of foods. Simplified information provided by a health consultant and adapted to cultural preferences seems to be useful but not at all sufficient. Implementing and maintaining a healthy diet and food choice on board is a huge challenge. Knowledge transfer along with individualized tips, strategies to overcome traditional dietary habits, and improved skills of the cooks, as well as logistical efforts to offer fresh food and free calcium-rich mineral water should be considered and addressed at the management level [7]. In the SeaNut study particularly Europeans suggest better training for cooks. Encouragement and continuous training of seafarers with food responsibilities will contribute better quality and taste to prepared meals, a frequently mentioned desire in both groups. In a pilot project from Finland special attention and information regarding healthier eating habits and less alcohol consumption was provided to seafarers at risk [29]. One year after the intervention alcohol consumption was reduced and an improvement in seafarers' perception of the meals prepared as being healthier was documented. Another study from Denmark clearly showed that, after a training was provided to cooks, significant changes, such as sugar reduction and more frequent use of vegetables were observed however, the results may not apply to multi-ethnic groups [7].

Interventions should take cultural preferences into consideration

Results from the SeaNut study indicate that cultural background markedly influences satisfaction with the food supply and individual food choice. Particularly Kiribati claimed that the cook did not consider culture-specific preferences when preparing meals. Despite high satisfaction with meat dishes, Kiribati predominately suggest more frequent preparation of fish dishes, reflecting the traditional diet in their home country. Instead of an often uncontrolled use of nutritional supplements, replacing meat by more fish on board will markedly reduce the intake of saturated fat and cholesterol and contribute to an improved and sufficient supply of iodine, vitamin D, and omega-3 fatty acids. In contrast, seafarers of European origin predominately cited the restricted food choice as one explanation for why they stored food twice as often in their cabins. Of course, in light of a sustainable intervention continuous training of seafarers responsible for food preparation should be considered. A shift towards a lighter, more plant-based nutrient-dense diet comprising higher amounts of fresh fruits and vegetables, fish instead of meat, less fat, salt and sugar will reduce the prevalence of overweight and obesity. In addition, a healthy, well-balanced diet will counteract micronutrient deficiency. The use of iodized table salt will contribute to an improved supply of iodine. Overall, the findings of the SeaNut study underline the need for continuous interventions taking into account multi-ethnic differences. The very rich food offerings on board seems particularly tempting for the Kiribati promoting overconsumption and weight gain.

Limitations

The present analysis of the SeaNut study has several limitations that need to be addressed. First, the sample size is rather small. In consequence differences between the two groups have to be large to reach significance. Second, the nutrient assessment was obtained from 24-h recalls and thus depended on self-reported data. Therefore, underreporting might have occurred, particularly in overweight and obese seafarers. However, if anything this is more likely to lead to an underestimation of the differences in intake. Thirdly, interpretation and comparison of anthropometry and clinical characteristics between the two groups are limited, because reference values for the Kiribati population are lacking. Despite these limitations, our data provide relevant hypotheses about food offerings on board, satisfaction with the food supply, and individual nutrition intake in light of cultural-specific differences that require further confirmation in a larger cohort.

Conclusion

The analysis of the SeaNut study clearly showed a mismatch between food supply, food choice and current recommendations in multi-ethnic ship crews. However, differences were more pronounced in Kiribati compared to European seafarers. In summary, a higher quality of food supply, training for the cook, improved logistics to offer more fresh food, increased awareness about the necessity of dietary improvements, and nutritional counseling delivered to all crew members with respect to cultural preferences and beliefs are highly justified. In the light of the increasing global labor migration the results of the SeaNut study may also provide specific information to enhance future interventions at multi-ethnic workings places.

Acknowledgments
We are indebted to all the study participants for their collaboration and to Dr. Claudia Terschüren for checking the statistical concept of this study. The authors thank the shipping company for their support and all seafarers for participating in this study.

Funding
The study was financially and logistically supported by the shipping company Hamburg Süd "COLUMBUS" Ship management, which made all four vessels available for on-board examination.

Authors' contributions
BCZ contributed to the concept of the study and wrote the paper. RK recruited participants and acquired all data, was responsible for the statistical analysis, was involved in drafting the manuscript and made a critical revision of the manuscript. BJ, JW, HJJ and VH contributed to the concept of the study and made critical revisions of the manuscript. MO suggested the study, contributed to the design and concept of the statistical analysis and made critical revisions of the manuscript. All authors read and approved the final manuscript.

Competing interests
The authors declare that they have no competing interests.

Author details
[1]Preventive Medicine and Nutrition, Institute for Health Services Research in Dermatology and Nursing (IVDP), University Medical Center Hamburg-Eppendorf, Martinistr. 52 - Bldg. O56 – D-20246, Hamburg, Germany. [2]Department of Maritime Medicine, Institute for Occupational and Maritime Medicine (ZfAM) Hamburg, University Medical Center Hamburg-Eppendorf, Hamburg, Germany. [3]I. Medical Clinic and Polyclinic; University Medical Center Hamburg-Eppendorf, Hamburg, Germany. [4]Competence Center Health, Faculty of Life Sciences, Hamburg University of Applied Sciences, Hamburg, Germany.

References
1. Oldenburg M, Jensen HJ, Latza U, Baur X. Coronary risks among seafarers aboard German-flagged ships. Int Arch Occup Environ Health. 2008;81:735–41.
2. Hansen HL, Hjarnoe L, Jepsen JR. Obesity continues to be a major health risk for Danish seafarers and fishermen. Int Marit Health. 2011;62:98–103.
3. Nas S, Fiskin R. A research on obesity among Turkish seafarers. Int Marit Health. 2014;65:187–91. https://doi.org/10.5603/IMH.2014.0036.
4. Oldenburg M, Jensen HJ, Latza U, Baur X. Seafaring stressors aboard merchant and passenger ships. Int J Public Health. 2009;54:96–105. https://doi.org/10.1007/s00038-009-7067-z.
5. Chen WQ, Wong TW, Yu TS. Influence of occupational stress on mental health among Chinese off-shore oil workers. Scand J Public Health. 2009;37:766–73. https://doi.org/10.1177/1403494809341097.
6. Fort E, Massardier-Pilonchery A, Bergeret A. Alcohol and nicotine dependence in French seafarers. Int Marit Health. 2009;60:18–28.
7. Hjarnoe L, Leppin A. What does it take to get a healthy diet at sea? A maritime study of the challenges of promoting a healthy lifestyle at the workplace at sea. Int Marit Health. 2014;2:79–86. https://doi.org/10.5603/IMH.2014.0018.
8. Babicz-Zielinska E, Zabrocki R. Assessment of nutrition of seamen and fishermen. Rocz Panstw Zakl Hig. 1998;49:499–505.
9. Lawrie T, Matheson C, Ritchie L, Murphy E, Bond C. The health and lifestyle of Scottish fishermen: a need for health promotion. Health Educ Res. 2004;19:373–9.
10. German Society for Nutrition (2017), http://www.dge-ernaehrungskreis.de/start. Accessed 25 June 2017.
11. Westenhoefer J, von Katzler R, Jensen HJ, Zyriax BC, Jagemann B, Harth V, Oldenburg M. Cultural differences in food and shape related attitudes and eating behavior are associated with differences of body mass index in the same food environment: crosssectional results from the seafarer nutrition study of Kiribati and European seafarers on merchant ships. BMC Obesity. 2018;5:1. https://doi.org/10.1186/s40608-018-0180-x.
12. Ngo J, Engelen A, Molag M, Roesle J, García-Segovia P, Serra-Majem L. A review of the use of information and communication technologies for dietary assessment. Br J Nutr. 2009;101(Suppl 2):S102–12. https://doi.org/10.1017/S0007114509990638.
13. Gibson RS. Principles of nutritional assessment: Oxford university press; 2005.
14. D-A-CH Referenzwerte für die Nährstoffzufuhr. Deutsche Gesellschaft für Ernährung (DGE), Österreichische Gesellschaft für Ernährung (ÖGE), Schweizerische Vereinigung für Ernährung (SGE). Frankfurt/ Main: Umschau/ Braus; 2015. 2015, ISBN-10: 3829571143
15. Hartmann B, Bell S, et al. Der Bundeslebensmittelschlüssel: Aktuelle Entwicklungen, Potential und Perspektiven; Ernährungs-Umschau : Forschung & Praxis, vol. 53; 2006. p. 124–9.
16. American Heart Association. Recommended dietary pattern to achieve

Food offerings on board and dietary intake of European and Kiribati seafarers - cross-sectional...

197

adherence to the American Heart Association/American College of Cardiology (AHA/ACC) guidelines: a scientific statement from the American Heart Association. Circulation. 2016;134:e505–29. https://doi.org/10.1161/CIR. 0000000000000462. Accessed at 27 Apr 2017

17. Jepsen JR, Rasmussen HB. The metabolic syndrome among Danish seafarers: a follow-up study. Int Marit Health. 2016;67:129–36. https://doi. org/10.5603/IMH.2016.0025.

18. Cassels S. Overweight in the Pacific: links between foreign dependence, global food trade, and obesity in the Federated States of Micronesia. Glob Health. 2006;2:10.

19. Micha R, Khatibzadeh S, Shi P, Fahimi S, Lim S, Andrews KG, et al. Global, regional, and national consumption levels of dietary fatsand oils in 1990 and 2010: a systematic analysis including 266 country-specific nutrition surveys. BMJ. 2014;348:g2272. https://doi.org/10.1136/bmj.g2272.

20. Charlton KE, Russell J, Gorman E, Hanich Q, Delisle A, Campbell B, et al. Fish, food security and health in Pacific Island countries and territories: a systematic literature review. BMC Public Health. 2016;16:285. https://doi.org/ 10.1186/s12889-016-2953-919.

21. Zyriax B-C, Boeing H, Windler E. Nutrition is a powerful independant risk factor for coronary heart disease in women - the CORA study: a population-based case-control study. Eur J Clin Nutr. 2005;59:1201–7.

22. Hjarnoe L, Leppin A. A risky occupation? (un)healthy lifestyle behaviors among Danish seafarers. Health Promot Int. 2013;29:720–9. https://doi.org/ 10.1093/heapro/dat024.

23. Oldenburg M. Risk of cardiovascular diseases in seafarers. Int Marit Health. 2014;65:53–7. https://doi.org/10.5603/IMH.2014.0012.

24. Kuo LE, Kitlinska JB, Tilan JU, Li L, Baker SB, Johnson MD, et al. Neuropeptide Y acts directly in the periphery on fat tissue and mediates stress-induced obesity and metabolic syndrome. Nat Med. 2007;13:803–11.

25. Marmot M. Social determinants of health inequalities. Lancet. 2005;365: 1099–104.

26. Møller Pedersen SF, Jepsen JR. The metabolic syndrome among Danish seafarers. Int Marit Health. 2013;64:183–90. https://doi.org/10.5603/IMH.2016.0025.

27. Wang D, Hawley NL, Thompson AA, Lameko V, Reupena MS, McGarvey ST, et al. Dietary patterns are associated with metabolic outcomes among adult Samoans in a cross-sectional study. J Nutr. 2017; https://doi.org/10.3945/jn. 116.243733.

28. Seakins JM, Elliott RB, Quested CM, Matatumua A. Lactose malabsorption in Polynesian and white children in the south west Pacific studied by breath hydrogen technique. Br Med J (Clin Res Ed). 1987;295:876–8.

29. Saarni H, Laine M, Niemi L. Health promotion in the Finnish shipping industry. Int Marit Health. 2001;52:44–58.

23

Mutagenic and DNA repair activity in traffic policemen

Caterina Ledda[1][*] [iD], Carla Loreto[2], Massimo Bracci[3], Claudia Lombardo[2], Gaetano Romano[1], Diana Cinà[4], Nicola Mucci[5], Sergio Castorina[2] and Venerando Rapisarda[1]

Abstract

Background: Emissions from vehicles are composed of heterogeneous mixtures of hazardous substances; several pollutants such as Polycyclic Aromatic Hydrocarbons (PAHs) are amongst the most dangerous substances detected in urban monitoring. A cohort of traffic policemen usually occupationally exposed to PAHs present in the urban environment were examined in order to assess the mutagenicity and DNA capacity repair.

Methods: Seventy-two urban traffic policemen working in Catania's metropolitan area were enrolled in the study. Two spot urine samples were collected from each subject during the whole working cycle as follows: sample 1 (S1), pre-shift on day 1; sample 2 (S2) post-shift on day 6. 1-hydroxypyrene (1-OHP) was measured to serve as an indirect exposure indicator. Urinary mutagenic activity was assessed through the plate incorporation pre-incubation technique with S9, using YG1024 Salmonella typhimurium strain over-sensitive to PAH metabolite. Concentrations of urinary 8-oxodG were measured using liquid chromatography tandem mass spectrometry.

Results: As regards the exposure to PAHs, results highlighted a statistically significant difference ($p < 0.001$) between pre-shift on day 1 and post-shift on day 6 levels. Mutagenic activity was detected in 38 (66%) workers on S1 and in 47 (81%) on S2. Also 8-oxodG analysis showed a statistically significant difference between S1 and S2 sampling.

Conclusions: This study demonstrated that occupational exposure to pollutants from traffic emission, assessed via 1-OHP measurements in urine, may lead to DNA repair and mutagenic activity, in line with other studies.

Keywords: PAHs, DNA damage, Oxidative stress, Air pollution, Urban traffic, Cancer, Worker, Salmonella typhimurium, 8-oxodG, 1-hydroxypyrene

Background

Urban traffic may impact on human health through various biological mechanisms and causes several health effects [1–5]. Moreover, the association between exposure to traffic-related air pollution and cause-specific mortality and morbidity has long been studied and dealt with in several epidemiological surveys [4, 6–9]. Emissions from vehicles are composed of heterogeneous mixtures of hazardous substances [10]; several pollutants such as Polycyclic Aromatic Hydrocarbons (PAHs) are amongst the most dangerous substances detected in urban monitoring [11–13].

PAHs are a large group of chemicals with 2 to 7 fused aromatic rings [14]. Benzo(a)pyrene (B(a)P) is one of the best-known PAHs, categorized by the International Agency for Research on Cancer (IARC) as carcinogenic to humans (group 1).

Besides, B(a)P is commonly used as indicator of PAHs global concentrations in environmental monitorings [15]. Many other PAHs are well known as cytotoxic, carcinogens, mutagens and teratogens and therefore represent a serious threat for the general population's health and well-being [5, 14, 16]. Mutagenicity of PAHs, associated with urban traffic, has been demonstrated only through in-vitro assays [17–22]. Epidemiological studies of the correlation between presence of urinary mutagens and exposure to PAHs have been previously conducted [23–26] and certainly contributed to adapting the law limits on air pollution. Presently in Europe, Directive

* Correspondence: cledda@unict.it
[1]Occupational Medicine, Department of Clinical and Experimental Medicine, University of Catania, 95100 Catania, Italy
Full list of author information is available at the end of the article

2004/107/EC provides the target values for PAHs and establishes that the threshold limit is 1 ng/m^3.

PAHs and other genotoxic chemicals are metabolized by humans and induce the expression of cytochrome P450 enzymes (i.e. CYP1A2) [27–29]. The CYP1A2 enzyme is involved in the metabolic activation of a wide range of chemicals and carcinogens like PAHs [28, 29]. Its activity has been shown to increase by smoking, ingestion of charbroiled meat, cruciferous vegetables, PAHs and PCBs exposures [28, 30–33]. The catalyzed metabolism by CYP1A2 can generate reactive oxygen species (ROS) which might lead to oxidative DNA damage [27, 34, 35]. This damage has been associated with an increased risk of cancer, generally ascribed to DNA adducts [36–38]. Oxidative DNA damage may be also important in carcinogenesis since the DNA base lesions, such as 8-oxo-7,8-dihydro-2′-deoxyguanosine (8-oxodG), are massive and highly mutagenic [39, 40]. However, DNA repair via nucleotide and base excision processes leads to elimination and excretion of 8-oxodG in urine quantitatively without metabolism [41–44]. Urinary excretion of 8-oxodG is the most widely used non-invasive urinary biomarker of oxidative stress and its measurement in urine has been proposed to assess whole-body DNA repair activity [43, 44].

In the present study, the authors investigated a cohort of traffic policemen usually occupationally exposed to PAHs present in the urban environment in order to assess the mutagenic and DNA repair activity.

Methods

Study designs, population and setting

In this case-crossover study the population comprised 72 urban traffic policemen working in Catania's metropolitan area and spend > 6 h outdoor, daily. A working cycle consisted of six consecutive working days followed by two days off. All subjects enrolled in the study were of Caucasian origin, living in the same work area. Subjects had been current non-smokers for at least 6 months, their age ranging between 20 and 60 years, being employed during at least the same period, had no history of chronic or recent illnesses (diabetes or influenza for example) and had not been taking any medication (omeoprazole, for instance) that could interfere with the study results. The study was conducted in a framework of regular occupational medical visits in April – July 2016.

Several haematological parameters tested in all these policemen, including haemoglobin, haematocrit, platelets, white blood-cell count, lymphocytes and neutrophils were analysed following standard methods.

Two spot urine samples were collected from each subject during the whole working cycle as follows: sample 1 (S1), pre-shift on day 1; sample 2 (S2) post-shift on day 6.

Prior to this, a diet had been prescribed, two weeks before, so that it did not affect this study results over the whole sampling period. In particular, subjects were asked to avoid charcoal-cooked or grilled foods.

Urine samples from workers were collected in polyethylene containers and stored in the dark at – 20 °C until analysis.

Creatinine analysis

Urine creatinine concentration was measured by spectrophotometry according to Jaffé (1885), using a commercial laboratory kit (Roche Diagnostics, Basel, Switzerland) [45].

1-hydroxypyrene analysis

The well-validated PAHs exposure biomarker 1-hydroxypyrene (1-OHP) was measured to serve as an indirect exposure indicator [46, 47]. Urinary 1-OHP was determined by HPLC (Agilent Technologies, Santa Clara, California, USA) with the fluorescence detection method, using a commercial laboratory kit (Chromsystems Instruments & Chemicals GmbH, Gräfelfing, Germany).

Briefly, after the enzymatic hydrolysis of each sample, carried out mixing 1 ml urine with 50 µl internal standard and 200 µl of the prepared enzyme solution in a reaction vial, a solid phase extraction was performed, by adding 1 ml of hydrolyzed urine to a Sample Clean Up Column and drawing through by centrifugation (2 min at 700 x g) or suction. Effluents were discarded. Then the sample was centrifuged (1 min at 700 x g) with 1000 µl Wash Buffer through the Sample Clean Up Column. Effluents were discarded. Then 300 µl of Elution Buffer were centrifuged (2 min at 700 x g) through the Sample Clean Up Column into a light-protected collection vessel. Finally, 10 µl eluate were injected into the HPLC system in isocratic flow rate (1.2 ml/min) at 35 ° C. Wave lengths were 242 and 388, for excitation and emission, respectively. The 1-OHP levels were adjusted by urinary creatinine excretion and expressed as µg/g creatinine. The method limit of quantification was 0.1 µg/l.

Mutagenic activity analysis

Urinary mutagenic activity was evaluated with the plate incorporation pre-incubation technique with S9, using YG1024 Salmonella typhimurium strain over-sensitive to PAH metabolite.

Urine samples (~ 50 ml) were thawed and filtered to remove urothelial cells. The exact volume of each sample was recorded and the samples enzymatically deconjugated in 0.2 M (10% v/v) sodium acetate buffer (pH 5.0) (Sigma–Aldrich, Missouri, USA), containing Helix pomatia β-glucuronidase (Sigma–Aldrich, Missouri, USA) 6 units/ml urine and 2 units/ml urine of sulphatase (Sigma–Aldrich, Missouri, USA) for 16 h at 37 °C. Solids were removed by centrifugation. Deconjugated urinary metabolites were then concentrated using solid-phase extraction on Mega Bond Elut Flash cartridge, C18, 2 g, 12 mL (Agilent Technologies, California, USA) with methanol elution (Sigma–Aldrich, Missouri, USA). The resulting extracts were reconstituted in dimethylsulphoxide (DMSO; Sigma–Aldrich, Missouri, USA) to produce urine extracts suitable for assessing mutagenicity. Extracts were stored at − 20 °C until use.

Urines were tested for mutagenic activity in the Salmonella assay mainly according to Maron and Ames [48].

Mutagenic activity was determined using the plate-incorporation pre-incubation technique on the YG1024 Salmonella typhimurium strain in the presence of Aroclor-induced rat liver S9 (50 µl per plate) [49]. The concentrations selected for mutagenicity testing were 0.3, 0.6, 1.2, 3.0 and 6.0 ml-equivalent urine per plate. 2-Aminofluorene (0.2 µg per plate) was used as a positive control and negative solvent checks (i.e. DMSO) were made on each day of mutagenicity testing.

Following a 72-h incubation at 37 °C, the frequency of mutant (i.e. revertant; rev) colonies was scored using a ProtoCol automated colony counter (Synbiosis Corporation, Exton, PA, USA).

Mutagenic activity was taken as positive when at least one of the tested doses was able to double the number of revertants compared to spontaneous ones and expressed as the slope of the linear portion of the dose–response curve calculated by the linear regression method, from at least two urine extract doses different from zero, as number of revertants/ml urine and number of revertants/mmol of creatinine.

Oxidative DNA lesions analysis

Concentrations of urinary 8-oxodG were measured using liquid chromatography tandem mass spectrometry (LC–MS/MS). Briefly, 5 pmol of internal standard, 15 N5-8-oxodG, were added to 200 µL of urine and then ultrapure water was added to a final volume of 1 mL, prior to solid-phase extraction (Oasis HLB column, 1 mL, 30 mg; Waters, Connecticut, USA). Quantitative analysis was performed using LC–MS/MS (6420, Agilent Technologies, California, USA).

The urine samples were processed and analyzed in duplicates on two occasions and the repeatability of the method expressed as the coefficient of variation was 10.5%. The 8-oxodG concentration was calculated as the mean of the two measurements. Two internal controls were included in each batch. Urinary 8-oxodG concentrations were adjusted to the average-specific urine gravity (1.015 g/ml) using the formula: 8-oxodG x [(1.015–1)/(measured specific gravity − 1)], as well as to nmol 8-oxodG/mmol creatinine.

Statistical analysis

Data were summarized as mean ± SD for continuous variables and frequencies for categorical variables. Normality was checked by Kolmogrov-Smirnov test and homogeneity of variance by Levene's test. Unpaired t test was used to compare the means of two groups. P values ≤0.05 were considered significant. Correlations were evaluated using simple regression analysis. Data analysis was performed using GraphPad Prism ver.7 (GraphPad Software, Inc. USA).

Results

Application of the exclusion criteria caused 14 workers to be ruled out of the sample because they admitted not having complied with the previously prescribed diet directives. Out of the 58 remaining subjects, 41 were males and 17 females, averagely aged 47 and with a mean working history of 17.6 years. Table 1 reports the main features of the subjects.

A routine occupational health examination revealed no alteration of any hematological parameters in any of the subjects. As regards the exposure to PAHs, results highlighted a statistically significant difference ($p < 0.001$) between pre-shift on day 1 and post-shift on day 6 in 1-OHP levels, that were 0.17 ± 0.09 and 0.38 ± 0.12 µg/g creatinine, respectively.

Mutagenic activity was detected in 38 (66%) workers on S1 and in 47 (81%) on S2, the mean levels of revertants/mmol creatinine being 21.26 ± 10.63 and 62.43 ± 20.91, respectively ($p < 0.001$).

Also 8-oxodG analysis showed a statistically significant difference ($p < 0.001$) between S1 and S2 sampling, the mean values being 2.73 ± 1.11 (nmol/mmol creatinine) and 4.52 ± 1.27 (nmol/mmol creatinine), respectively.

Figure 1 reports the graphic results.

No statistically different variation was detected between males and females for 1-OHP, mutagenic and repair activity.

Correlation between 1-OHP with mutagenic activity and 8-oxodG showed a statistically significant difference ($p > 0.05$).

Table 1 Main features of samples and main results

	Results
Gender (Male)	41 (71%)
Age (yrs)	47 ± 10.2
BMI (kg/m²)	22.7 ± 2.1
Working age (yrs)	17.6 ± 8.4
No smokers	58 (100%)
Alcohol consumption (g/die)	12.4 ± 2.7

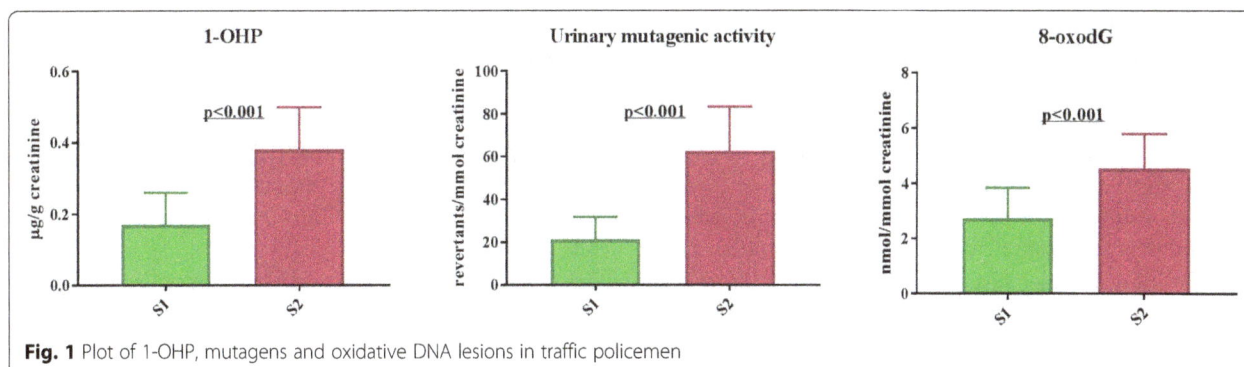

Fig. 1 Plot of 1-OHP, mutagens and oxidative DNA lesions in traffic policemen

Discussion

Air pollution is a constant problem the world over and it has given rise to many different health problems [50]. As described by World Health Organization, traffic is the most important contributor to outdoor air pollution, because it is associated with negative effects on human health [51]. Traffic pollution contains high proportions of PAHs which is a group of over a hundred different organic compounds [10]. The main source of PAHs in the environment is incomplete combustion of organic substances; however, they are mainly released from vehicle exhaust pipes during diesel and petrol incomplete combustion [52, 53].

PAHs have drawn the scientific community's attention because of their persistence and carcinogenic properties [54]. They enter the human body via lungs, ingestion and cutaneous paths of absorption [55]. In the urban environment, traffic pollution can be observed in traffic jams, while many studies provided evidence that owing to these events, traffic police workers, bus drivers and other cohorts exposed to traffic pollution are highly exposed to PAHs [56–58]. In human biomonitoring studies, the urinary 1-OHP, a metabolite of pyrene is a most widely used PAH internal dose biomarker and represents an internal dose of PAHs [59]. 1-OHP is also a biomarker of exposure to mixtures of PAHs [60]. A good correlation between PAH concentration in the air and urine 1-OHP has been observed in several occupational studies. Urinary levels of 1-OHP are often greatly increased in the population of polluted areas compared to those of less polluted ones [58, 60]. In addition to direct occupational exposure, indirect exposure to the outdoor environment is also a cause of increased urinary 1-OHP concentration [61].

In the present study, increased 1-OHP values were analyzed from S1 sample to S2 sample, that is after 6 working days following vehicle traffic in the streets. 1-OHP values turned out to be borderline compared to those provided by the law (0.3 μg/g creatinine).

1-OHP values were higher than those detected by Hansen et al. [58] in bus drivers (mean 0.19 μmol/mol creat) and mail carriers (mean 0.11 μmol/mol creat). The same authors, referring to a preliminary survey, had described an increased mutagenic activity in these categories of workers, although the numeric value was not comparable, as it was not reported. [58].

A study conducted by Hu et al. [57] on vehicle traffic environmental PHAs monitoring confirms that street policemen are highly exposed, even more than cooks, their levels of exposures being comparable to workers in the black carbon manufacturing industries and coke plants.

A study conducted by Burgaz et al. [56] on Ankara policemen revealed high concentrations of 1-OHP among non-smoking policemen. Comparing the data obtained with another control study, the authors concluded that occupational exposure to vehicle traffic PAHs is most evident.

Scientific past literature showed that PAHs present in traffic pollution may cause significant oxidative stress, which is characterized by an increased synthesis of free radicals [60]. Oxidative stress occurs during the imbalance between the syntheses of free radicals and antioxidants [62]. It seems that PAHs may be considered as major risk factors present in the automobile exhausts, which induce oxidative stress, as exposure to PAHs is associated with the increased production of free radicals [63]. Oxidative stress, on the other hand, may be one of the mechanisms behind many adverse health effects related to air pollution [64].

The health risks associated with exposure to PAHs is the consequence of a disturbance in the anti-oxidants defense system, resulting in significant oxidative stress [64], which is one of the major mechanisms behind the onset of cancer [65]. Large amounts of reactive oxygen species and many electrophiles are generated during the activation of PAHs by CYP450, which bind covalently with DNA and disturb cell homeostasis [66].

High antioxidants' activity in exposed subjects shows that they suffer from oxidative stress, because PAHs are known for their potential to cause oxidative stress [67, 68].

As reported by Chao et al. [69], PAHs exert their biological effects probably through the generation of ROS. These excess ROSs can lead to oxidative DNA damage. Amongst the most abundant oxidatively damaged DNA is 8-oxodG, which was found to induce mutation through G to T transversion [70].

In this study, the 8-oxodG level in S2 sample, after 6 working days, was significantly greater than S1 (day 1).

In the past decade, several studies using 8-oxodG as an oxidative injury biomarker found significantly higher 8-oxodG levels in leukocyte DNA or urine of workers exposed to PAHs deriving from coke oven emissions compared to those of non-exposed workers [71, 72]. A previous study showed a significant correlation between urinary 1-OHP and 8-oxodG in coke oven workers [73].

In the present study 8-oxodG well correlated with urinary 1-OHP concentrations.

The urinary 8-oxodG levels were also highly correlated with urinary 1-OHP and not confounded by other variables. Zang et al. [74] measured leukocyte 8-oxodG levels in workers and found that high-exposed workers had even lower levels of 8-oxodG than low-exposed workers.

Urine sampling at the end of the working week was widely used for the policemen because urinary 1-OHP excretion levels were found to rise during a working week and its half-life ranges from 6 to 35 h [75].

Besides, the urinary 8-oxodG at the end of the working week (S2) showed relatively higher levels compared to day 1 (S1), as the biomarker of effect (e.g., 8-oxodG) not only reflects the exposure during a week-shift but also a much longer period of exposure [76].

There are some limitations to the present study. Firstly, the number of workers investigated was small because strict inclusion criteria to select the participants were applied. A second limitation was that there was no environmental sampling. Thirdly, no benzene determination was carried out either in the environment or amongst the biological exposure indicators. The benzene action shall be analyzed in a further study. Finally, biological monitoring of the study should also take other seasons than spring into due consideration [77–82]. As a matter of fact, a previous study, conducted in Catania, revealed greater concentrations of PAHs during winter time.

Conclusions

From the result analysis of this study, it can be observed that 1-OHP urine concentration increases significantly in street policemen, after one week work shift. This reveals a certain exposure to PAHs. In the same way, the mutagenic activity initially observed (S1) in 66% of the sample turns out to be increased, as it involves over 80% of it.

The DNA repair activity, computed by measuring 8-oxidG concentrations, significantly increased between the S1 and S2 periods. Besides, 8-oxidg values significantly correlated with 1-OHP concentrations.

The analysis of other risk factors such as benzene, also emitted into the atmosphere through exhaust pipes, will further contribute to better understanding such phenomenon.

In conclusion, this study demonstrated that occupational exposure to pollutants from traffic emission is correlated to DNA repair and mutagenic activity.

Acknowledgments

The participation of the workers is this study is gratefully acknowledged. The authors thank Dr. Ermanno Vitale for the support given during the revision phase of the manuscript.

Authors' contributions

CLe, Clo and VR contributed to the concept of the study, performed the experiments, statistical analysis and wrote the paper. CIL and GR recruited participants and acquired all data. NM was involved in drafting the manuscript and made a critical revision of the manuscript. DC, MB and SC contributed to the concept of the study and made critical revisions of the manuscript. All authors read and approved the final manuscript.

Competing interests

The authors declare that they have no competing interests.

Author details

[1]Occupational Medicine, Department of Clinical and Experimental Medicine, University of Catania, 95100 Catania, Italy. [2]Human Anatomy and Histology, Department of Biomedical and Biotechnology Sciences, University of Catania, 95100 Catania, Italy. [3]Occupational Medicine, Department of Clinical and Molecular Sciences, Polytechnic University of Marche, 60100 Ancona, Italy. [4]Clinical Pathology Unit, "Garibaldi Centro" Hospital of Catania, 95100 Catania, Italy. [5]Occupational Medicine, Department of Experimental and Clinical Medicine, University of Florence, 50100 Florence, Italy.

References

1. Baccarelli A, Wright RO, Bollati V, Tarantini L, Litonjua AA, Suh HH, Zanobetti A, Sparrow D, Vokonas PS, Schwartz J. Rapid DNA methylation changes after exposure to traffic particles. Am J Respir Crit Care Med. 2009;179(7):572–8.
2. Chuang KJ, Chan CC, Su TC, Lee CT, Tang CS. The effect of urban air pollution on inflammation, oxidative stress, coagulation, and autonomic dysfunction in young adults. Am J Respir Crit Care Med. 2007;176(4):370–6.
3. Fischer PH, Hoek G, Van Reeuwijk H, Briggs DJ, Lebret E, Van Wijnen JH, Kingham S, Elliott PE. Traffic-related differences in outdoor and indoor concentrations of particles and volatile organic compounds in Amsterdam. Atmos Environ. 2000;34(22):3713–22.
4. Le Tertre A, Medina S, Samoli E, Forsberg B, Michelozzi P, Boumghar A, Vonk JM, Bellini A, Atkinson R, Ayres JG, Sunyer J, Schwartz J, Katsouyanni K. Short-term effects of particulate air pollution on cardiovascular diseases in eight european cities. J Epidemiol Community Health. 2002;56(10):773–9.
5. Nielsen T, Jørgensen HE, Larsen JC, Poulsen M. City air pollution of polycyclic aromatic hydrocarbons and other mutagens: Occurrence, sources and health effects. Sci Total Environ. 1996;189–90. 41–9
6. Hoek G, Fischer P, Van Den Brandt P, Goldbohm S, Brunekreef B. Estimation of long-term average exposure to outdoor air pollution for a cohort study on mortality. J Expos Anal Environ Epidemiol. 2001;11(6):459–69.
7. Brauer M, Hoek G, Van Vliet P, Meliefste K, Fischer PH, Wijga A, Koopman LP, Neijens HJ, Gerritsen J, Kerkhof M, Heinrich J, Bellander T, Brunekreef B. Air pollution from traffic and the development of respiratory infections and asthmatic and allergic symptoms in children. Am J Respir Crit Care Med. 2002;166(8):1092–8.
8. Nyberg F, Gustavsson P, Järup L, Bellander T, Berglind N, Jakobsson R, Pershagen G. Urban air pollution and lung cancer in Stockholm. Epidemiology. 2000;11(5):487–95.
9. Nyberg F, Pershagen G. Epidemiologic studies on the health effects of ambient particulate air pollution. Scand J Work Environ Health. 2000; 26(SUPPL. 1):49–88.
10. Kleeman MJ, Schauer JJ, Cass GR. Size and composition distribution of fine particulate matter emitted from motor vehicles. Environ Sci Technol. 2000; 34(7):1132–42.
11. Vardar N, Noll KE. Atmospheric PAH concentration in fine and coarse particles. Environ Monit Assess. 2003;87(1):81–92.
12. Zhu X, Fan Z, Wu X, Jung KH, Ohman-Strickland P, Bonanno LJ, Lioy PJ. Ambient concentrations and personal exposure to polycyclic aromatic hydrocarbons (PAH) in an urban community with mixed sources of air pollution. J Expos Sci Environ Epidemiol. 2011;21(5):437–49.
13. de Guidi G, Librando V, Minniti Z, Bolzacchini E, Perrini G, Bracchitta G, Alparone A, Catalfo A. The PAH and nitro-PAH concentration profiles in size-segregated urban particulate matter and soil in traffic-related sites in Catania, Italy. Polycycl Aromat Compd. 2012;32(4):439–56.
14. Kim KH, Jahan SA, Kabir E, Brown RJC. A review of airborne polycyclic aromatic hydrocarbons (PAHs) and their human health effects. Environ Int. 2013;60:71–80.
15. IARC Working Group on the Evaluation of Carcinogenic Risks to Humans. Some non-heterocyclic polycyclic aromatic hydrocarbons and some related exposures. IARC Monogr Eval Carcinog Risks Hum. 2010;92:1–853.
16. Boström CE, Gerde P, Hanberg A, Jernström B, Johansson C, Kyrklund T, Rannug A, Törnqvist M, Victorin K, Westerholm R. Cancer risk assessment, indicators, and guidelines for polycyclic aromatic hydrocarbons in the ambient air. Environ Health Perspect. 2002;110(SUPPL. 3):451–88.
17. Ciganek M, Neca J, Adamec V, Janosek J, Machala M. A combined chemical and bioassay analysis of traffic-emitted polycyclic aromatic hydrocarbons. Sci Total Environ. 2004;334–5. 141–8
18. Masiol M, Hofer A, Squizzato S, Piazza R, Rampazzo G, Pavoni B. Carcinogenic and mutagenic risk associated to airborne particle-phase polycyclic aromatic hydrocarbons: a source apportionment. Atmos Environ. 2012;60:375–82.
19. Monarca S, Crebelli R, Feretti D, Zanardini A, Fuselli S, Filini L, Resola S, Bonardelli PG, Nardi G. Mutagens and carcinogens in size-classified air particulates of a northern italian town. Sci Total Environ. 1997;205(2–3):137–44.
20. Škarek M, Janošek J, Čupr P, Kohoutek J, Novotná-Rychetská A, Holoubek I. Evaluation of genotoxic and non-genotoxic effects of organic air pollution using in vitro bioassays. Environ Int. 2007;33(7):859–66.
21. Oh SM, Kim HR, Park YJ, Lee SY, Chung KH. Organic extracts of urban air pollution particulate matter (PM2.5)-induced genotoxicity and oxidative stress in human lung bronchial epithelial cells (BEAS-2B cells). Mutat Res Genet Toxicol Environ Mutagen. 2011;723(2):142–51.
22. Topinka J, Rossner P, Milcova A, Schmuczerova J, Svecova V, Sram RJ. DNA adducts and oxidative DNA damage induced by organic extracts from PM2.5 in an acellular assay. Toxicol Lett. 2011;202(3):186–92.
23. Clonfero E, Jongeneelen F, Zordan M, Levis AG. Biological monitoring of human exposure to coal tar urinary mutagenicity assays and analytical determination of polycyclic aromatic hydrocarbon metabolites in urine. IARC Sci Publ. 1990;104:215–22.
24. Moller M, Dybing E. Mutagenicity studies with urine concentrates from coke plant workers. Scand J Work Environ Health. 1980;6(3):216–20.
25. Granella M, Clonfero E. Sensitivity of different bacterial assays in detecting mutagens in urine of humans exposed to polycyclic aromatic hydrocarbons. Mutat Res Fundam Mol Mech Mutagen. 1992;268(1):131–7.
26. Černà M, Pastorková A, Myers SR, Rössner P, Binková B. The use of a urine mutagenicity assay in the monitoring of environmental exposure to genotoxins. Mutat Res Genet Toxicol Environ Mutagen. 1997;391(1–2):99–110.
27. Szeliga J, Dipple A. DNA adduct formation by polycyclic aromatic hydrocarbon dihydrodiol epoxides. Chem Res Toxicol. 1998;11(1):1–11.
28. Landi MT, Sinha R, Lang NP, Kadlubar FF. Human cytochrome P4501A2. IARC Sci Publ. 1999;148:173–95.
29. Rundle A, Tang D, Zhou J, Cho S, Perera F. The association between glutathione S-transferase M1 genotype and polycyclic aromatic hydrocarbon-DNA adducts in breast tissue. Cancer Epidemiol Biomark Prev. 2000;9(10):1079–85.
30. Sinha R, Rothman N, Mark SD, Hoover RN, Caporaso NE. Pan-fried meat containing high levels of heterocyclic aromatic amines but low levels of polycyclic aromatic hydrocarbons induces cytochrome P4501A2 activity in humans. Cancer Res. 1994;54(23):6154–9.
31. Safe SH. Modulation of gene expression and endocrine response pathways by 2,3,7,8-tetrachlorodibenzo-p-dioxin and related compounds. Pharmacol Ther. 1995;67(2):247–81.
32. Kall MA, Clausen J. Dietary effect on mixed function P450 1A2 activity assayed by estimation of caffeine metabolism in man. Hum Exp Toxicol. 1995;14(10):801–7.
33. Li W, Harper PA. Tang B-, Okey AB. Regulation of cytochrome P450 enzymes by aryl hydrocarbon receptor in human cells. CYP1A2 expression in the LS180 colon carcinoma cell line after treatment with 2,3,7,8-tetrachlorodibenzo-p-dioxin or 3-methylcholanthrene. Biochem Pharmacol. 1998;56(5):599–612.
34. Loft S, Deng X-, Tuo J, Wellejus A, Sørensen M, Poulsen HE. Experimental study of oxidative DNA damage. Free Radic Res 1998;29(6):525–539.
35. Bonvallot V, Baeza-Squiban A, Baulig A, Brulant S, Boland S, Muzeau F, Barouki R, Marano F. Organic compounds from diesel exhaust particles elicit a proinflammatory response in human airway epithelial cells and induce cytochrome p450 1A1 expression. Am J Resp Cell Mol Biol. 2001;25(4):515–21.
36. Cheng YW, Chen CY, Lin P, Chen C-, Huang KH, Lin TS, Wu MH, Lee H. DNA adduct level in lung tissue may act as a risk biomarker of lung cancer. Eur J Cancer 2000;36(11):1381–1388.
37. Loft S, Poulsen HE. Cancer risk and oxidative DNA damage in man. J Mol Med. 1996;74(6):297–312.
38. Kasai H. Analysis of a form of oxidative DNA damage, 8-hydroxy-2'-deoxyguanosine, as a marker of cellular oxidative stress during carcinogenesis. Mutat Res Rev Mutat Res. 1997;387(3):147–63.
39. Loft S, Poulsen HE. Antioxidant intervention studies related to DNA damage, DNA repair and gene expression. Free Radic Res. 2000; 33(SUPPL):S67–83.
40. Nishimura S. Involvement of mammalian OGG1(MMH) in excision of the 8-hydroxyguanine residue in DNA. Free Radic Biol Med. 2002;32(9):813–21.
41. Bjelland S, Seeberg E. Mutagenicity, toxicity and repair of DNA base damage induced by oxidation. Mutat Res Fundam Mol Mech Mutagen. 2003;531(1–2):37–80.
42. Møller P, Vogel U, Pedersen A, Dragsted LO, Sandström B, Loft S. No effect of 600 grams fruit and vegetables per day on oxidative DNA damage and repair in healthy nonsmokers. Cancer Epidemiol Biomark Prev. 2003;12(10):1016–22.
43. Loft S, Poulsen HE. Markers of oxidative damage to DNA: antioxidants and molecular damage; 1998. 166 p.

44. Olinski R, Rozalski R, Gackowski D, Foksinski M, Siomek A, Cooke MS. Urinary measurement of 8-OxodG, 8-OxoGua, and 5HMUra: a noninvasive assessment of oxidative damage to DNA. Antioxid Redox Signal. 2006;8(5–6):1011–9.

45. Costa C, Rapisarda V, Catania S, Di Nola C, Ledda C, Fenga C. Cytokine patterns in greenhouse workers occupationally exposed to α-cypermethrin: an observational study. Environ Toxicol Pharmacol. 2013;36(3):796–800.

46. Loreto C, Rapisarda V, Carnazza ML, Musumeci G, D'Agata V, Valentino M, Martinez G. Bitumen products alter bax, bcl-2 and cytokeratin expression: an in vivo study of chronically exposed road pavers. J Cutaneous Pathol. 2007; 34(9):699–704.

47. Rapisarda V, Carnazza ML, Caltabiano C, Loreto C, Musumeci G, Valentino M, Martinez G. Bitumen products induce skin cell apoptosis in chronically exposed road pavers. J Cutaneous Pathol. 2009;36(7):781–7.

48. Maron DM, Ames BN. Revised methods for the salmonella mutagenicity test. Mutat Res Environ Mutagen Relat Subj. 1983;113(3–4):173–215.

49. Ledda C, Cocuzza S, Salerno M, Senia P, Matera S, Rapisarda V, Loreto C. Occupational exposure to Mount etna's basaltic dust: assessment of mutagenic and cytotoxic effects. Mol Med Rep. 2017;15(5):3350–4.

50. Oakes M, Baxter L, Long TC. Evaluating the application of multipollutant exposure metrics in air pollution health studies. Environ Int. 2014;69:90–9.

51. Krzyzanowski M, Kuna-Dibbert B, Schneider J. Health Effects of Transport-Related Air Pollution. 2005.

52. HEI International Scientific Oversight Committee. Outdoor air pollution and health in the developing countries of asia: A comprehensive review. In: Outdoor Air Pollution and Health in the Developing Countries of Asia: A Comprehensive Review; 2010.

53. Valavanidis A, Fiotakis K, Vlachogianni T. Airborne particulate matter and human health: toxicological assessment and importance of size and composition of particles for oxidative damage and carcinogenic mechanisms. J Environ Sci Health Part C Environ Carcinog Ecotoxicol Rev. 2008;26(4):339–62.

54. Oanh NTK, Reutergårdh LB, Dung NT. Emission of polycyclic aromatic hydrocarbons and particulate matter from domestic combustion of selected fuels. Environ Sci Technol. 1999;33(16):2703–9.

55. Unwin J, Cocker J, Scobbie E, Chambers H. An assessment of occupational exposure to polycyclic aromatic hydrocarbons in the UK. Ann Occup Hyg. 2006;50(4):395–403.

56. Burgaz S, Cakmak Demircigil G, Karahalil B, Karakaya AE. Chromosomal damage in peripheral blood lymphocytes of traffic policemen and taxi drivers exposed to urban air pollution. Chemosphere. 2002;47(1):57–64.

57. Hu Y, Bai Z, Zhang L, Wang X, Zhang L, Yu Q, Zhu T. Health risk assessment for traffic policemen exposed to polycyclic aromatic hydrocarbons (PAHs) in Tianjin, China. Sci Total Environ. 2007;382(2–3):240–50.

58. Hansen ÅM, Wallin H, Binderup ML, Dybdahl M, Autrup H, Loft S, Knudsen LE. Urinary 1-hydroxypyrene and mutagenicity in bus drivers and mail carriers exposed to urban air pollution in Denmark. Mutat Res Genet Toxicol Environ Mutagen. 2004;557(1):7–17.

59. JBouchard M, Viau C. Urinary 1-hydroxypyrene as a biomarker of exposure to polycyclic aromatic hydrocarbons: Biological monitoring strategies and methodology for determining biological exposure indices for various work environments. Biomarkers. 1999;4(3):159–87.

60. Li Z, Sandau CD, Romanoff LC, Caudill SP, Sjodin A, Needham LL, Patterson DG Jr. Concentration and profile of 22 urinary polycyclic aromatic hydrocarbon metabolites in the US population. Environ Res. 2008;107(3):320–31.

61. Hansen ÅM, Raaschou-Nielsen O, Knudsen LE. Urinary 1-hydroxypyrene in children living in city and rural residences in Denmark. Sci Total Environ. 2005;347(1–3):98–105.

62. Terada LS. Specificity in reactive oxidant signaling: think globally, act locally. J Cell Biol. 2006;174(5):615–23.

63. Rossner P Jr, Svecova V, Milcova A, Lnenickova Z, Solansky I, Sram RJ. Seasonal variability of oxidative stress markers in city bus drivers. Part II. Oxidative damage to lipids and proteins. Mutat Res Fundam Mol Mech Mutagen. 2008;642(1–2):21–7.

64. Singh VK, Patel DK, Jyoti RS, Mathur N, MKJ S. Blood levels of polycyclic aromatic hydrocarbons in children and their association with oxidative stress indices: an indian perspective. Clin Biochem. 2008;41(3):152–61.

65. Garçon G, Zerimech F, Hannothiaux M-, Gosset P, Martin A, Marez T, Shirali P. Antioxidant defense disruption by polycyclic aromatic hydrocarbons-

coated onto Fe2O3 particles in human lung cells (A549). Toxicology 2001; 166(3):129–137.

66. Cavalieri EL, Rogan EG. Central role of radical cations in metabolic activation of polycyclic aromatic hydrocarbons. Xenobiotica. 1995;25(7):677–88.

67. Bravo CF. Biomarker responses and disease susceptibility in juvenile rainbow trout oncorhynchus mykissfeda high molecular weight PAH mixture. Environ Toxicol Chem. 2010;884–93.

68. Bae S, Pan XC, Kim SY, Park K, Kim YH, Kim H, Hong YC. Exposures to particulate matter and polycyclic aromatic hydrocarbons and oxidative stress in schoolchildren. Environ Health Perspect. 2010;118(4):579–83.

69. Chao MR, Wang CJ, Wu MT, Pan CH, Kuo CY, Yang HJ, Chang LW, Hu CW. Repeated measurements of urinary methylated/oxidative DNA lesions, acute toxicity, and mutagenicity in coke oven workers. Cancer Epidemiol Biomark Prev. 2008;17(12):3381–9.

70. Cheng KC, Cahill DS, Kasai H, Nishimura S, Loeb LA. 8-hydroxyguanine, an abundant form of oxidative DNA damage, causes G → T and a → C substitutions. J Biol Chem. 1992;267(1):166–72.

71. Liu AL, Lu WQ, Wang ZZ, Chen WH, Lu WH, Yuan J, Nan PH, Sun JY, Zou YL, Zhou LH, Zhang C, Wu T. Elevated level of urinary 8-hydroxy-2'-deoxyguanosine, lymphocytic micronuclei, and serum glutathione S-transferase in workers exposed to coke oven emissions. Environ Health Perspect. 2006;114(5):673–7.

72. Marczynski B, Rihs HP, Rossbach B, Hölzer J, Angerer J, Scherenberg M, Hoffmann G, Brüning T, Wilhelm M. Analysis of 8-oxo-7,8-dihydro-2'-deoxyguanosine and DNA strand breaks in white blood cells of occupationally exposed workers: comparison with ambient monitoring, urinary metabolites and enzyme polymorphisms. Carcinogenesis. 2002;23(2):273–81.

73. Hu CW, Wu MT, Chao MR, Pan CH, Wang CJ, Swenberg JA, Wu KY. Comparison of analyses of urinary 8-hydroxy-2'-deoxyguanosine by isotope-dilution liquid chromatography with electrospray tandem mass spectrometry and by enzyme-linked immunosorbent assay. Rapid Commun Mass Spectrom. 2004;18(4):505–10.

74. Zhang J, Ichiba M, Hanaoka T, Pan G, Yamano Y, Hara K, Takahashi K, Tomokuni K. Leukocyte 8-hydroxydeoxyguanosine and aromatic DNA adduct in coke-oven workers with polycyclic aromatic hydrocarbon exposure. Int Arch Occup Environ Health. 2003;76(7):499–504.

75. Jongeneelen FJ. Benchmark guideline for urinary 1-hydroxypyrene as biomarker of occupational exposure to polycyclic aromatic hydrocarbons. Ann Occup Hyg. 2001;45(1):3–13.

76. Manzella N, Bracci M, Strafella E, Staffolani S, Ciarapica V, Copertaro A, Rapisarda V, Ledda C, Amati M, Valentino M, Tomasetti M, Stevens RG, Santarelli L. Circadian modulation of 8-oxoguanine DNA damage repair. Sci Rep. 2015;5

77. Rapisarda V, Ledda C, Matera S, Fago L, Arrabito G, Falzone L, Marconi A, Libra M, Loreto C. Absence of t(14;18) chromosome translocation in agricultural workers after short-term exposure to pesticides. Mol Med Rep. 2017;15(5):3379–82.

78. Ledda C, Fiore M, Santarelli L, Bracci M, Mascali G, D'agati MG, Busà A, Ferrante M, Rapisarda V. Gestational hypertension and organophosphorus pesticide exposure: a cross-sectional study. Biomed Res Int. 2015;2015

79. Lovreglio P, De Palma G, Barbieri A, Andreoli R, Drago I, Greco L, Gallo E, Diomede L, Scaramuzzo P, Ricossa MC, Fostinelli J, Apostoli P, Soleo L. Biological monitoring of exposure to low concentrations of benzene in workers at a metallurgical coke production plant: new insights into S-phenylmercapturic acid and urinary benzene. Biomarkers. 2017:1–8.

80. Lovreglio P, Doria D, Fracasso ME, Barbieri A, Sabatini L, Drago I, Violante FS, Soleo L. DNA damage and repair capacity in workers exposed to low concentrations of benzene. Environ Mol Mutagen. 2016;57(2):151–8.

81. Lovreglio P, Maffei F, Carrieri M, D'Errico MN, Drago I, Hrelia P, Bartolucci GB, Soleo L. Evaluation of chromosome aberration and micronucleus frequencies in blood lymphocytes of workers exposed to low concentrations of benzene. Mutat Res Genet Toxicol Environ Mutagen. 2014;770:55–60.

82. Lovreglio P, Carrieri M, Barbieri A, Sabatini L, Fracasso ME, Doria D, Iavicoli S, Drago I, D'Errico MN, Imbriani M, Violante FS, Bartolucci GB, Soleo L. Applicability of urinary benzene to biological monitoring of occupational and environmental exposure to very low benzene concentrations. G Ital Med Lav Ergon. 2011;33(1):41–6.

24

Long-term effect of hand-arm vibration on thermotactile perception thresholds

Ronnie Lundström[1,3]* (iD), Adnan Noor Baloch[2], Mats Hagberg[2], Tohr Nilsson[3] and Lars Gerhardsson[2]

Abstract

Background: Occupational exposure to hand-transmitted vibration (HTV) is known to cause neurological symptoms such as numbness, reduced manual dexterity, grip strength and sensory perception. The purpose of this longitudinal study was to compare thermotactile perception thresholds for cold (TPT_C) and warmth (TPT_W) among vibration exposed manual workers and unexposed white collar workers during a follow-up period of 16 years to elucidate if long-term vibration exposure is related to a change in TPT over time.

Methods: The study group consisted of male workers at a production workshop at which some of them were exposed to HTV. They were investigated in 1992 and followed-up in 2008. All participants were physically examined and performed TPT bilaterally at the middle and distal phalanges of the second finger. Two different vibration exposure dosages were calculated for each individual, i.e. the individual cumulative lifetime dose (mh/s^2) or a lifetime 8-h equivalent daily exposure (m/s^2).

Results: A significant mean threshold difference was found for all subjects of about 4–5 °C and 1–2 °C in TPT_W and TPT_C, respectively, between follow-up and baseline. No significant mean difference in TPT_C between vibration exposed and non-exposed workers at each occasion could be stated to exist. For TPT_W a small but significant difference was found for the right index finger only. Age was strongly related to thermotactile perception threshold. The 8-h equivalent exposure level (A (8)) dropped from about 1.3 m/s^2 in 1992 to about 0.7 m/s^2 in 2008.

Conclusions: A lifetime 8-h equivalent daily exposure to hand-transmitted vibration less than 1.3 m/s^2 does not have a significant effect on thermotactile perception. Age, however, has a significant impact on the change of temperature perception thresholds why this covariate has to be considered when using TPT as a tool for health screening.

Keywords: Hand-arm vibration, Hand-transmitted vibration, Hand, Thermotactile perception

Background

Hand-transmitted vibration (HTV) may lead to neurological, vascular, and musculoskeletal disorders in the upper extremity. The symptoms, that may occur singly or in different combinations, are collectively denoted as the hand-arm vibration syndrome (HAVS) [1]. The neurological component of HAVS is characterized by diffusely distributed peripheral neuropathy with predominant symptoms of sensory impairment, The most common symptoms are subjective experience of digital paraesthesia and numbness, deterioration of sensory perception (i.e. vibration, cold, warmth, pain), and loss of manipulative dexterity [2, 3].

Hand intensive work, including exposure to HTV, is associated with an increased risk of impaired thermal perception (eg. [4–7]). Interestingly, exposure to vibration seems to affect perception of cold more compared with warmth [8, 9]. Moreover, an exposure-response relationship between HTV and thermal perception has been suggested in some studies (eg. [5, 10]. For vibration-induced thermotactile impairment the conceivable target structures are the end organs, the thinly myelinated (A-delta), and the small calibre non-myelinated (C) fibres [11]. Experiments addressing temporary thermotactile threshold shift induced by vibration indicate an effect, especially on cold compared with warmth (eg. [8, 12]). Hypoaesthesia of the sensation of warmth is

* Correspondence: ronnie.lundstrom@umu.se
[1]Department of Radiation Sciences, Umeå University, SE-901 87 Umeå, Sweden
[3]Department of Occupational and Environmental Medicine, Umeå University, SE-901 87 Umeå, Sweden
Full list of author information is available at the end of the article

claimed to be more prevalent at the early stages of vibration disease whereas hypoesthesia to cold occurs at more advanced stages of hand-arm vibration disease [9]. The diversity of symptoms expressed by long-term vibration exposed workers implies that different pathophysiological mechanisms may affect the degeneration of small fibre neuropathy [13]. Some workers may develop quite severe neurophysiological symptoms and signs within a few years, while others with similar exposure for decades develop no or only minor disturbances. The reason for this is still unclear. The prevalence of peripheral sensorineural disorders among vibration-exposed workers varies from a few per cent to more than 80% [14]. The awareness of the importance as well as relatively high prevalence of sensory neuropathy has entailed an increasing interest to get a deeper knowledge of the causes of small fibre neuropathy as well as the underlying pathophysiological mechanisms. Quantitative sensory testing is a psychophysical neurological test battery that can examine subgroup changes in different nerve fibre functions, mainly linked to A-delta and C-nerve fibres, and thus useful for screening and diagnosis of vibration induced neuropathy (eg. [2, 3, 15–17]).

The aim of the present longitudinal study is to explore whether a long-term occupational exposure to HTV lead to a deterioration of the thermotactile sense among a group of workers employed at a heavy production workshop.

Methods

Study group

This longitudinal study is based on a sample from a cohort consisting of male white- and blue-collar workers at a plant that produces heavy equipment for paper and pulp mills that was investigated in 1992 ($n = 229$) and followed-up in 2008 ($n = 228$). At both occasions basic information about age, work assignment, years at work, general state of health, previous and present exposure to vibration and more was collected in a questionnaire. All participants were physically examined by one and same occupational physician. The inclusion criteria for this study were; 1) Participation at both or any occasions with thermotactile perception threshold (TPT) measurements on the volar side of the index finger, and 2) Not having symptoms of diseases known to cause sensory neuropathies, such as diabetes, metabolic disturbances, and carpal tunnel syndrome. For more information about the criteria for inclusion, see Nilsson and Lundström 2001 [5]. At baseline (1992) 140 study (out of 229) participants had TPT measurements, and at follow-up (2008) 142 study participants (out of 228) had TPT measurements. Among these, 119 study participants had TPT measurements at both occasions, 21 only at the baseline (1992) and 23 only at follow-up. Our

study is approved by the Regional Ethics Review Board at Umeå University (Registration number 97–76 and 2007-161 M) and conducted accordingly. All subjects signed an informed consent before entering the study.

Thermotactile perception thresholds

Thermotactile perception thresholds for cold (TPT_C) and warmth (TPT_W) was at both occasions in 1992 and 2008 determined using a modification of the Marstock method [18] with computer assisted automatic exposure and response recording (Thermotest; Somedic, Sales AB, Sweden). A thermostimulator, i.e. a Peltier element-based contact thermode (25×50 mm), was applied to the skin on the volar surface of the two distal phalanges (i.e. the middle and distal phalanx) of the second digit (lengthways along the finger). The TPT_C and TPT_W induced by contact temperature were assessed by the method of limits. The rate of the temperature change was linear and about 1 °C/s. For TPT measurement conducted 1992 the skin temperature, measured by contact thermometry, was used as the start temperature. In this way a neutral starting temperature was accomplished that was perceived as indifferent, i.e. nor warm nor cold. For measurement conducted 2008 the start temperature was however fixed and set to 32 °C. The subject was instructed to press a button on a hand switch when a sensation of warmth or cold was perceived. The operating temperature range was set to 10–52 °C. After the subject's response the temperature of the thermostimulator returned to the pre-set starting temperature. The measurement of warmth and cold was repeated 10 times. The threshold was taken as the mean of the measurements. The interstimulus interval for all threshold measurements was randomly distributed within 2 s.

Assessment of vibration exposure

Personal vibration doses were estimated 1992 and 2008 for all exposed workers through measurement on all types of tools used at all relevant job stations. Hand transmitted vibration most often occurred from use of grinders that was used for grinding, polishing, and cutting. Hammers and nut wrenches were used for finishing welding seams and assembly of machinery. The vibration magnitudes, in terms of frequency-weighted acceleration level (SI: m/s^2), were measured in accordance with the international standard ISO 5349-1 [19]. A detailed description of measurement conducted in 1992 is reported elsewhere [20]. Measurement conducted in 2008 was done accordingly. The daily duration of exposure to vibration for each individual was estimated through observation at the workstation. The observer noted the kind of tool the operator was handling, whether the machine was working, and which hand that was exposed during an observation time of 150 min. Furthermore, all workers were interviewed in order to obtain information about their entire lifetime exposures, about the number of years in different work, types of exposure, and duration of exposure per day. On that basis two different lifetime vibration doses (LTVD1 and LTVD2) was calculated for each individual worker using the following formulas;

$$LTVD1 = \sum_{i}^{n} a_{wi} t_{Ti}$$

(mh/s^2), and

$$LTVD2 = A_{w(8)} = \left(\Sigma \left(a_{wi}^2 \cdot t_i \right) / \left(60 \cdot T_{(8)} \right) \right)^{1/2}$$

(m/s^2) where; a_{wi} is the frequency weighted acceleration level for vibrating tool i, t_i is the exposure time for tool i, and t_{Ti} the total lifetime exposure (i.e. hours/workday · workdays/year · years; workdays/year was set to 200) for tool i.

LTVD1 thus reflects an individual's cumulative lifetime dose based on the total number of hours with vibration exposure where as LTVD2 reflects a lifetime 8-h equivalent daily exposure. For more information, see [21].

The study group (ALL) was dichotomized in to sub-groups, i.e. exposed to HTV (EHTV) and not exposed to HTV (NEHTV). For statistical calculation based on LTDV1 and LTVD2, EHTV is defined as those workers having LTDV1 > 1600 mh/s^2 and LTDV2 > 0.5 m/s^2, respectively. The rationale for the LTDV1 dichotomization is discussed elsewhere [20]. The dichotomization level for LTDV2 was set to one fifth of the daily exposure action value of 2.5 m/s^2 specified in the current EU Directive [22].

Statistical analysis

Descriptive statistics of variables of interest was performed separately for exposed and referents at both time point, i.e. 1992 and 2008. We used longitudinal regression models to investigate the relationship between the outcomes and explanatory variables. By using SAS procedure PROC MIXED one can use all available data in analysis instead of ignoring subjects with missing data, hence having more statistical power [23–25]. We have used PROC MIXED and used all available data in our analysis, which resulted in different number of data points (subjects) in tables for descriptive statistics at baseline and follow-up. We assumed fixed effects, i.e. the model holds true across the sample and with the same slope. In other words, exposure will affect all persons in the same way. These models study both between- and within-subject changes over time.

First simple longitudinal regression models were used to investigate the relationship between one outcome and

one predictor variable at a time. Finally multivariate longitudinal regression models were built partly based on the results of simple regression analyses and partly on the researchers clinical experience. The longitudinal regression analyses yielded beta values (regression coefficients) with standard error and p-values. It also yielded least square means (LSM) and differences in LSM to compare Categorical variable's means adjusted for other variables and averaged across the repeated measures. Statistical significance, alpha was set at 0.05. All statistical analyses were performed with SAS 9.4 for windows (SAS Institute Inc., Cary, NC, USA).

Results

Descriptive statistics for age, height, temperature perception thresholds and vibration dosages for all included workers as well as for the two sub-groups, i.e. EHTV and NEHTV, are presented in Table 1. At baseline and follow-up, there was a mean difference of 3.7 years (CI 95%; 0.1–7.4) and 5.6 years (CI 95%; 1.8–9.3) for the two sub-groups. There was no significant difference in height between the two groups at baseline and at follow-up.

Simple longitudinal regression analyses showed that all predictor variables had a significant relationship with all temperature perception thresholds. We investigated the following predictor variables; age, height, LTVD1, LTVD2, ELTVD1 (binary exposure variables based on LTVD1), ELTVD2 (binary exposure variables based on LTVD2) and Year (1992 and 2008) (Table 2).

For left index finger, vibration exposed workers (ELTVD1) had a mean level of 26.1 °C and non-vibration exposed workers had a mean level of 26.0 °C for TPT$_C$ during the follow-up period. The difference in these means was not significant, see column 1 in Table 2. There were not any significant mean difference in TPT$_C$ and TPT$_W$ (left index finger) between vibration exposed and non-exposed workers based on LTVD1 and LTVD2, respectively. For TPT$_W$ on the right index finger a small but significant difference was however found.

As can be seen in Table 2 there was a significant mean difference in TPT$_C$ and TPT$_W$ for both fingers between the two occasions. As an example, the mean TPT$_C$ for left index finger among all workers in 1992 was 25.2 °C compared to 26.9 °C in 2008, i.e. a mean difference of about 1.7 °C. Corresponding figures for TPT$_W$ was 33.7 °C and 38.4 °C, i.e. a mean difference of about 4.7 °C. Similar figures is valid for the right index finger. This means that subjects need more heat stimuli and less cold stimuli for thermotactile perception at follow-up.

To further elucidate the influence of vibration exposure on the temperature perception thresholds, multivariate analyses were performed with TPT$_C$ and TPT$_W$ as outcome variables. We built four multivariate models with one exposure variable adjusted for age and height

Table 1 Descriptive statistics for study group and its sub-groups during the follow-up period 1992–2008. Mean thermotactile perception thresholds for cold (TPT$_C$) and warmth (TPT$_W$) measured on the volar side of two distal phalanges on the right and left index finger among vibration exposed (ETHV) and un-exposed (NETHV) workers during the follow-up period. LTVD1 and LTVD2 are two different lifetime vibration doses. For more information, see text

	1992			2008		
	ALL ($n = 140$)	NEHTV ($n = 41$)	EHTV ($n = 99$)	ALL ($n = 142$)	NEHTV ($n = 35$)	EHTV ($n = 107$)
	Mean (95% CI)	Mean (95% CI)	Mean (95% CI)	Mean (95% CI)	Mean (95% CI)	Mean (95% CI)
Age (years)	41 (39, 42)	43 (40, 46)	39 (38, 41)	55 (53, 57)	59 (56, 62)	54 (52, 56)
Height (cm)	179 (178, 180)	179 (178, 181)	179 (178, 180)	179 (178, 180)	179 (177, 181)	179 (178, 180)
LTVD1 (mh/s^2)× 10^3	21.0 (16.7, 25.3)	0	29.7 (24.5, 35.0)	28.4 (23.7, 33.2)	0.0 (0, 0.0)	37.7 (32.6, 42.9)
LTVD2 (m/s^2)	0.9 (0.7, 1.2)	0	1.3 (1.1, 1.6)	0.6 (0.4, 0.7)	0	0.7 (0.6, 0.9)
Right hand						
TPT$_W$ (°C)	34.1 (33.6, 34.6)	33.1 (32.5, 33.7)	34.5 (33.8, 35.2)	38.8 (38.3, 39.4)	38.5 (37.5, 39.6)	38.9 (38.3, 39.6)
TPT$_C$ (°C)	25.0 (24.4, 25.5)	25.3 (24.3, 26.2)	24.9 (24.2, 25.5)	26.6 (26.0, 27.2)	25.7 (24.1, 27.3)	26.9 (26.3, 27.5)
Left hand						
TPT$_W$ (°C)	33.7 (33.2, 34.2)	33.2 (32.5, 34.0)	33.9 (33.2, 34.5)	38.4 (37.9, 38.9)	38.3 (37.1, 39.4)	38.5 (37.8, 39.1)
TPT$_C$ (°C)	25.2 (24.6, 25.8)	25.7 (24.8, 26.7)	25.0 (24.2, 25.7)	26.9 (26.2, 27.5)	26.6 (24.8, 28.5)	27.0 (26.3, 27.6)

for each outcome (Table 3). The model including the dichotomous exposure variable ELTVD1 based on LTVD1 and adjusting for age and height resulted in similar beta-coefficients for exposed and not-exposed workers for all TPT-indices (Table 3). Comparison of LSM reveals significant differences between exposed and not exposed for TPT$_W$ but not for TPT$_C$. These differences

were between 1.5–2.0 °C. A similar result was noted when using dichotomous exposure variable ELTVD2 based on LTVD2 and adjusting for Age and Height in the models.

When adjusting the vibration doses LTVD1 and LTVD2 for age and height in Model 1 and 3, respectively, the association between vibration doses and TPT$_C$

Table 2 Univariate analyses of thermotactile perception thresholds for cold (TPT$_C$) and warmth (TPT$_W$) measured on the volar side of the two distal phalanges on the right and left index finger with four explanatory variables, vibration exposure (LTVD1 and LTVD2), age and height

	Left index finger				Right index finger			
	TPT$_C$		TPT$_W$		TPT$_C$		TPT$_W$	
	β	SE	β	SE	β	SE	β	SE
Age	.5	0.01	0.7	0.001	0.5	0.01	0.7	0.01
Height	.1	0.002	0.2	0.001	0.1	0.001	0.2	0.001
LTVD1	.0002	0.00003	0.0004	0.00004	0.0002	0.00003	0.0005	0.00004
LTVD2	−0.6	0.2	−1.0	0.4	−2.0	0.2	1.1	0.3
ELTVD1								
(Exp)	26.1	0.3	36.3	0.3	26.0	0.3	36.8	0.25
(Not-Exp)	26.0	0.5	35.6	0.4	25.4	0.5	35.6	0.42
Mean difference	0.04 (0.6)		0.7 (0.5)		0.5 (0.5)		**1.2 (0.5)**	
ELTVD2								
(Exp)	25.5	0.4	36.0	0.4	25.3	0.4	36.2	0.37
(Not-Exp)	26.4	0.3	36.1	0.3	26.1	0.3	36.6	0.28
Mean difference	−0.9 (0.5)		−0.1 (0.5)		−0.8 (0.4)		−0.4 (0.5)	
Year								
(1992)	25.2	0.3	33.7	0.3	25.1	0.3	34.1	0.27
(2008)	26.9	0.3	38.4	0.3	26.6	0.3	38.8	0.27
Mean difference	**−1.7 (0.3)**		**−4.7 (0.3)**		**−1.5 (0.3)**		**−4.7 (0.3)**	

Significant differences in bold

Table 3 Results from longitudinal regression analysis of four multivariate models (Model 1 to 4). Thermotactile perception thresholds for cold (TPT$_C$) and warmth (TPT$_W$) are outcome variables, and vibration doses (LTVD1 and LTVD2, respectively), age and height are explanatory variables. All available data is included in the analysis. For more information, see text

	Left index finger						Right index finger					
	TPT$_C$			TPT$_W$			TPT$_C$			TPT$_W$		
Model 1	ß (SE)	p	LSM	ß (SE)	p	LSM	ß (SE)	p	LSM	ß (SE)	p	LSM
LTVD1	−0.00001 (0.00001)	.25		0.00002 (0.00001)	.027		0.000007 (0.00001)	.5		0.00002 (0.00001)	.04	
Age	0.07 (0.02)	<.0001		0.2 (0.02)	<.0001		0.04 (0.02)	.01		0.19 (0.017)	<.0001	
Height	0.13 (0.004)	<.0001		0.1 (0.004)	<.0001		0.1 (0.004)	<.0001		0.15 (0.005)	<.0001	
Model 2												
LTVD1 Exp	23.6 (8.3)	.02	26.1	14.9 (7.4)	.003	**36.5**	26.1 (7.4)	.001	26.0	15.7 (6.6)	<.0001	**37.0**
LTVD1 NExp	23.4 (8.3)	.02	25.9	13.4 (7.4)	.003	**35.0**	25.4 (7.4)	.001	25.4	13.7 (6.6)	<.0001	**35.0**
Age	0.1 (0.02)	<.001		0.2 (0.02)	<.0001		0.03 (0.02)	.05		0.2 (0.02)	<.0001	
Height	−0.002 (0.05)	.97		0.1 (0.04)	0.1		−0.01 (0.04)	.8		0.1 (0.04)	.1	
Model 3												
LTVD2	−0.2 (0.2)	.41		0.7 (0.2)	.003		−0.5 (0.2)	.03		0.8 (0.21)	.0003	
Age	0.1 (0.02)	<.001		0.2 (0.02)	<.0001		0.03 (0.02)	.08		0.2 (0.02)	<.0001	
Height	0.1 (0.01)	<.0001		0.1 (0.01)	<.0001		0.1 (0.01)	<.0001		0.1 (0.01)	<.0001	
Model 4												
LTVD2 Exp	23.9 (8.3)	.02	25.7	15.1 (7.3)	.004	**37.0**	26.4 (7.4)	.004	25.4	15.3 (6.8)	.002	**37.5**
LTVD2 NExp	24.5 (8.3)	.02	26.3	13.6 (7.3)	.004	**35.5**	27.0 (7.4)	.004	26.1	13.7 (6.8)	.002	**35.9**
Age	0.1 (0.02)	<.002		0.2 (0.02)	<.0001		0.02 (0.02)	.2		0.2 (0.02)	<.0001	
Height	−0.004 (0.05)	.94		0.1 (0.04)			−0.01 (0.04)	.8		0.1 (0.04	.07	

Significant differences between LSM in bold

disappeared. However, we observed a significant association between vibration doses and TPT$_W$ even after adjusting for age and height but with a smaller magnitude.

As an example, from Model 1 for TPT$_W$ of right index finger we have the following regression equation;

$$\text{TPT}_W = 1.7 \times 10^{-5}\left(\text{mh/s}^2\right) + 0.2 \times \text{Age} + 0.2 \times \text{Height} \quad (1)$$

This means that the thermotactile threshold for warmth (TPT$_W$) is estimated to increase by 1.7 °C for every 100,000 h of vibration exposure (i.e. 12,500 days with 8 h daily exposure) if the effect of age and height was kept constant.

Discussion

A significant difference in thermotactile perception thresholds when comparing baseline and follow-up has been found. For TPT$_W$ a small but significant difference was found for the right index finger only (unadjusted). Significant differences in thermotactile perception thresholds for warmth were found for both hands after adjusting

for age and height. However, no significant differences in this respect were found for cold. The majority of the workers (96% in 1997), were right-handed. Smaller and lighter vibrating tools are usually held in the dominant hand, in this case mainly in the right hand. Larger and heavier vibrating tools are usually held in both hands. Thus, the right hand will have a higher vibration exposure than the left hand in right handed workers. Accordingly, the right hand will have a lower temperature perception threshold for cold and a higher temperature perception threshold for warmth than the left hand as shown in our study. Age, however, had a strong impact on the change of temperature perception thresholds and is therefore an important covariate in this context.

The vibration exposure has decreased during the follow-up period as shown in Table 1. This is supported by the fact that the mean current life-time 8-h equivalent exposure level (A (8)), that was about 1.3 m/s^2 among the workers in 1992 dropped to about 0.7 m/s^2 in 2008. The main reasons for the reduction of vibration exposure are technical preventive measures (e.g. usage of isolation gloves and less vibrating tools), improved medical surveillance and the replacement of manual tasks with robotic controlled processes. A reason for not finding a significant impact from the vibration exposure at follow-up may thus be that the general exposure after 1992 was reduced to a level considerably lower than the action level of 2.5 m/s^2 specified in EU:s health and safety directive [22].

It is clear that the magnitude of an individual's thermotactile threshold is depending on the starting temperature of the test. In 1992 the starting temperature was adjusted to the individuals actual skin temperature. In 2008, however, a fixed starting temperature of 32 °C was used. This shift in methodology is of course not optimal but was due to a modification of the standardized protocol for TPT measurements in our country. We know that the thermotactile sense is sensitive to a sudden change in temperature within a relatively narrow range, approximately less than ±3–4 °C, and more or less independent of starting point. So, an individual's absolute TPT level will thus differ if a test and re-test TPT measure is taken using different starting temperatures. A starting temperature of 29 °C in 1992 would thus yield an approximate TPT span between 25 °C and up to 33 °C for cold and warmth, respectively. A corresponding span from a starting temperature of 32 °C would then be approximately 28 °C to 36 °C. Due to this methodological difference the absolute TPT values measured in 1992 and 2008 cannot be directly compared. As it now looks in Table 1, the sensitivity to cold had improved during the follow-up period while the sensitivity to warmth had deteriorated. This pattern is common for both sub-groups, i.e. for vibration-exposed workers as well as for non-vibration exposed workers. This does not affect our findings when comparing TPT values between vibration-exposed workers with non-vibration exposed workers.

In Table 3, the β (regression)-coefficients for the explanatory variables with temperature perception thresholds as outcome variables are listed. If assuming a mean vibration exposure dose of 8000 mh/s^2 during the follow-up period (Table 1) an increase of 0.14 degrees of the warmth threshold in dig 2 right hand would be expected while keeping the effect of age and height constant (Table 3). Using the mean values from the descriptive statistics in Table 1 in regression eq. (1), we will have a LSM of 35.1 °C at baseline and 37.9 °C at follow-up, with an expected increase of 2.8 °C for the ALL group. This is a fair estimate of the real difference of 4.7 °C shown in Table 2. As seen in this example, a length of + 10 cm from 180 cm to 190 cm would give an increase of TPT$_W$ of 1.5 °C (Table 3) while keeping the vibration dose and age constant. An explanation for this effect is that a longer peripheral nerve pathway also led to a longer transmission time from end organ to cortex.

This extra transmission time enables the continuously increasing or decreasing stimulus to increase a little bit further before it is perceived. Also in other studies, age has shown an impact on thermal thresholds of quantitative sensory testing [26–31]. In a study of 484 normal subjects, Lin and co-workers [27] found that age was consistently and significantly correlated with sensory thresholds of all tested modalities and had a stronger impact on the multivariate model compared to other factors such as gender, body height, body weight and body mass index. The authors concluded that age had the strongest impact on sensory thresholds compared with other factors of gender and anthropometric parameters. Separate tests are recommended for cold and warm determinations and these measurements should not be replaced by a single measurement such as the neutral-zone gap [5, 16]. On the contrary, Seah and Griffin [32] show a small and insignificant effect and conclude that an age correction may not be needed for persons aged between 20 to 65 years.

Not only the size but also the position of the finger on the thermode can influence the level of TPT. In this study we have chosen to measure perception with the two distal phalanxes of one finger in contact with the thermode in order to cover the major part of the stimulus area. It can be questioned whether this is a good or bad arrangement. In this longitudinal study we have used the same thermode and methodological arrangement at both occasions that enables direct comparisons.

One problem with longitudinal studies with follow-up periods of 10 to 15 years or longer is that it is difficult to use the same equipment during the whole study period. The measuring equipment is "aging" and may need to be replaced. Sometimes it also becomes increasingly difficult to find spare parts. Even if the original equipment is available it might not be comparable to the one that was used 15–20 years ago. During such a long study period there will also be improved technological changes that may be desirable to use. It can be difficult to compare the new equipment with the measures from the old one. These problems are growing with the length of the study period. In this study the measuring equipment has however been basically the same both at baseline and at follow-up.

Moreover, no generally accepted reference materials for the determination of temperature perception thresholds are available when the thermometry equipment is bought. This means that all users will have to collect their own reference values for TPT cold and warmth, respectively. Accordingly there may be some differences in reference values when comparing different research centres in different parts of the world. We have collected a reference sample with a normal range between 23 and 42 °C for male subjects less or equal to 44 years and between 20 and 45 °C for subjects 45 years and older.

There seems to be a breaking point around 45 years of age. After that point we can see a slight deterioration of the neurosensori sensitivity. If using these criteria almost all subjects in the study group and in the reference group will fall within the normal range in this study. Hafner and co-workers found a clear effect of age on thermal thresholds in a study of 101 normal volunteers but no significant effect on gender was noted [26]. They also found some differences between the three operators that performed the testing.

It is also important that the examiner is experienced with the test and can understand and respond if the test subject doesn't understand the instructions or is conducting the testing in an improper way. At both occasions in this study the test were performed by a qualified examiner.

Another factor that must be considered is the thickness of the nerve fibres. A-delta fibres are thicker than the C-fibres giving an estimated velocity of 12–30 m/s versus 0.5–2 m/s, which may affect the response time. Also, the cognitive set of the subject may influence the response to cold or warm stimuli. The subjects are asked to respond when they feel a temperature shift from neutral to cold or from neutral to warm. A careful and meticulous person may wait a little longer with the response compared to a subject with another type of personality. In this study, however, all workers and referents were their own controls, investigated the same way in 1992 and in 2008. Thus, we don't think that any of these facts would have influenced the final results.

Conclusions

A lifetime 8-h equivalent daily exposure to hand-transmitted vibration less than 1.3 m/s^2 does not have a significant effect on thermotactile perception. Age, however, has a significant impact on the change of temperature perception thresholds why this covariate has to be considered when using TPT as a tool for diagnosis or health screening.

Abbreviations

ALL: All individuals in the study group; EHTV: Individuals exposed to hand-transmitted vibration; ELTVD1: Binary exposure variables based on LTVD1; ELTVD2: Binary exposure variables based on LTVD2; HAVS: Hand-arm vibration syndrome; HTV: Hand-transmitted vibration; LSM: Least square means; LTVD1: Reflects an individual's cumulative lifetime dose based on the total number of hours with vibration exposure; LTVD2: Reflects an individual's lifetime 8-h equivalent daily vibration exposure; NEHTV: Individuals not exposed to hand-transmitted vibration; TPT: Thermotactile perception threshold; TPT$_C$: Thermotactile persception threshold for cold; TPT$_W$: Thermotactile perception threshold for warmth

Acknowledgements
Financial support from the Swedish Work Environment Fund and Swedish Council for Working Life and Social research are gratefully acknowledged.

Funding
Swedish Work Environment Fund (Project 1991:1640) and Swedish Council for Working Life and Social research (Project 2006:0968).

Authors' contributions
RL wrote the manuscript, contributed to the design of the study and to the outcome measurements, participated in the collection of thermotactile perception threshold and vibration exposure data, and in the statistical analyses and the interpretation of the data. AN performed the statistical analysis, discussed and contributed to the manuscript. MH, TN and LG contributed to the design of the study and to the outcome measurements, participated as examining physicians and discussed and contributed to the manuscript. All authors have read and approved the final manuscript.

Competing interests
The authors declare that they have no competing interests.

Author details
[1]Department of Radiation Sciences, Umeå University, SE-901 87 Umeå, Sweden. [2]Department of Occupational and Environmental Medicine, University of Gothenburg and Sahlgrenska University Hospital, Gothenburg, Sweden. [3]Department of Occupational and Environmental Medicine, Umeå University, SE-901 87 Umeå, Sweden.

References
1. Gemne G. Diagnostics of hand-arm system disorders in workers who use vibrating tools. Occup Environ Med. 1997;54:90–5.
2. Lundström R. Neurological disorders - aspects of quantitative sensory testing methodology in relation to hand-arm vibration syndrome. Int Arch Occup Environ Health. 2002;75:68–77.
3. Nilsson T. Neurological diagnosis: aspects of bedside and electrodiagnostic examinations in relation to hand-arm vibration syndrome. Int Arch Occup Environ Health. 2002;75(1–2):55–67.
4. Lindsell CJ, Griffin MJ. Thermal thresholds, vibrotactile thresholds and finger systolic blood pressures in dockyard workers exposed to hand-transmitted vibration. Int Arch Occup Environ Health. 1999;72(6):377–86.
5. Nilsson T, Lundström R. Quantitative thermal perception thresholds relative to exposure to vibration. Occup Environ Med. 2001;58(7):472–8.
6. Virokannas H, Virokannas A. Temparature and vibration perception thresholds in workers exposed to hand-arm vibration. Cent Eur J Public Health. 1995;3(Suppl):66–9.
7. Nilsson T, et al. Thermal perception thresholds among young adults exposed to hand-transmitted vibration. Int Arch Occup Environ Health. 2008;81(5):519–33.
8. Hirosawa I, Nishiyama K, Watanabe S. Temporary threshold shift of temperature sensation caused by vibration exposure. Int Arch Occup Environ Health. 1992;63:531–5.
9. Hirosawa I, et al. Availability of temparature sense indices for diagnosis of vibration disease. Int Arch Occup Environ Health. 1983;52:215–22.
10. Bovenzi M, Ronchese F, Mauro M. A longitudinal study of peripheral sensory function in vibration-exposed workers. Int Arch Occup Environ Health. 2011; 84(3):325–34.
11. Hoitsma E, et al. Small fiber neuropathy: a common and important clinical disorder. J Neurol Sci. 2004;227(1):119–30.
12. Burström L, et al. Acute effects of vibration on thermal perception thresholds. Int Arch Occup Environ Health. 2008;81(5):603–11.
13. Üçeyler N. Small fiber pathology – a culprit for many painful disorders? Pain. 2016;157:S60–6.
14. Bovenzi M. Exposure-response relationship in the hand-arm vibration syndrome: an overview of current epidemiology research. Int Arch Occup Environ Health. 1998;71(8):509–19.
15. Seah SA, Griffin MJ. Thermotactile thresholds at the fingertip: effect of contact area and contact location. Somatosens Mot Res. 2010;27(3):82–92.
16. Shukla G, Bhatia M, Behari M. Quantitative thermal sensory testing - value of testing for both cold and warm sensation detection in evaluation of small fiber neuropathy. Clin Neurol Neurosurg. 2005;107(6):486–90.
17. Mucke M, et al. Quantitative sensory testing (QST). English version. Schmerz. 2016; https://doi.org/10.1007/s00482-015-0093-2.
18. Fruhstorfer H, Lindblom U, Schmidt WG. Method for quantative estimation of thermal threshold in patients. J Neurol Neurosurg Psychiatry. 1976;39(11): 1071–5.
19. ISO 5349-1. Mechanical vibration - Measurement and evaluation of human

exposure to hand-transmitted vibration - Part 1: General guidelines. Geneva: International Organization for Standardization; 2001.

20. Burström L, et al. Exposure to vibrations among platers within a heavy engineering production workshop. Arbete och Hälsa (Work and Health). 1994;8:1–16. (In Swedish with a summary in English)

21. Griffin, MJ. and M. Bovenzi, Risks of Occupational Vibration Exposures (VIBRISKS). European Commission FP5 Project No. QLK4–2002-02650. Annex 1 to Final Technical Report. Protocol for epidemiological studies of hand-transmitted vibration. 2007: http://www.humanvibration.com/eu-projects/vibrisks.

22. EU Directive (Eng). Directive 2002/44/EC of the European Parliament and of the Council of 25 June 2002 on the minimum health and safety requirements regarding the exposure of workers to the risks arising from physical agents (vibration) (sixteenth individual Directive within the meaning of Article 16(1) of Directive 89/391/EEC). Off J Eur Communities. 2002;L 177:13–9.

23. SAS Institute Inc. SAS/STAT® 14.2 User's Guide The MIXED procedure. NC, USA: SAS Institute Inc., Cary; 2016.

24. Verbeke G, Molenberghs G. Linear Mixed models for longitudinal data. New York: Springer; 2001.

25. Wolfinger, R. And M. Chang, Comparing the SAS® GLM and MIXED procedures for repeated measures. Proceedings of the 20th annual SAS® users group international conference, Cary, NC: SAS Institute, Inc., 1995.

26. Hafner J, et al. Thermal quantitative sensory testing: a study of 101 control subjects. J Clin Neurosci. 2015;22(3):588–91.

27. Lin YH, et al. Influence of aging on thermal and vibratory thresholds of quantitative sensory testing. J Peripher Nerv Syst. 2005;10(3):269–81.

28. Lindsell C, Griffn M. Normative data for vascular and neurological tests of the hand-arm vibration syndrome. Int Arch Occup Environ Health. 2002; 75(1–2):43–54.

29. Harju E. Cold and warmth perception mapped for age, gender and body area. J Somatosens Mot Res. 2002;19(1):61–75.

30. Doeland H, et al. The relationship of cold and warmth cutaneous sensation to age and gender. Muscle Nerve. 1989;12:712–5.

31. Bartlett G, et al. Normal distributions of thermal and vibration sensory thresholds. Muscle Nerve. 1998;21(3):67–374.

32. Seah S, Griffin MJ. Normal values for thermotactile and vibrotactile thresholds in males and females. Int Arch Occup Environ Health. 2008;81:535–43.

25

Work related injuries in Qatar: a framework for prevention and control

Amber Mehmood[1*] ⓘ, Zaw Maung[1], Rafael J. Consunji[2,3,5], Ayman El-Menyar[3,8], Ruben Peralta[4,5], Hassan Al-Thani[5] and Adnan A. Hyder[1,6,7]

Abstract

Work related injuries (WRIs) are a growing public health concern that remains under-recognized, inadequately addressed and largely unmeasured in low and middle-income countries (LMIC's). However, even in high-income countries, such as those in Gulf Cooperating Council (GCC) like Qatar, there are challenges in assuring the health and safety of its labor population. Countries in the GCC have been rapidly developing as a result of the economic boom from the petrochemical industry during the early seventies. Economic prosperity has propelled the migration of workers from less developed countries to make up for the human resource deficiency to develop its infrastructure, service and hospitality industries. Although these countries have gradually made huge gains in health, economy and human development index, including improvements in life expectancy, education, and standard of living, there remains a high incidence of work-related injuries especially in jobs in the construction and petrochemical sector. Currently, there is scarcity of literature on work-related injuries, especially empirical studies documenting the burden, characteristics and risk factors of work injuries and the work injured population, which includes large numbers of migrant workers in many GCC countries. This paper will focus on the current understanding of WRIs in those countries and identify the gaps in current approaches to workplace injury prevention, outlining current status of WRI prevention efforts in Qatar, and propose a framework of concerted action by multi-sectoral engagement.

Keywords: Work-related injuries, Occupational injuries, Qatar, Injury prevention, Migrant workers, Middle East, Labor migration

Background

Work-related (or occupational) injuries (WRI) are a significant cause of death worldwide, whereas non-fatal WRIs result in long-term disability or prolonged leave from work [1]. WRI is defined by the International Labor Organization (ILO) as "an unanticipated and un-planned occurrence including acts of violence result-ing from and in connection with work which cause one or more workers to incur a personal injury, disease or death" [2]. The Occupational Safety and Health Administration of the United States, also deems an injury to be work-related if an event or exposure in the work environment either caused, or

contributed to, the resulting condition or significantly aggravated a pre-existing injury [3].

WRI result not only in fatalities and disabilities, but also leads to decreased productivity from lost work-days and loss of skilled workers. The average economic costs of work-related illnesses and injuries is 4% of gross do-mestic product (GDP) but varies between countries with an estimated 1.8% to 6% in places such as United States, Australia, and Singapore [4]. According to the ILO, 7600 people die every day as a result of work-related injuries or illnesses, with 15% of deaths directly attributable to WRI [1, 5]. About 6 of every 1000 workers will be fatally injured on the job during a 40 year work span in the United States [6]. Despite underreporting, the Global Estimates of Occupational Accidents and Work-related Illnesses (2014) reported that approximately 289 out of 313 million (92%) cases of WRIs occurred in low- and middle-income countries [5, 7].

* Correspondence: amehmoo2@jhu.edu
[1]Johns Hopkins International Injury Research Unit, Health Systems Program, Department of International Health, Johns Hopkins Bloomberg School of Public Health, 615 N Wolfe St, Baltimore, MD 21205, USA
Full list of author information is available at the end of the article

According to the ILO, certain occupations and industries are known to have a higher risk for WRIs because the nature of the job and the conditions where the work is performed increase the risk of injuries or exposure to hazardous agents. In high income countries, the rate of WRI has dramatically declined due to investment in interventions focusing on hazard mitigation, occupational safety and health. In the United States, work-related fatalities between 1933 and 1997 decreased from 37 to four per 100,000 workers, and work-related road traffic injuries declined from 18 to 1.7 per 100 million vehicle miles traveled. These successes were dubbed as two of the top ten leading public health achievements in the United States [6, 8].

Some countries in the Middle East, such as members of the Gulf Cooperating Council (GCC) have rapidly developing economies after the boom in the oil industry during the early 1970s and have adopted a policy of hiring an expatriate labor force to make up for their human resource deficiency to support the infrastructure, service and hospitality businesses. Although these countries have gradually made considerable gains in health, economy and human development index (Table 1) [9], there is a concern about high incidence of WRIs especially in construction and oil-industry related jobs, and related economic losses [9–11]. Currently there is scarcity of literature on WRIs, especially empirical studies documenting the burden, characteristics and risk factors for WRIs and the work injured population, which includes large numbers of migrant workers in many GCC countries like Qatar [10–12].

This paper will focus on the current understanding of WRIs in Gulf states, specifically Qatar, and identify the gaps in current approaches to WRI prevention, outlining the current status of WRI prevention efforts in Qatar; and propose a framework of concerted action through multi-sectoral engagement.

The burden of WRIs in the GCC and neighboring countries

Economic prosperity and job opportunities in the middle east, particulary in gulf countries where the demand for hydrocarbon products has fueled economic growth and, along with it, infrastructure development has propelled the migration of workers from LMICs [13]. In a study published in 2006 from Turkey, Egypt, Morocco, and Tunisia, the fatal occupational "accident" rate was estimated to be 21.2 per 100,000 employees in agriculture, 21.2 per 100,000 in industry, and 12.4 per 100,000 employees in service [4]. While in Jordan, the fatality rate was estimated to be 25.5 per 100,000 [14].

In a recent study from Oman, the injury rate amongst oil field workers was reported to be 1980 per 100,000 [11], and the mortality rate of WRIs in the United Arab Emirates was estimated to be 136 per 100,000 workers per year in 2009, where unintentional injuries are the second leading cause of death among the expatriate population and 21% of all non-fatal injuries were a result of WRIs [10, 15–17]. Morbidity and mortality related to WRIs and other illnesses among migrant workers are disproportionately higher when compared to native workers in the GCC [18]. With the lack of proper surveillance systems, these numbers are likely to be gross underestimates of the true number of WRIs and their consequences. Therefore, not only WRIs are a major public health issue in this region, but also affecting a large vulnerable population.

Qatar: Current status of labor force and WRIs

Qatar is a rapidly developing, oil rich, small gulf country within GCC with a total population of 2,569,804 in 2016 [19, 20]. Development across different sectors has attracted a large migrant or "expatriate" (expat) worker population (Fig. 1), who are now employed in diverse industries; from highways, rail networks, seaports, airports, oil facilities, chemical factories, residential and commercial facilities to the construction of stadiums [21].

Table 1 Human development indicators for Gulf Cooperating Council countries, 2016

	Human development Index (HDI)[a]	Average HDI growth (%) 1990–2015	GDP per capita PPP $ (2015)[c]	Life expectancy at birth (years)	Expected years of schooling	Under-five mortality rate (per 1000 live births)
Bahrain	0.824	40	44,182	76.7	14.5	6.2
Kuwait	0.8	46	67,113	74.5	13.3	8.6
Oman	0.796	121[b]	35, 983	77	13.7	11.6
Qatar	0.856	51	135,322	78.3	13.4	8
Saudi Arabia	0.847	77	50,284	74.4	16.1	14.5
United Arab Emirates	0.84	58	66,102	77.1	13.3	6.8

[a]Human Development Index integrates life expectancy at birth, mean years of schooling and gross national income per capita
[b]Data available from 2000 to 2015 for Oman
[c]Gross domestic Product (GDP) estimated using the purchasing power parity (PPP)

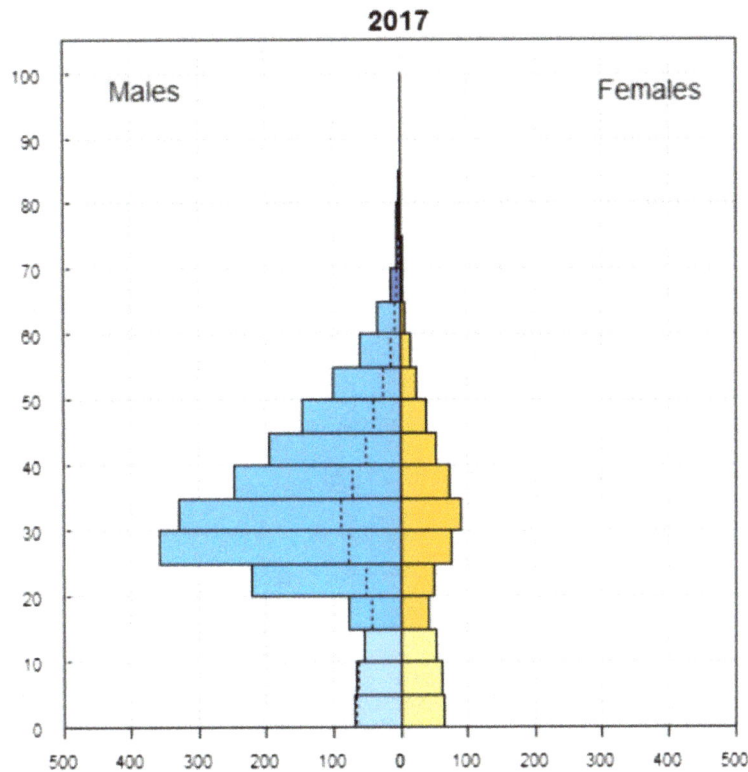

Fig. 1 Qatar 2017 demographic profile. Source: United Nations, Department of Economic and Social Affairs, Population Division (2017). World Population Prospects: The 2017 Revision (On X-Axis, Numbers expressed in × 1000 for each age group; on Y- axis: age in years. The dotted line indicates the excess male or female population in certain age groups)

Qatar has witnessed rapid population growth from just 373,392 in 1986, which stems largely from the influx of migrant workers that is estimated to make up approximately 85.7% of population, or 94.1% of the employed population in 2013 [20, 22]. Expat workers are largely of South Asian origin with other nationalities such as Filipino and Egyptians also making modest contributions [23]. Within this foreign labor population, men exceeded women by a ratio of 8 to 1 (Fig. 1). The largest proportion (39.2%) were employed in the construction industry, primarily to fulfill the requirements of rapid infrastructure development for the much anticipated 2022 FIFA World Cup [20]. Ensuring the health and safety of the working migrant population is challenging since the majority work in what is known as the "3D" sector - the dangerous, dirty, and difficult jobs [24].

Most current information on WRIs in Qatar is based on hospital-based studies capturing moderate to severe injuries (Table 2). A study based on trauma registry data in Qatar reported that a significant proportion of severe WRI affected construction workers (42%) [25]. Fall from height was the major contributor for WRIs [12]. Another study reported that the incidence of fall injuries for a period of one year was 86.7 per 100,000 workers with fatality rate of 8.44 per 100,000 workers. The annual cost

of providing care to these patients was estimated to be over 4.4 million USD, with a mean cost of $15,735 per patient [26].

The case fatality rate for WRIs in Qatar is much higher when compared to other high-income countries like the United Kingdom and United States. Many international organizations have voiced concerns about construction workers exposed to other risks such as high temperature, humidity, noise and long works hours, some of which have been documented previously in scientific papers [27–30]. These concerns have served as an impetus for the government to follow these recommendations, in order to minimize the risks to worker health and take steps towards a safer work environment, mandated by tough policies and robust monitoring systems [31].

The incidence of WRIs in Qatar is similar to rates seen in other low- and middle-income countries and partly attributable to lack of a cohesive occupational health and safety infrastructure, as well as regulations and enforcement of policies [18]. There is limited data available in the GCC as to whether identified risk factors and proven mitigation strategies from other high-income countries were applicable in the local context [32]. There are additional challenges in GCC countries for occupational

Table 2 Selected studies describing epidemiology of WRIs in Qatar

Author and year	Title of the study	Major finding
Consunji et al. 2017 [54]	Epidemiologic and temporal trends of work-related injuries in expatriate workers in a high-income rapidly developing country: Evidence for preventive programs.	Although there was a 37% reduction of the incidence of injury per 100,000 workers, from 2008 to 16, the proportion of falls from height decreased and that from RTIs increased.
Al-Thani et al. 2015 [12]	Epidemiology of occupational injuries by nationality in Qatar: Evidence for focused occupational safety programmes	Most of the workers experiencing WRIs were from Nepal (28%), India (20%) and Bangladesh (9%). Fatal WRIs were predominately among Indians (20%), Nepalese (19%), and Filipinos/Bangladeshis (both 8%)
Al-Thani et al. 2014 [25]	Workplace-Related Traumatic Injuries: Insights from a Rapidly Developing Middle Eastern Country	WRI patients are mainly laborers involved in industrial work (43%), transportation (18%), installation/repair (12%), carpentry (9%), and housekeeping (3%). A vast majority of workers (64%) did not use protective devices
Tuma et al. 2013 [26]	Epidemiology of workplace-related fall from height and cost of trauma care in Qatar	Incidence of fall related WRI was 86.7 per 100,000 and associated death rate was 8.44 per 100,000 workers.
Bener et al. 2011. [41]	Trends and characteristics of head and neck injury from falls: A hospital based study, Qatar	Among 1952 patients who were treated at a major trauma center for head and neck injuries, nearly half of them suffered from falls during work
Bener et al. 2012 [34]	Trends and characteristics of injuries in the State of Qatar: hospital-based study	This 5-year study demonstrated that overwhelming majority were non-Qatari males and over 50% of 46,701 injuries were related to WRIs. Common injuries included injuries of head and neck, extremities, and back.
Khan et al. 2005 [30]	Study of Patients with Heat Stroke Admitted to the Intensive Care Unit of Hamad General Hospital, Doha, Qatar During Summer 2004.	This case series highlighted the WRIs resulting from heat stroke and its medical complications during the hot summer months

health and safety that largely stem from the culturally, economically, ethnically, and socially heterogeneous nature of the worker population. More focused research is needed to better understand the nature of WRIs, and understanding of workers' skills and training, job experience, use of protective equipment and risk perceptions [33].

Employing large numbers of migrant workers could also stress the existing healthcare infrastructure. In a study published in 2012 from Qatar, a high burden of WRIs on their health system was reported. Of 53,366 patients visiting the hospital over year period, 88% were migrant workers and road traffic injuries, occupational falls and construction work were among the top three causes of WRIs [34].

A model approach to address WRI burden

The most promising strategy for WRIs is a public health approach that incorporates policy and research into practice, interventions, and training. Such a process would have its foundations in collecting up-to-date and credible data on workplace hazards, environment and workers' health policies, assessment of risks, education for employers and workers, participation in prevention campaigns, and referral to necessary services [35]. A public health framework (Fig. 2) often utilized in injury prevention could be adapted for WRI control and prevention [6]. This framework builds upon the relationship of problem identification, analytical injury research to facilitate development and implementation

of strategies, and continuous monitoring and evaluation of interventions.

The most successful economies have demonstrated that workplaces designed according to the principles of occupational health, safety and ergonomics are also the most sustainable and productive [36, 37]. At the core of these principles, lies the foundation of all effective public health strategies and interventions: good data that can be used to develop, implement and monitor evidence-based policies, specific to the community. Active surveillance systems provide up-to-date information on WRI's, this could be achieved through the development of a unified WRI database to quantify the WRI burden and identification of risk factors and work place hazards.

Risk factor identification and hazard mitigation is facilitated by government's policies that address workers' protection, environmental safety, and maintaining safety standards in industrial and domestic sectors. To put the methods in practice, education and training of the labor force is integral, combined with guidelines and supervision to promote safe behavior at work tailored to the needs of workers' population. Engagement, encouragement, and incentivization of different stakeholders including representatives of labor work force to integrate and expand injury prevention activities must be prioritized.

Based on the injury prevention framework outlined above, we propose a comprehensive framework integrating WRI prevention and care for injured workers in Qatar (Fig. 3), that is largely based on World

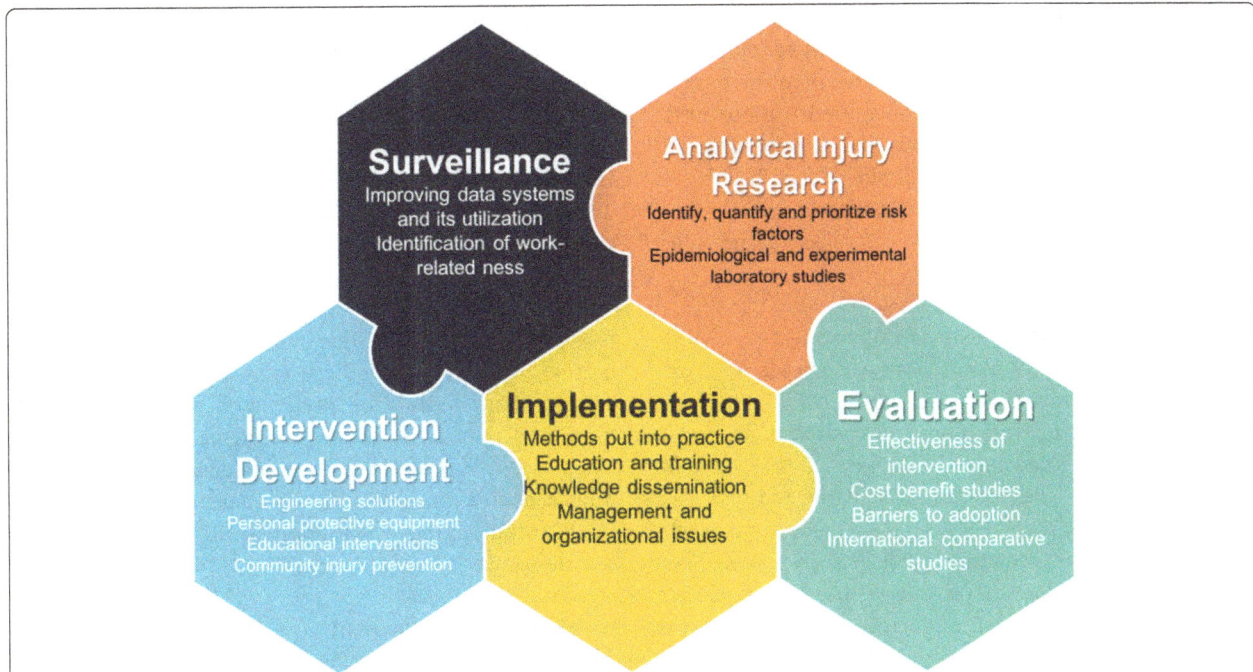

Fig. 2 The public health approach to occupational injury prevention. Adopted from G. S. Smith – Public health approaches to occupational injury prevention: do they work?[6]

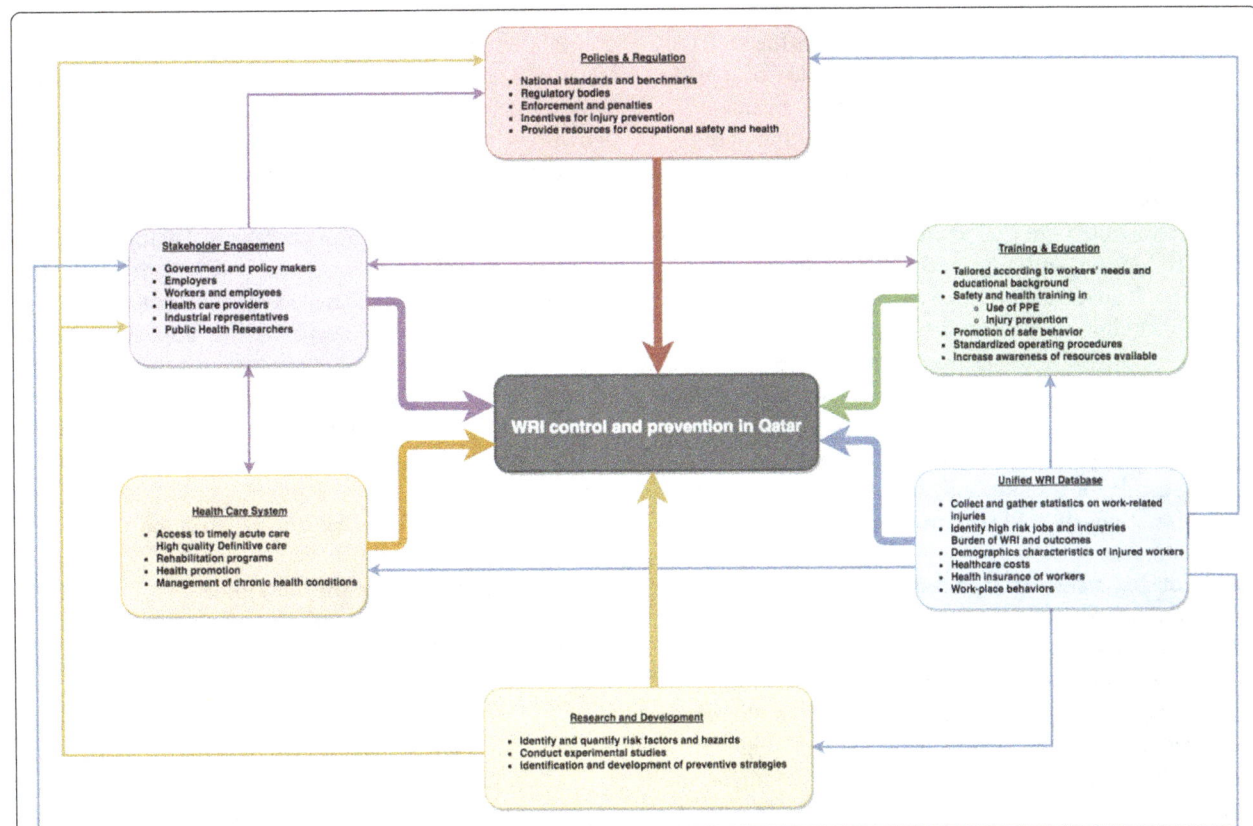

Fig. 3 A comprehensive framework for WRI prevention and control in Qatar. Adopted from WHO Injury Surveillance Guidelines [38]

Health Organization injury surveillance guidelines [38]. This framework incorporates the principles of injury control into the context of Qatar and builds upon the seminal work already undertaken to improved work place safety and systematic reforms to promote injury control by different organizations. Each entity (stakeholders, health system, research and development) is linked with others through a common path of active surveillance and information sharing.

Identification and engagement of stakeholders

WRI prevention and control involves a multitude of players and stakeholders. Identifying and engaging with important players, and using a participatory approach to policy development and implementation is the key to ensure buy-in and collaboration, and may necessitate the creation of a dedicated forum or high-level committee. Government officials, ministry representatives, industrial representatives, contractors and employers provide support and resources for implementation. Epidemiological knowledge, international safe practices, evidence based strategies, advocacy, and monitoring the impact of policies and interventions are best represented by the academics, employees, health professionals, legal experts, and international organizations.

Health informatics: Unified database on occupational injuries

Effective injury prevention is contingent on the development of good data systems. A unified database of injuries, where every entity that employs workers is mandated to submit details of incidents and injuries in a standard format, could potentially create the most robust platform of WRI surveillance. Existing data are often not collected for this purpose, often not shared and thus different databases are disconnected and frequently remain uncoordinated. WRI surveillance would require data input across different sectors including ministries of public health, labor, social affairs, etc., private and government health care providers, small and large companies, and corporations. Regular data analysis and dissemination of findings to all stakeholders will help develop evidence-based policies, set research priorities, agenda for training and education and monitor the cost implications of WRI burden.

Laws, policies, standards, and regulatory bodies

A comprehensive policy framework for occupational health and safety is needed to support education, training, research and healthcare services to prevent WRIs. A central regulatory body could facilitate the implementation and monitoring of these policies, ensuring adherence with international standards of safety. Judicial use of incentives by government could expedite the uptake of policies and interventions by different sectors and improve adherence with international safety standards.

Introduction of on-site health teams, inspections of safety practices, mandatory reporting of adverse incidents and injuries could promote organizational safety culture. Empowering and training the workers to be on-site inspectors will bolster the power and impact of regulatory bodies through a bottom up approach [39]. They can also be used to address common complaints, claims and concerns of the employees, or refer them to higher authorities through well-defined channels.

Efforts could also be directed towards strengthening bilateral treaties with the migrant workers' states of origin. Frameworks of official communication and information sharing could be streamlined through clear policies, and redress processes should be made easier and transparent. Workers' access to policies, procedures, and official documents produced by relevant ministries must be ensured, along with improved interpretation and translation services.

Research and Development

The epidemiology of injuries in Qatar demonstrate a higher burden of WRIs in construction jobs, falls and RTIs. Research addressing hazard identification in construction sector, research to mitigate risk of fall related WRIs, and identification of modifiable injury risk factors is needed. Ergonomic interventions, environmental protection, and human resource management are only some of a long list of broad research topics that could provide essential and contextual information on how to protect health and improve safety without compromising productivity in the context of Qatar [36, 37, 40]. As reported previously, many WRIs result in head and neck, extremity and back injuries (Table 2) [41]. Short- and long- term consequences of these injuries including cumulative economic cost of treatment, loss of productivity, rehabilitation and replacement have not been studied. Priority should be placed on improving health outcomes, prevention of disability, psychological and mental health impact of WRIs among workers who frequently live without family support [42]. Cost benefit analyses could help determine effectiveness of WRI control strategies vs. cost of treatment, decreased productivity from lost work-days, and repatriation.

Education and training of the workforce

The hierarchy of hazard control is often utilized across industries to minimize or eliminate exposure to workplace hazards [43]. Personal protective equipment is at the bottom of the hierarchy and is the least effective measure of hazard control but is also the minimum protection provided to all workers. Workers should receive the education and training for identifying workplace hazards and provided with appropriate equipment and training for its operation and/or use.

Qatar where the majority of the workforce are from different backgrounds, may show variability in knowledge and behavior about workplace safey. Other countries with the same issue have developed and incorporated educational and training materials for safety and health targeting migrant workers [44, 45]. Education and training programs would require specific customizations that would increase comprehension of material to the migrant population. This may necessitate offering programs that are linguistically and culturally appropriate, in languages that are understood and spoken fluently by the workers.

Healthcare system: Access to care and rehabilitation

Injured workers seek medical care at different points throughout the healthcare infrastructure depending on the severity of the injury. Medical care provided at the trauma centers is likely to reflect more severe injuries; for workers with less severe injuries, treatment may be sought at primary care facilities, through private healthcare providers, or they may not receive any care at all. Recent studies have shown that WRIs are a leading cause of hospital visits in Qatar; less is known about the burden and outcome outside of hospitals [41]. Currently, all expatriates and migrant workers are provided with a heath card that provides access to all public hospitals and clinics. Additionally, the Qatar Red Crescent has been providing therapeutic services to workers for some years. However, accessing acute care in a timely manner remains difficult for many migrant workers [46]. The barriers to access care may include fear of losing job or part of the wage, inadequate knowledge of the use of health card, long travel to reach the tertiary care medical center, which may be undesirable for employer, or puts the employee at the peril of using extra resources, such as service fee and transportation charges. [47].

State of policy environment for WRIs in Qatar

The legislative and regulatory framework for work-related injuries is still developing in Qatar [48]. The current legislations governing workplace injuries are laid out in the Qatar Labor Laws [31]. Qatari labor law requires employers to inform their workers of hazards associated with the work and safety precautions that should be exercised, to protect the workers from injuries, disease and accident, provide personal protective equipment and gear, hygiene and good ventilation, first aid box and periodical medical checkup [49]. Failure to comply with these procedures or violation of standard safety measures may result in possible closure of the work site, or fine or imprisonment or both. A Decree by the Ministry of Civil Service and Housing Affair prohibits working on areas exposed to the sun between 1130 and 1500 h during the hottest months of the year. Although this seems very promising in ensuring

workers' welfare, the implementation of these laws has not been effective or uniform across sectors [29]. With recent reforms in the Qatari labor laws, the government has taken steps to further strengthen policies to protect the rights of domestic workers [50].

The National Occupational Health and Safety Committee was established in 2011 under the Ministry of Labor and Social Affairs, and the Supreme Council of Health, as part of the National Health Strategy to improve governance and regulation of WRIs. Current legislation does dictate that the employer assume responsibility for medical expenses and salary for work-related injuries. Despite the existence of such legislations and regulations, many migrant workers may not be aware of it, which calls for better dissemination of information. Trade unions or committees for foreign workers are prohibited in Qatar and the Qatari government only allows Qatari workers to "to strike, form committees, and join international labor organizations, pending ministerial approval" [51].

Recently, the Qatar Red Crescent in agreement with the Ministry of Public Health [formerly the Supreme Council of Health] established a health center dedicated to expatriate health care needs, with a capacity to receive 32,000 visitors per month [52]. So far, there is one government state-of-the-art rehabilitation institution operating in Qatar, which started functioning in 2016 to offer five rehabilitation programs [53]. It is unclear at this point, if the services would be expanded to include occupational therapy and rehabilitation for WRIs.

Under the Qatar Foundation National Priority Research Programs, a research project was launched in 2015 to initiate and implement a targeted unified workplace injury surveillance system to inform policies and programs to reduce the health burden, and the healthcare costs from WRI's in Qatar. Under this collaborative project, a stakeholder network was established to discuss the WRI problem, engage and exchange ideas, prioritize research agenda, as well as push the efforts towards identification, evaluation, and integration of WRI data sources. New efforts are currently under way at Red Crescent and Hamad Medical Center to place an electronic tag in medical records, on all patients attending their outpatient and inpatient facilities with WRI. Additionally, empirical data on risk factors and vulnerable populations is being collected and analysis of health care data to measure the burden, risk factors, hospital outcome and cost of treatment has been conducted [54].

Discussion

Work-related injuries are debilitating not only to the injured worker, but also to the country's productivity and economy. Despite economic growth, GCC nations like Qatar, have their own challenges in assuring the health and safety of its migrant worker population. Currently, there is a dearth of data from Qatar and other neighboring states, with media reports of increased incidence of WRIs in migrant workers [27, 28]. WRI related information is fragmented among different industries, governmental bodies, healthcare system and is collected mainly for legal or care related documentation. A concerted effort by all stakeholders, guided by evidence collected through a unified database registry, that gives a strategic direction to preventive efforts, effective interventions and evaluation of impact of different policies will steer the country towards the common goal of WRI prevention and control.

While there are well established safety practices that should be adopted in all work environments, some risk factors are variable across different industries, dependent on individual worker characteristics, and affected by workplace organizational policies and practices [55–58]. The most recent example is from Chile, where Fatal Work Accidents Registry captured work related mortality, high risk occupations, vulnerable population and characteristics of industry with high fatality risk [59]. Thus, blind adoption of strategies to prevent workplace injuries may not be effective, could be costly and such efforts may fail or be inadvertently harmful. Some of the core principles incorporated in the policies of the countries with the strongest occupational health and safety traditions include primary prevention and use of safe technology; governance and stewardship to monitor and regulate working conditions. Integration of production and healthy activities enhances employees' own interest in health and safety at work.

Given a complex environment and upkeep of WRI prevention agenda, priorities for Qatar include establishing and enforcing legislation that protects the health of workers in the construction industry. Using our proposed framework (Fig. 3), WRI control and prevention can be achieved through a multi-strategy approach that (1) empowers employers and workers to share responsibility for the safety and health of all; (2) acknowledges that government have the authority and responsibility to develop and roll out appropriate policies and create and an equitable environment that places workers safety and health on priority; (3) highlights the importance of research and development to advance the agenda of evidence informed policy making; (4) recognizes that training and education of employees in a multicultural and multilinguistic context, especially unskilled labor workforce requires customization; (5) places a priority on health care needs of the WRI patients, both in acute phase and during rehabilitation and finally (6) the foundation of this framework lies on a good and up-to-date WRI surveillance systems that provides necessary input for policy, training, and monitoring and evaluation of interventions to control WRI. This approach could

become the pioneering effort within Qatar and an example for the neighboring countries with a similar economic environment and rapidly changing labor force.

Funding

The work in this paper is supported through Qatar National Research Fund, National Priorities Research Program, grant # 7–1120 - 3 - 288, titled "A Unified Registry for Occupational Injury Prevention in Qatar". The content is solely the responsibility of the authors and does not necessarily represent the official views of the Qatar National Research Fund.

Authors' contributions

AM, ZM, conducted literature review, developed the framework and prepared the draft manuscript; RC, AE, RP, HA, provided contextual local input; AAH provided critical review for the final draft of manuscript. All authors read and approved the final manuscript.

Competing interests

The authors declare that they have no competing interests.

Author details

[1]Johns Hopkins International Injury Research Unit, Health Systems Program, Department of International Health, Johns Hopkins Bloomberg School of Public Health, 615 N Wolfe St, Baltimore, MD 21205, USA. [2]HMC Injury Prevention Program, Hamad General Hospital, Hamad Medical Corporation, Doha, Qatar. [3]Trauma Surgery Section, Hamad General Hospital, Hamad Medical Corporation, and Weill Cornell Medical College, Doha, Qatar. [4]Universidad Nacional Pedro Henriquez Urena (UNPHU), Santo Domingo, Dominican Republic. [5]Department of Surgery, Hamad General Hospital, Hamad Medical Corporation, Doha, Qatar. [6]Johns Hopkins Berman Institute of Bioethics, Baltimore, MD, USA. [7]George Washington University Milken Institute School of Public Health, Washington, DC, USA. [8]Weill Cornell Medical College, Doha, Qatar.

References

1. International Labor Organization. Safety and health at work. 2013. http://www.ilo.org/global/topics/safety-and-health-at-work/lang%2D%2Den/index.htm. Accessed 2 Nov 2017.
2. Organization for Economic Co-operation and Development. OECD Glossary of Statistical Terms - Occupational injury Definition. https://stats.oecd.org/glossary/detail.asp?ID=3565. Accessed 16 Sep 2017.
3. Occupational Safety and Health Administration. Occupational safety and health standards: Occupational health and environmental control (Standard No. 1904.5). 1970.
4. Takala J, Hamalainen P, Saarela KL, Yun LY, Manickam K, Jin TW, et al. Global estimates of the burden of injury and illness at work in 2012. J Occup Environ Hyg. 2014;11:326–37.
5. Nenonen N, Saarela KL, Takala J, Manickam K. Global estimates of occupational accidents and work-related illnesses 2014. Singapore: Workplace Safety & Health Institute; 2014. Available at: https://www.researchgate.net/publication/265214122_Global_Estimates_of_Occupational_Accidents_and_Work-related_Illnesses_2014_made_for_the_ILO_Report_at_XX_World_Congress_Frankfurt.
6. Smith GS. Public health approaches to occupational injury prevention: do they work? Inj Prev. 2001;7(suppl 1):3–11. https://doi.org/10.1136/ip.7.suppl_1.i3
7. Azaroff LS, Levenstein C, Wegman DH. Occupational Injury and Illness Surveillance: Conceptual Filters Explain Underreporting. Am J Public Health. 2002;92:1421–9.
8. Centers for Disease Control and Prevention. Our History - Our Story. 2017. https://www.cdc.gov/about/history/index.html. Accessed 10 Jan 2018.
9. United Nations Development Programme. Human Development Report 2016. 2016. doi:eISBN: 978-92-1-060036-1.

10. Barss P, Addley K, Grivna M, Stanculescu C, Abu-zidan F. Occupational injury in the United Arab Emirates: epidemiology and prevention. Occup Med. 2009;59(7):493–8.

11. Al-rubaee FR, Al-maniri A. Work Related Injuries in an Oil field in Oman. Oman Med J. 2011;26:315–8.

12. Al-Thani H, El-Menyar A, Consunji R, Mekkodathil A, Peralta R, Allen KA, et al. Epidemiology of occupational injuries by nationality in Qatar: evidence for focused occupational safety programmes. Injury. 2015;46:1806–13.

13. Kapiszewski A. Arab Versus Asian Migrant Workers in the Gcc Countries. United Nations Expert Gr Meet Int. 2006:1–21.

14. Rabi AZ, Jamous LW, AbuDhaise BA, Alwash RH. Fatal occupational injuries in Jordan during the period 1980 through 1993. Saf Sci. 1998;28:177–87.

15. Gomes J, Lloyd O, Norman N. The health of the workers in a rapidly developing country: effects of occupational exposure to noise and heat. Occup Med. 2002;52:121–8.

16. Barss P, Addley K, Grivna M, Stanculescu C, Abu-zidan F. Occupational injury in the United Arab Emirates: epidemiology and prevention. Occup Med. 2017;2009:493–8.

17. Health Authority of Abu Dhabi. Health Statistics 2015. 2016. https://www.haad.ae/HAAD/LinkClick.aspx?fileticket=gzx_WUkD27Y%3D&tabid=1516. Accessed 29 Jan 2018.

18. Schenker MB. A Global Perspective of Migration and Occupational Health Am J Ind Med 2010;337:329–37.

19. World Development Indicators. Country Profile: Qatar. 2017;:1.

20. De Bel-Air F. Demography, Migration, and Labour Market in Qatar. Gulf Labour Markets and Migration. 2014;:19. http://cadmus.eui.eu/bitstream/handle/1814/32431/GLMM_ExpNote_08-2014.pdf?sequence=1. Accessed 29 Jan 2018.

21. Gardner A, Pessoa S, Diop A, Al-ghanim K, Trung KLE, Harkness L. A Portrait of Low-Income Migrants in Contemporary Qatar. J Arabian Studies. 2013;3(1):1–17.

22. Ministry of Development and Planning Statistics. Labor Force Survey: The second quarter (April – June 2017). 2017.

23. Snoj J. Population of Qatar by nationality - 2017 report. 2017. http://priyadsouza.com/population-of-qatar-by-nationality-in-2017/.

24. International Labor Organization. Hazardous Work. http://www.ilo.org/safework/areasofwork/hazardous-work/lang%2D%2Den/index.htm. Accessed 10 Jan 2018.

25. Al-thani H, El-menyar A, Abdelrahman H, Zarour A, Consunji R, Peralta R, et al. Workplace-Related Traumatic Injuries: Insights from a Rapidly Developing Middle Eastern Country. J Environ Public Health. 2014;2014(430832):8. https://doi.org/10.1155/2014/430832.

26. Tuma MA, Acerra JR, El-menyar A, Al-thani H, Al-hassani A, Recicar F, et al. Epidemiology of workplace-related fall from height and cost of trauma care in Qatar Statistical Analysis: Results: Conclusions. Int J Crit Illn Inj Sci. 2013;3:3–7.

27. International Trade Union Confederation. The Case Against Qatar, Host of FIFA 2022 World Cup. Brussels, Belgium; 2014. International Trade Union Confederation. https://www.ituc-csi.org/IMG/pdf/the_case_against_qatar_en_web170314.pdf. Accessed 15 Jan 2018.

28. Human Rights Watch. Qatar: Take Urgent Action to Protect Construction Workers. 2017. qatar: Take Urgent Action to Protect Construction Workers. Accessed 2 Nov 2017.

29. DLA Piper. Migrant labour in the construction sector in the State of Qatar. 2014. http://www.engineersagainstpoverty.org/documentdownload.axd?documentresourceid=58. Accessed 29 Jan 2018.

30. Khan FY, Kamha A, A EH. Study of Patients with Heat Stroke Admitted to the Intensive Care Unit of Hamad General Hospital , Doha , Qatar During Summer 2004. 2005;14:40–43.

31. Qatar Labor Law. Law No (14) of the Year 2004 – Qatar Labor Law. https://qatarlaborlaw.com/qatar-labor-law/. Accessed 29 Jan 2018.

32. Fass S, Yousef R, Liginlal D, Vyas P. Understanding causes of fall and struck-by incidents: what differentiates construction safety in the Arabian gulf region? Appl Ergon. 2017;58:515–26. https://doi.org/10.1016/j.apergo.2016.05.002.

33. Hassan HA, Houdmont J. Health and safety implications of recruitment payments in migrant construction workers. 2014:331–336.

34. Bener A, Abdul Rahman YS, Abdel Aleem EY, Khalid MK. Trends and characteristics of injuries in the State of Qatar: hospital-based study. Int J Inj Control Saf Promot. 2012;19:368–72.

35. World Health Organization. Global strategy on occupational health for all: the way to health at work, recommendation of the Second Meeting of the WHO Collaborating Centres in Occupational Health, 11–14 October 1994, Beijing, China. Beijing. Geneva: World Health Organization; 1995.

36. Niu S. Ergonomics and occupational safety and health: an ILO perspective. Appl Ergon. 2010;41:744–53. https://doi.org/10.1016/j.apergo.2010.03.004.

37. Zacharatos A, Barling J, Iverson RD. High-Performance Work Systems and Occupational Safety. 2005;90:77–93.

38. Holder Y, Peden M, Krug EG, Lund J, Gururaj G, Kobusingye O. Injury surveillance guidelines. Geneva: World Health Organization; 2001.

39. Dejoy DM. Behavior change versus culture change : Divergent approaches to managing workplace safety q. 2005;43:105–29.

40. Nuwayhid IA. Occupational Health Research in Developing Countries: A Partner for Social Justice. Am J Public Health. 2004;94:1916–21.

41. Bener A, Rahman YSA, Aleem EYA, Khalid MK. Trends and characteristics of head and neck injury from falls: a hospital based study. Qatar Sultan Qaboos Univ Med J. 2011;11(2):244–51.

42. MacDonald LA, Karasek RA, Punnett L, Scharf T. Covariation between workplace physical and psychosocial stressors: evidence and implications for occupational health research and prevention. Ergonomics. 2001;44:696–718. https://doi.org/10.1080/00140130119943.

43. The National Institute for Occupational Safety and Health (NIOSH). Workplace Safety & Health Topics - Hierarchy of Controls. CDC. 2016. https://www.cdc.gov/niosh/topics/hierarchy/. Accessed 29 Jan 2018.

44. Brunette MJ. Development of educational and training materials on safety and health: targeting Hispanic Workers in the Construction Industry. Fam Community Health. 2005;28(3):253–66.

45. McGlothlin J, Hubbard B, Aghazadeh F, Hubbard S. Case study: safety training issues for Hispanic construction workers. J Occup Environ Hyg. 2009;6:D45–50. https://doi.org/10.1080/15459620903106689.

46. Bener A. Health status and working condition of migrant workers: major public health problems. Int J Prev Med. 2017;8:68. https://doi.org/10.4103/ijpvm.IJPVM_396_16.

47. Joshi S, Simkhada P, Prescott GJ. Health problems of Nepalese migrants working in three gulf countries. BMC Int Health Hum Rights. 2011;11:3–13. https://doi.org/10.1186/1472-698X-11-3.

48. Clyde & Co LLP. Managing Workplace Injuries and Fatalities in Qatar and the UAE: What do employers need to know? 2017. https://www.lexology.com/library/detail.aspx?g=d1f1a2db-eaf3-43f5-bab5-f91f2ada3dd2. Accessed 2 Nov 2017.

49. Qatar Labor Law. Qatar Labor Law Part 10 - Safety, Vocational Health, and Social Care. http://qatarlaborlaw.com/qatar-labor-law/#safety-vocational-health-and-social-care. Accessed 2 Nov 2017.

50. Qatar Labor Law. Amendments to Law No (14) of the Year 2004. https://qatarlaborlaw.com/amendments/. Accessed 29 Jan 2018.

51. Sultan Z. High-rise and high risk: Spotlight on Qatar's safety standards. Nature Middle East [Internet]. 2013. Available from: https://www.natureasia.com/en/nmiddleeast/article/10.1038/nmiddleeast.2013.62. Accessed 8 Jan 2018.

52. Gulf Times. Health minister inaugurates Medical Centre in Industrial Area Doha, Qatar. 2016. [Available from: https://www.gulf-times.com/story/505372/Health-minister-inaugurates-Medical-Centre-in-Indu. Accessed 2 Nov 2017].

53. Hamad Medical Corporation. HMC Welcomes the First Inpatients to Qatar Rehabilitation Institute. 2017. https://www.hamad.qa/EN/news/2017/March/Pages/HMC-Welcomes-the-First-Inpatients-to-Qatar-Rehabilitation-Institute.aspx. Accessed 2 Nov 2017.

54. Consunji R, Mehmood A, Hirani N, El-Menyar A, Abeid A, Hyder A, et al. Epidemiologic and temporal trends of work-related injuries in expatriate workers in a high-income rapidly developing country: Evidence for preventive programs. In: Prevention of Accidents at Work. Prague: Taylor and Francis Group. 2017. p. 55–9. https://doi.org/10.1201/9781315177571-11.

55. Saurin TA, Formoso CT, Cambraia FB. An analysis of construction safety best practices from a cognitive systems engineering perspective. Safety Science. 2008;46(8):1169–83.

56. Teo EAL, Ling FYY, Chong AFW. Framework for project managers to manage construction safety. Int J Proj Manag. 2005;23:329–41.

57. Robson LS, Clarke JA, Cullen K, Bielecky A, Severin C, Bigelow PL, et al. The effectiveness of occupational health and safety management system interventions : A systematic review. Safety Science. 2007;45:329–53.

58. Brenner MD, Fairris D, Ruser J. "Flexible work practices" and occupational safety and health: exploring the relationship between cummalitive trauma disorders and workplace transformation. Ind Relat (Berkeley). 2004;43:242–67. https://doi.org/10.1111/j.0019-8676.2004.00325.x.

59. Bachelet VC. Work-related injuries resulting in death in Chile : a cross-sectional study on 2014 and 2015 registries. BMJ Open. 2018:1–8.

Permissions

List of Contributors

Jan Bauer and David A.Groneberg
Institute of Occupational, Social and Environmental Medicine, Goethe-University Frankfurt, Theodor-Stern-Kai 7, 60329 Frankfurtam Main, Germany

Xiali Zhong, Ming Zeng, Caigao Zhong and Fang Xiao
Department of Health Toxicology, Xiangya School of Public Health, Central South University, NO. 238 Shangmayuanling Road, Kaifu District, Changsha 410078, Hunan, People's Republic of China

Huanfeng Bian
Shajing Institution of Health Supervision of Baoan District, Shenzhen 518104, People's Republic of China

Menen E. Mund, Christoph Gyo, David Quarcoo and David A. Groneberg
Institute of Occupational Medicine, Social Medicine and Environmental Medicine, Departments of Female Health and Preventive Medicine, Goethe University, Frankfurt am Main, Theodor-Stern-Kai 7, Frankfurt 60590, Germany

Dörthe Brüggmann
Institute of Occupational Medicine, Social Medicine and Environmental Medicine, Departments of Female Health and Preventive Medicine, Goethe University, Frankfurt am Main, Theodor-Stern-Kai 7, Frankfurt 60590, Germany
Department of Obstetrics and Gynecology, Keck School of Medicine, University of Southern California, Los Angeles, CA, USA

Sanja Stopinšek, Alojz Ihan and Saša Simčič
Institute of Microbiology and Immunology, Faculty of Medicine, University of Ljubljana, Zaloška 4, SI-1000 Ljubljana, Slovenia

Barbara Salobir and Marjeta Terčelj
Department for Respiratory and Allergic Diseases, University Medical Centre, Zaloška 2, SI-1000 Ljubljana, Slovenia

Steven E. Mischler, Emanuele G. Cauda and Linda J. McWilliams
National Institute for Occupational Safety and Health, Office of Mine Safety and Health Research, 626 Cochrans Mill Road, Pittsburgh, PA 15236, USA

Michelangelo Di Giuseppe and Luis A. Ortiz
Department of Environmental and Occupational Health, University of Pittsburgh, Pittsburgh, PA, USA

Claudette St. Croix
Center for Biological Imaging, Environmental and Occupational Health, University of Pittsburgh, Pittsburgh, PA, USA

Ming Sun and Jonathan Franks
Center for Biological Imaging, University of Pittsburgh, Pittsburgh, PA, USA

Sebsibe Tadesse, Bikes Destaw and Yalemzewod Assefa
Institute of Public Health, the University of Gondar, Gondar, Ethiopia

Kassahun Bezabih
City Government of Addis Ababa Health Bureau, Addis Ababa, Ethiopia

Peter Koch, Jan Felix Kersten and Johanna Stranzinger
Centre of Excellence for Epidemiology and Health Services Research for Healthcare Professionals (CVcare), University Medical Centre Hamburg-Eppendorf, Martinistrasse 52, 20246 Hamburg, Germany

Albert Nienhaus
Centre of Excellence for Epidemiology and Health Services Research for Healthcare Professionals (CVcare), University Medical Centre Hamburg-Eppendorf, Martinistrasse 52, 20246 Hamburg, Germany
Health Protection Division (FBG), Institution for Statutory Accident Insurance and Prevention in the Health and Welfare Services (BGW), Pappelallee 33, 22089 Hamburg, Germany

Monica Lamberti, Mariarosaria Muoio, Antonio Arnese, Sharon Borrelli, Teresa Di Lorenzo and Elpidio Maria Garzillo
Department of Experimental Medicine, Section of Hygiene, Occupational Medicine and Forensic Medicine, Second University of Naples, Via dei Crecchi 16, 80133 Naples, Italy

Giuseppe Signoriello, Stefania De Pascalis and Nicola Coppola
Department of Mental Health and Public Medicine, Section of Infectious Diseases, Second University of Naples, Naples, Italy

Albert Nienhaus
Institute for Health Services, Research in Dermatology and Nursing, Germany, Institution for Statutory Accident Insurance and Prevention in Healthcare and Welfare Services, University Medical Centre Hamburg-Eppendorf, Hamburg, Germany

Solomon Tesfa Tezera, Daniel Haile Chercos and Awrajaw Dessie
Department of Environmental and Occupational Health and Safety, Institute of Public Health, University of Gondar, Gondar, Ethiopia

David Schneberger, Gurpreet Aulakh, Shankaramurthy Channabasappa and Baljit Singh
Department of Veterinary Biomedical Sciences, Western College of Veterinary Medicine, University of Saskatchewan, 52 Campus Drive, Saskatoon, SK S7N 5B4, Canada

Kaitlin Merkowsky and Baljit Singh
Department of Veterinary Biomedical Sciences, Western College of Veterinary Medicine, University of Saskatchewan, 52 Campus Drive, Saskatoon, SK S7N 5B4, Canada

Ram S. Sethi
School of Animal Biotechnology, Guru Angad Dev Veterinary and Animal Sciences University, Ludhiana, India

Jatinder P. S. Gill
School of Veterinary Public Health, Guru Angad Dev Veterinary and Animal Sciences University, Ludhiana, India

Praveen Chokhandre and Gyan Chandra Kashyap
International Institute for Population Sciences, Govandi Station Road Donor, Mumbai 400088, India

Shrikant Singh
Department of Mathematical Demography and Statistics, International Institute for Population Sciences, Govandi Station Road Deonar, Mumbai 400088, India

Mónica Villalba-Campos, Sandra Rocío Ramírez-Clavijo, Magda Carolina Sánchez-Corredor, Milena Rondón-Lagos and Lilian Chuaire-Noack
Facultad de Ciencias Naturales y Matemáticas, Universidad del Rosario, Carrera 26 63B-48, Bogotá, DC, Colombia

Milcíades Ibáñez-Pinilla and Marcela Eugenia Varona-Uribe
Escuela de Medicina y Ciencias de la Salud, Universidad del Rosario, Bogotá, DC, Colombia

Ruth Marien Palma
Instituto Nacional de Salud, Bogotá, DC, Colombia

Sebsibe Tadesse
Institute of Public Health, the University of Gondar, Gondar, Ethiopia

Dagnachew Israel
City Government of Addis Ababa Health Bureau, Addis Ababa, Ethiopia

Kristina L. Bailey and Debra J. Romberger
Research Service, Veterans Administration Nebraska Western Iowa Health Care System, Omaha, NE 68105, USA
Pulmonary, Critical Care, Sleep and Allergy Division, Department of Internal Medicine, University of Nebraska Medical Center, 985910 The Nebraska Medical Center, Omaha, NE 68198-5910, USA

Todd A. Wyatt
Research Service, Veterans Administration Nebraska Western Iowa Health Care System, Omaha, NE 68105, USA
Pulmonary, Critical Care, Sleep and Allergy Division, Department of Internal Medicine, University of Nebraska Medical Center, 985910 The Nebraska Medical Center, Omaha, NE 68198-5910, USA
Department of Environmental, Agricultural and Occupational Health, University of Nebraska Medical Center, 985910 The Nebraska Medical Center, Omaha, NE 68198-5910, USA

David Schneberger and Jane M. DeVasure
Pulmonary, Critical Care, Sleep and Allergy Division, Department of Internal Medicine, University of Nebraska Medical Center, 985910 The Nebraska Medical Center, Omaha, NE 68198-5910, USA

Prajjwal Pyakurel, Anup Ghimire and Paras Kumar Pokharel
School of Public Health and Community Medicine, B.P.Koirala Institute of Health Sciences, Postal Address: 56705, Dharan, Nepal

Prahlad Karki
Department of Internal Medicine, B.P.KoiralaInstitue of Health Sciences, Dharan, Nepal

Madhab Lamsal
Department of Bio-chemistry, B.P.KoiralaInstitue of Health Sciences, Dharan, Nepal

Lygia Therese Budnik
Division of Translational Toxicology and Immunology, Institute for Occupational and Maritime Medicine (ZfAM), University Medical Center Hamburg-Eppendorf (UKE), Hamburg, Germany

Balazs Adam
Faculty of Public Health, Department of Preventive Medicine, University of Debrecen, Debrecen, Hungary

Maria Albin
Division of Occupational and Environmental Medicine, University of Lund, Lund, Sweden
Karolinska Institutet, Institute of Environmental Medicine (IMM), Stockholm, Sweden

Karin Broberg and Per Gustavsson
Karolinska Institutet, Institute of Environmental Medicine (IMM), Stockholm, Sweden

Barbara Banelli
Tumor Epigenetics Unit, Ospedale Policlinico San Martino, National Cancer Institute, IRCCS and University of Genoa, DISSAL, Genoa, Italy

Xaver Baur
European Society for Environmental and Occupational Medicine, Berlin, Germany

Fiorella Belpoggi and Fabiana Manservisi
Cesare Maltoni Cancer Research Center, Ramazzini Institute, Bentivoglio, Bologna, Italy

Claudia Bolognesi
San Martino-IST Environmental Carcinogenesis Unit, IRCCS, Ospedale Policlinico San Martino, National Cancer Institute, Genoa, Italy

Thomas Göen
Social and Environmental Medicine, Institute and Outpatient Clinic of Occupational, Friedrich-Alexander-University Erlangen-Nurnberg, Erlangen, Germany

Axel Fischer
Institute of Occupational Medicine, Charité Universitäts Medizin, Berlin, Germany

Dorota Jarosinska and Elizabet Paunovic
WHO European Centre for Environment and Health, Bonn, Germany

Richard O'Kennedy
Biomedical Diagnostics Institute, Dublin City University, Dublin, Ireland

Johan Øvrevik and Per E. Schwarze
Norwegian Institute of Public Health, Oslo, Norway

Beate Ritz
Center for Occupational and Environmental Health, Fielding School of Public Health (FSPH), University of California Los Angeles (UCLA), Los Angeles, USA

Paul T. J. Scheepers
Radboud Institute for Health Sciences, Radboudumc (Radboud university medical center), Nijmegen, the Netherlands

Vivi Schlünssen
National Research Center for the Working Environment, Copenhagen, Denmark
Department of Public Health, Section Environment, Occupation and Health and Danish Ramazzini Centre Aarhus, Aarhus University, Aarhus, Denmark

Torben Sigsgaard
Department of Public Health, Section Environment, Occupation and Health and Danish Ramazzini Centre Aarhus, Aarhus University, Aarhus, Denmark

Heidi Schwarzenbach
Department of Tumor Biology, University Medical Center Hamburg-Eppendorf (UKE), Hamburg, Germany

Orla Sheils
Department of Histopathology, Central Pathology Laboratory, St James's Hospital, Trinity translational Medicine Institute, Dublin, Ireland

Karel Van Damme and Ludwine Casteleyn
Center for Human Genetics, University of Leuven, Leuven, Belgium

Ruonan Chai, Hua Xie, Junli Zhang and Zhuang Ma
Department of Respiratory Medicine, General Hospital of Shenyang Military Command, No. 83 Wenhua Road, Shenhe District, Shenyang 110016, China

Jennifer D. Sisler, Justine Shaffer and Yong Qian
Pathology and Physiology Research Branch, Health Effects Laboratory Division, National Institute for Occupational Safety and Health, Centers for Disease Control and Prevention, 1095 Willowdale Road, Morgantown, West Virginia 26505, USA

Jhy-Charm Soo and Taekhee Lee
Exposure Assessment Branch, Health Effects Laboratory Division, National Institute for Occupational Safety and Health, Centers for Disease Control and Prevention, 1095 Willowdale Road, Morgantown, West Virginia 26505, USA

Martin Harper
Exposure Assessment Branch, Health Effects Laboratory Division, National Institute for Occupational Safety and Health, Centers for Disease Control and Prevention, 1095 Willowdale Road, Morgantown, West Virginia 26505, USA
Zefon International, Inc., 5350 SW 1st Lane, Ocala, FL, USA
Department of Environmental Engineering Sciences, University of Florida, Gainesville, FL, USA

Ryan F. LeBouf
Field Study Branch, Respiratory Health Division, National Institute for Occupational Safety and Health, Centers for Disease Control and Prevention, 1095 Willowdale Road, Morgantown, West Virginia 26505, USA

Khalil H. Al Ali and Waleed H. Mahallawi
Department of Clinical Laboratory Sciences, Taibah University, Al-Madinah 41477, Saudi Arabia

Omar F. Khabour
Department of Clinical Laboratory Sciences, Taibah University, Al-Madinah 41477, Saudi Arabia
Department of Medical Laboratory Sciences, Jordan University of Science and Technology, Irbid, Jordan

Yehia Z. Alami and Beesan T. Ghanim
Department of Medicine, College of Medicine and Health Sciences, An-Najah National University, Nablus 44839, Palestine

Sáed H. Zyoud
Poison Control and Drug Information Center (PCDIC), College of Medicine and Health Sciences, An-Najah National University, Nablus 44839, Palestine
Department of Clinical and Community Pharmacy, Department of Pharmacy, College of Medicine and Health Sciences, An-Najah National University, Nablus 44839, Palestine

Birgit-Christiane Zyriax
Preventive Medicine and Nutrition, Institute for Health Services Research in Dermatology and Nursing (IVDP), University Medical Center Hamburg-Eppendorf, Martinistr. 52 - Bldg. O56 – D-20246, Hamburg, Germany

Robert von Katzler, Hans-Joachim Jensen, Volker Harth and Marcus Oldenburg
Department of Maritime Medicine, Institute for Occupational and Maritime Medicine (ZfAM) Hamburg, University Medical Center Hamburg-Eppendorf, Hamburg, Germany

Bettina Jagemann
I. Medical Clinic and Polyclinic; University Medical Center Hamburg-Eppendorf, Hamburg, Germany

Joachim Westenhoefer
Competence Center Health, Faculty of Life Sciences, Hamburg University of Applied Sciences, Hamburg, Germany

Caterina Ledda, Gaetano Romano and Venerando Rapisarda
Occupational Medicine, Department of Clinical and Experimental Medicine, University of Catania, 95100 Catania, Italy

Carla Loreto, Claudia Lombardo and Sergio Castorina
Human Anatomy and Histology, Department of Biomedical and Biotechnology Sciences, University of Catania, 95100 Catania, Italy

Massimo Bracci
Occupational Medicine, Department of Clinical and Molecular Sciences, Polytechnic University of Marche, 60100 Ancona, Italy

Diana Cinà
Clinical Pathology Unit, "Garibaldi Centro" Hospital of Catania, 95100 Catania, Italy

Nicola Mucci
Occupational Medicine, Department of Experimental and Clinical Medicine, University of Florence, 50100 Florence, Italy

Ronnie Lundström
Department of Radiation Sciences, Umeå University, SE-901 87 Umeå, Sweden
Department of Occupational and Environmental Medicine, Umeå University, SE-901 87 Umeå, Sweden

Adnan Noor Baloch, Mats Hagberg and Lars Gerhardsson
Department of Occupational and Environmental Medicine, University of Gothenburg and Sahlgrenska University Hospital, Gothenburg, Sweden

Tohr Nilsson
Department of Occupational and Environmental Medicine, Umeå University, SE-901 87 Umeå, Sweden

Amber Mehmood and Zaw Maung
Johns Hopkins International Injury Research Unit, Health Systems Program, Department of International Health, Johns Hopkins Bloomberg School of Public Health, 615 N Wolfe St, Baltimore, MD 21205, USA

Adnan A. Hyder
Johns Hopkins International Injury Research Unit, Health Systems Program, Department of International Health, Johns Hopkins Bloomberg School of Public Health, 615 N Wolfe St, Baltimore, MD 21205, USA
Johns Hopkins Berman Institute of Bioethics, Baltimore, MD, USA
George Washington University Milken Institute School of Public Health, Washington, DC, USA

Rafael J. Consunji
HMC Injury Prevention Program, Hamad General Hospital, Hamad Medical Corporation, Doha, Qatar
Trauma Surgery Section, Hamad General Hospital, Hamad Medical Corporation, and Weill Cornell Medical College, Doha, Qatar

Department of Surgery, Hamad General Hospital, Hamad Medical Corporation, Doha, Qatar

Ayman El-Menyar
Trauma Surgery Section, Hamad General Hospital, Hamad Medical Corporation, and Weill Cornell Medical College, Doha, Qatar
Weill Cornell Medical College, Doha, Qatar

Ruben Peralta
Universidad Nacional Pedro Henriquez Urena (UNPHU), Santo Domingo, Dominican Republic
Department of Surgery, Hamad General Hospital, Hamad Medical Corporation, Doha, Qatar

Hassan Al-Thani
Department of Surgery, Hamad General Hospital, Hamad Medical Corporation, Doha, Qatar

Index